HIV and AIDS

A Strategy for Nursing Care

HIV and AIDS

A Strategy for Nursing Care

Robert J. Pratt
RN BA MSc RNT DN(Lond)

Professor of Nursing, Director, The Centre for Sexual Health and HIV Studies, Wolfson School of Health Science, Thames Valley University, London

Fourth Edition

Edward Arnold
A member of the Hodder Headline Group
LONDON SYDNEY AUCKLAND

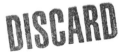

Fourth edition published in Great Britain 1995 by
Edward Arnold, a division of Hodder Headline PLC,
338 Euston Road, London NW1 3BH

First edition published 1986
AISE edition published 1988

Whilst the advice and information in this book is believed to be
true and accurate at the date of going to press, neither the author
nor the publisher can accept any legal responsibility or liability
for any errors or omissions that may be made. In particular
(but without limiting the generality of the preceding disclaimer)
every effort has been made to check drug dosages; however
it is still possible that errors have been missed. Furthermore,
dosage schedules are constantly being revised and new side
effects recognized. For these reasons the reader is strongly
urged to consult the drug companies' printed instructions before
administering any of the drugs recommended in this book.

British Library Cataloguing in Publication Data
A catalogue record for this book is available from the British
Library

ISBN 0 340 59233 8

1 2 3 4 5 95 96 97 98 99

Typeset in 10/11 pt Times by Anneset, Weston-super-Mare, Avon.
Printed and bound in Great Britain by J. W. Arrowsmith Ltd, Bristol.

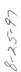

Contents

Foreword to the Fourth Edition	vii
Acknowledgements	x
Introduction	xi
1. The Evolution of a Pandemic	1
2. The Biology of HIV – The Cause of AIDS	11
3. HIV Transmission	28
4. Understanding Immunology	39
5. Pathways of Destruction in HIV Disease	64
6. The Clinical Consequences of HIV Infection	72
7. A Dangerous Liaison – Tuberculosis and HIV Disease	107
8. HIV Disease and the Nervous System	145
9. Acute Viral Hepatitis and HIV Disease	167
10. The Impact of HIV Infection on Women	175
11. Children and HIV Disease	188
12. A Strategy for Infection Control in Nursing Practice	202
13. The Risk of Occupational Exposure to HIV	220
14. The Individualized Care of Patients with HIV Disease	233
15. Nutrition and HIV Disease	265
16. Discharge Planning and Community Care	288
17. The Nurse as a Health Educator	302
18. The Management of Strategic Nursing Care	316
19. Nursing Issues Related to Medical Management	327

Appendices

Appendix 1:	Revision of the CDC Surveillance Case Definition for Acquired Immunodeficiency Syndrome	344
Appendix 2:	Interim Proposed World Health Organization Clinical Staging System for HIV Infection and Disease	368
Appendix 3:	Recommendations for Prevention of HIV Transmission in Health Care Settings	370

Appendix 4: Guidelines for Preventing the Transmission
of Tuberculosis in Health-Care Settings, with
Special Focus on HIV-related Issues   393
Appendix 5   Social History Form   421
Appendix 6: Model AIDS Educational Strategy for
Pre-registration Nursing Programmes   427
Appendix 7: Model Philosophy for Nursing   432
Appendix 8: Model Policy Statements   437
Appendix 9: Technical Guidance on HIV Counseling   446

Index   453

Foreword to the Fourth Edition

We are now well into the second decade of our experience of caring for individuals with AIDS and HIV-related health problems. In the United Kingdom, the North Thames Region in London is at the very epicentre of this global pandemic and, as such, we are caring for large numbers of individuals who are unwell as a result of HIV infection, in our hospitals and clinics, and who are dependent on our community health care services. Although our knowledge of the underlying science and pathology driving this epidemic has increased, there still has not emerged a biomedical 'cure' for this disease. **The need for nurses to 'care' is as urgent now as when the disease first surfaced.**

Since its first edition in 1986, this book has established itself as the definitive reference text in Europe on the nursing care of individuals with HIV disease. Now, completely rewritten and updated, the 4th Edition includes important new chapters reflecting the changing focus and instability of the epidemic.

A dangerous liaison, the 'cursed duet', has developed, uniting HIV infection and tuberculosis. All over the world, nurses caring for patients with HIV disease are having to acquire new knowledge and competencies in caring for patients with tuberculosis. A significant new chapter comprehensively describes the background to this oldest of human diseases, now returning as the terrible twin of HIV infection, and once again becoming a major threat to public health. The treatment and care of HIV-infected patients with TB is described, along with important infection control issues, especially in relation to multi-drug resistant tuberculosis.

Using the latest research and epidemiological studies available, Robert Pratt outlines a new understanding of the science driving the epidemic, describing more comprehensively, both the biology of HIV and a changing perception of the immunological responses to infection, in a language familiar to health care professionals. The changing epidemiology of HIV infection, risk behaviours and transmission models are extensively described. The evolving concept of how HIV infection causes disease is discussed, reflecting new advances in scientific thinking. Difficult subjects are made understandable and new staging systems and case definitions are linked to a detailed description of the clinical consequences of HIV infection.

A new chapter describes the impact of this disease on women, and summarizes their differing vulnerabilities and nursing care needs. An additional new chapter discusses the critical significance of nutrition in HIV disease and outlines the nursing care implications of patients requiring enteral or parenteral nutrition.

As in previous editions, the focus is firmly on the unique role of the nurse in caring for individuals infected with HIV. A strategic behavioural model of nursing sets the scene for an in-depth description of the actual and potential care requirements of an ever-escalating population of patients affected by HIV. Chapters on caring for children and for patients with neuropsychiatric illnesses secondary to HIV infection have been comprehensively updated. Advances in medical treatments and the nursing implications of new anti-HIV drugs are described.

Chapters on infection control have been rewritten to include the most current government (UK and USA) guidelines on 'Universal Infection Control Precautions' and 'Body Substance Isolation'.

Chapters on community care, health education, discharge planning and nursing management issues have been expanded and updated. Ethical issues associated with nursing care are explored and model policies are suggested for developing 'HIV-aware' health care facilities, positioned to manage effectively a professional service for both clients and health care staff. I share the author's belief that the nursing care of patients with HIV disease is no different from the nursing care of patients with any other chronic, ultimately fatal disease; it is the issues that are different, not the practice of nursing. This text provides reasoned models of care which grew out of more than 15 years of experience in major London teaching hospitals, in developing the procedural and policy base to caring for patients with HIV disease.

As in previous editions, the text is fully and comprehensively referenced.

Robert Pratt has been associated with the issues surrounding the nursing care of patients with AIDS since the very beginning of the pandemic and has made a major national and local contribution in facilitating the nursing profession's early, effective response to the challenges of AIDS in the United Kingdom. He has worked as a consultant to the World Health Organization's Global Programme on AIDS, conducting training for nurses in Africa, India, Eastern Europe and Asia. He is an adviser to a variety of government and non-governmental organizations and, drawing on his experience at working in the very epicentre of the HIV epidemic in London, he offers a clear, easy to understand, yet comprehensive reference text for nurses who need to acquire a new understanding of caring for patients with HIV disease. Having been published in five different languages, the continuing popularity of this book reflects how effectively it meets the needs of nurses, and other health care professionals, around the world.

Effective nursing care is based on research, knowledge, skill, compassion and integrity. I commend this text to you as the definitive reference guide for professional nurses and other health care professionals, striving to deliver confident, competent and compassionate care within the arena of AIDS patient care.

Chris Beasley
Director of Nursing, NHS Executive – North Thames, Nurse
Member, UK Department of Health Expert Advisory Group on
AIDS (EAGA)

Acknowledgements

I am grateful to Dr John M. Grange (Reader in Clinical Microbiology, National Heart & Lung Institute, London), Carole Fry (Senior Nurse for Infection Control, Chelsea & Westminster Hospital, London) and Dr Clive Loveday (Senior Clinical Lecturer and honarary consultant in Virology, Medical School, University College, London) for their professional advice and guidance on the preparation of specialist sections for this edition. I am also indebted to George Tregaskis for his patient proofreading and advice on style, and to Ian O'Reilly for preparing the artwork in this text. Not least of all, I am obliged to Maurice Jeffery, for his advice encouragement and support.

This text is dedicated to all my friends, colleagues and students, whose lives have been affected by AIDS, principally remembering Werner, David, John and Michael, who were my friends, my patients and, ultimately, my teachers. Finally, remembering always the contribution made to our profession by the late Richard Wells FRCN, at the Royal College of Nursing, I especially dedicate this text to his memory.

Introduction

> In the face of intense and immediate crisis, when an outbreak of
> plague implanted fear of imminent death in an entire community,
> ordinary routines and customary restraints broke down. Rituals
> arose to discharge anxiety and local panic often provoked bizarre
> behavior. The first efforts at ritualizing responses to the plague took
> extreme and ugly forms.
>
> *Plagues and Peoples*, W. H. McNeill

Shortly before Christmas in 1981, the first patient with AIDS in the
United Kingdom lay dying in a London hospital. Medical and nursing
experts, casting a nervous glance at the United States where over
three hundred cases of this new disease had been identified, probably
knew from the beginning that the UK would not escape this evolving
pandemic.

As 1982 and 1983 came and went, more cases were seen and, in a
sense, our worst fears were realized. Cases of AIDS were no longer
being imported into the UK but rather, we had our own endemic
brand, which was quickly spreading. Certain aspects of this particular
disease were especially alarming; its cause was unknown, as was its
means of spread. Treatment of the various infections and cancers seen
in this disease was ineffective, no one surviving once the disease took
hold. Almost all of the affected were young adults, mostly men, and
fear of the disease became a parallel epidemic in its own right.

The heady months of 1984 brought both good news and bad news.
Brilliant research work by French scientists the year before had
uncovered the causative agent of AIDS. This was now confirmed
by researchers in America. With this discovery, the different ways
in which the epidemic was spreading also became clear and it
seemed only a matter of time before a vaccine would be available
to stop, once and for all, this ferocious disease. Nurses, however,
noticed that increasing numbers of patients, either with AIDS or
under investigation for AIDS-related conditions, continued to be
admitted, and, thanks to the hysteria and panic whipped up by a
sensation-seeking media, health care workers became as confused

and frightened as everyone else. As always, the twenty-four hour care of these patients, like all other patients, was the paramount responsibility of nurses and they often seemed surrounded by frightened and sometimes hostile ancillary staff; domestics refusing to clean patients' rooms, catering staff refusing to serve meal trays to patients with AIDS, porters refusing to transport patients with this disease and undertakers refusing to accept the bodies of patients who had died form AIDS. Even some medical staff (notably surgeons) would refuse to treat patients who had AIDS. Draconian infectious disease control procedures, bearing no logical relationship to the known facts of transmission, were often implemented, regardless of cost either in nursing time or in the further, deepening sense of isolation of these patients, frightened of becoming ever more abandoned. In time, AIDS would bring out the best and the worst in people, including health care professionals.

In 1985, 165 new cases brought the total number of individuals in the UK with AIDS to 273. The Communicable Disease Surveillance Centre suggested that as the numbers continued to increase, in 1988, 2000 new cases might reasonably be expected[1].

This year (1985) also saw the introduction of a blood test which could detect infection with HIV, the virus which causes AIDS. The Chief Medical Officer at the Department of Health estimated that there might be over 10 000 HIV-infected individuals in the UK (estimates of asymptomatic infected individuals in the USA ranged from 500 000 to one and a half million)[2]. Not only were these large numbers of infected individuals now able to escalate the epidemic dramatically, but also suspicion grew that these thousands of asymptomatic carriers might not remain asymptomatic as the years went by. It was known by 1985 that HIV attacked not only the immune system, but also cells in the brain, leading, in many cases, to severe neurological disease, including dementia[3]. It seemed reasonable to speculate that everyone infected with this virus would eventually suffer some form of ill health as a consequence of that infection. No health care system, in any part of the world, including the National Health Service in the UK, seemed prepared for even the present number of cases of people with fully expressed AIDS. How they would cope with the 'worst case' scenario of caring for increased numbers of currently asymptomatic, infected individuals was not a pleasant thought to contemplate.

By 1986, there was not the least doubt that AIDS and HIV-related conditions posed the most significant public health issue of our time. Not only were there the American and European epidemics, but major epidemics were also occurring in Central Africa, South America and in Australia. AIDS had become of truly pandemic proportions. It was clear that this disease would be with us, in our hospitals and in our communities, for years to come.

By the end of 1988, over 2000 individuals in the UK had been diagnosed as having AIDS. The number of AIDS cases continued to increase until, by the beginning of 1995, over 10 000 AIDS cases had been reported in the UK, of which more than 66 per cent were then dead. In addition, of those coming forward for HIV testing, more than 20 000 persons were found to be infected[4].

Dealing with the disease one day at a time, and one patient at a time, professional nurses have built up considerable expertise in developing individualized nursing care strategies, designed to deliver compassionate, non-judgemental, confident and competent nursing care to large numbers of relatively young people, suffering and dying in fear and confusion. This text has been written to provide guidance and support, to share collective expertise, to reassure and to inform. Like our predecessors in the great epidemics of the past, nurses must be brave in the face of this current epidemic. We cannot abandon any of our patients, nor would we wish to do so. With accurate information, planned nursing care can be designed to safely and effectively meet the needs of patients suffering from one of the most devastating diseases seen in recent times. On the eve of the Second World War, the American President, Franklin D. Roosevelt, told the American people, 'we have nothing to fear except fear itself'. For health care workers confronting the calamity of AIDS in the 1990s, the same is equally true. The enemy is not only a virus, but equally, fear, ignorance and prejudice. If in a small way this text neutralizes some of these factors, it will have been worth the effort.

References

1. Acheson, E.D. (1985). The CMO's briefing on AIDS. *THS Health Summary*, August, **2**(VIII): 6–7.
2. Acheson, E.D. (1986). AIDS: A challenge for the public health. *Lancet*, 22 March, **i**(8482): 662–6.
3. Sattaur, O. (1985). More evidence for brain disease in AIDS. *New Scientist*, 10 October, p. 26.
4. PHLS Communicable Disease Surveillance Centre (1994). AIDS and HIV-1 infection in the United Kingdom: monthly report. *Communicable Disease Report*, 18 March, **4**(11): 51–2.

1

The Evolution of a Pandemic

> The Plague had swallowed up everything and everyone. No longer
> were there individual destinies, only a collective destiny, made
> of plague and the emotions shared by all. Strongest of these
> emotions was the sense of exile and of deprivation, with all the
> crosscurrents of revolt and fear set up by these.
>
> *The Plague*, Albert Camus

AIDS was to enter the world's consciousness, and become part of the
vocabulary of the human soul, as a result of a dawning awareness of
the advent of a strange, new disease, first reported in California in
1981.

United States of America

In the early months of 1981, five young men were admitted to
various hospitals in Los Angeles, suffering from an unusual type
of pneumonia caused by a commonly occurring protozoa known
as *Pneumocystis carinii*. Previously, pneumonia caused by *P. carinii*
had only been seen in patients who were immunocompromised,
such as infants born with a primary immune deficiency (e.g. severe
combined immune deficiency – SCID) or in adults whose immune
system became deficient due to other causes, i.e. secondary immune
deficiency states. Most cases of pneumonia caused by *P. carinii* had
been observed in renal transplant units, where patients had received
immunosuppressant chemotherapy following kidney transplants, or
in oncology units, where patients had been immunosuppressed as a
result of receiving anti-cancer chemotherapy. Most individuals have
been exposed to this microbe and it is part of the normal flora of many
people. It is harmless in individuals with a competent immune system.
Only in persons with a faulty immune system can it cause disease,
in which case the treatment of choice was a little-used antibiotic,

manufactured in the United Kingdom and known as pentamidine isethionate.

The physician in charge of the first cases in Los Angeles was puzzled. These five patients were all young men who had evidence of a widespread immunodeficiency without any apparent reason. They had evidence of other infections and, coincidentally, they were all homosexual. The Centers for Disease Control (CDC) in Atlanta, Georgia, was notified and supplies of pentamidine were requested, although, by this time, two of the five patients had died. The CDC, which has as part of its function the task of monitoring the trend of infectious diseases throughout the United States and its territories, published an account of these five cases in its weekly bulletin, the *Morbidity and Mortality Weekly Report (MMWR)* on 5 June 1981 and noted that the occurrence of pneumonia caused by *P. carinii* ('pneumocystosis') in five previously healthy individuals, who had no known reason for their defective immune status, was unusual, and questioned whether their homosexual lifestyle, or a disease acquired through sexual contact, could be associated with the development of the defects in the immune system which led to pneumocystosis[1].

Probably then no one actually suspected the magnitude of the epidemic that was in the making. However, evidence of the gathering storm was soon starting to arrive.

At about the same time as physicians in Los Angeles had reported the cluster of cases of pneumocystosis, physicians in New York City and California notified the CDC of the occurrence of a severe form of Kaposi's sarcoma in twenty-six young men. Kaposi's sarcoma is a vascular neoplasm, uncommon in the United States and in Western Europe, being seen mainly in elderly men, where it is manifested by skin lesions and a chronic clinical course (mean survival time is 8–13 years). However, in 1978 Kaposi's sarcoma had been described in patients who had undergone renal transplants and had received immunosuppressant therapy and in others who were iatrogenically immunosuppressed.

Of the twenty-six patients reported to the CDC in July of 1981, all had evidence of an immunodeficiency not related to any known cause and several had other serious infections (four having pneumocystosis). All were homosexual[2].

Simultaneously, an additional ten cases of pneumocystosis in healthy young gay men in Los Angeles and San Francisco were reported, two of whom also had Kaposi's sarcoma. All these patients had evidence of immunodeficiency with no known underlying cause. The following month saw an additional seventy cases of these two conditions[3]. It was then clear that an epidemic was brewing.

This was an epidemic in which death would be caused by one or more unusual, opportunistic infections or by cancer, present only because the immune system had broken down due to unknown reasons.

Extremely alarmed, the CDC instituted a nationwide surveillance programme in July 1981. The new disease was termed the **Acquired Immune Deficiency Syndrome (AIDS)** and it was characterized as the occurrence of unusual infections or cancers in previously healthy individuals, due to an immunodeficiency of unknown cause.

ARC, PGL and LAS

In addition to cases of fully expressed AIDS, many individuals in the same groups as those 'at risk' of developing fully expressed AIDS (e.g. gay men) were presenting for investigation or treatment with a lesser form of AIDS, which came to be referred to as the **AIDS-Related Complex (ARC)**. Individuals with ARC frequently had a combination of various indicators of ill health without having frank opportunistic infections or other conditions described in the surveillance definition of AIDS. Frequently, they presented with unexplained, persistent and generalized swollen lymph glands (this by itself became known as either **persistent, generalized lymphadenopathy – PGL**, or, in France, the **lymphadenopathy syndrome' – LAS**), almost always including cervical and axillary lymph nodes[4]. Individuals with ARC frequently complained of fever, profuse night sweats, fatigue and weight loss. All these patients showed abnormalities in tests for cell-mediated immunity. For every case of AIDS, there would be ten cases of ARC. The numbers started to look astronomical.

Data coming into the CDC from investigators all over the United States showed that the incidence of AIDS was roughly doubling every 6 months. In September 1982, more than two cases were being diagnosed every day and by March 1983, an average of 4–5 cases per day were being reported to the CDC. In 1993, a total of 103 500 new cases were reported for that year alone[5]. By the beginning of 1995, somewhere between 415 000 and 535 000 individuals in the USA will have been diagnosed with AIDS and between 73 and 78 per cent of them will have died of this disease[6]. The number of adolescent and adult persons in the USA infected with HIV is estimated as being over 1 million[7].

United Kingdom

Towards the end of 1981, the first patient diagnosed as suffering from AIDS was seen in a London hospital[8] – AIDS had arrived in Great Britain.

Data released from the Communicable Disease Surveillance Centre (CDSC) at Colindale (London) reflected a similar pattern of spread to that seen in the United States. Over the next 13 years, AIDS would become a significant threat to the health of the nation. From 1982 (when reporting in the UK began) to the end of June 1994, a total of 9436 AIDS cases would be reported to the CDSC; more than 68 per cent of these patients (i.e. 6388) having died[9]. By July 1994, over 22 000 persons were known to be infected with HIV-1[9] and undoubtedly many thousands more were infected but had not yet been tested. Short-term projections[10] for the UK predict that there will be:

- 2375 **new** AIDS cases in 1995;
- 2430 **new** AIDS cases in 1996;
- 2440 **new** AIDS cases in 1997; and
- at the end of 1997, 4190 AIDS cases still alive, plus an additional 4205 cases of other forms of severe HIV disease.

Trends observed and being predicted in the UK include an expected levelling off in the overall incidence of AIDS in 1996 and 1997. AIDS incidence in homosexual men was expected to peak during 1993/4. However, the incidence in those exposed heterosexually is expected to increase steadily. The incidence of HIV infection among injecting drug users seems to have peaked around 1985[10].

Europe

AIDS was destined to become a major public health issue for all Western European countries during the latter half of the 1980s. By the end of 1993, a cumulative total of almost 118 000 AIDS cases (and 58 808 deaths) were recorded. This included 4505 children and 2250 women. HIV infection in women, and HIV infection as a result of heterosexual exposure to the virus, continues to account for an increasing number of new infections[11]. By the year 2000, somewhere between 1 188 000 and 2 331 000 individuals in Western Europe, and between 2000 and 20 000 additional people in Eastern Europe will have become infected with HIV[12].

AIDS in the world

AIDS is now seen in virtually every country in the world. The cumulative number of AIDS cases reported to the World Health Organization's Global Programme on AIDS (WHO/GPA) by the end of 1993 was 851 628. However, taking into account underdiagnosis, underreporting, and delays in reporting, the real figure is more likely to be at least 3 million AIDS cases worldwide (Fig. 1.1)[13]. Three-quarters of current AIDS cases are in developing countries. The numbers of adults currently infected with HIV throughout the world is shown in Fig. 1.2. Projections for the year 2000[14] include:

HIV infection

- a total of 30–40 million persons will have been infected with HIV;

of these infections:

- 42 per cent will have occurred in Asia and Oceania;
- 31 per cent will have occurred in Africa;
- 14 per cent will have occurred in the Caribbean;
- 90 per cent will have occurred in the developing world.

AIDS cases

- 8–24 million adults will have developed AIDS;
- 85 per cent of the cumulative number of AIDS cases will have died by the year 2000 (somewhere between 5.9 and 20.4 million adults).

The major pandemic wave of HIV infection and AIDS will occur from 1995 onwards. This increase is a combined result of two forces: the continued spread in already affected areas (e.g. North America, Latin America, the Caribbean, Western Europe, sub-Saharan Africa) and the accelerating incidence of HIV infection in the most densely populated regions of the world, i.e. South-East and North-East Asia[12].

'At risk' of infection

Although in both the United States and the United Kingdom, AIDS was first recognized in young, male homosexuals, it became clear from the early months of the epidemic that AIDS was not confined to either group. Most individuals in whom AIDS has been diagnosed were men with either homosexual or bisexual lifestyles. Also at risk were injecting drug users, persons with haemophilia, the heterosexual

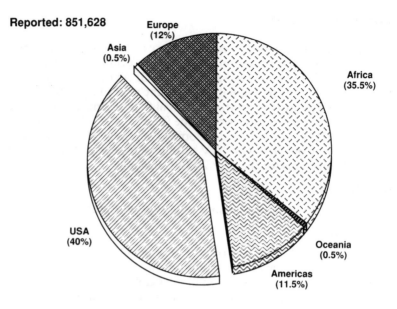

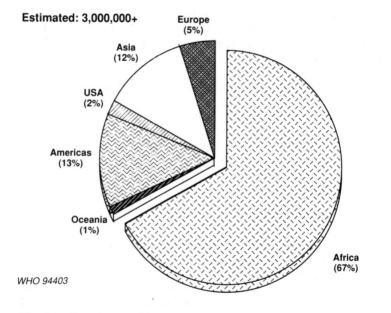

WHO 94403

Fig. 1.1   Cumulative AIDS cases in adults and children at end of 1993

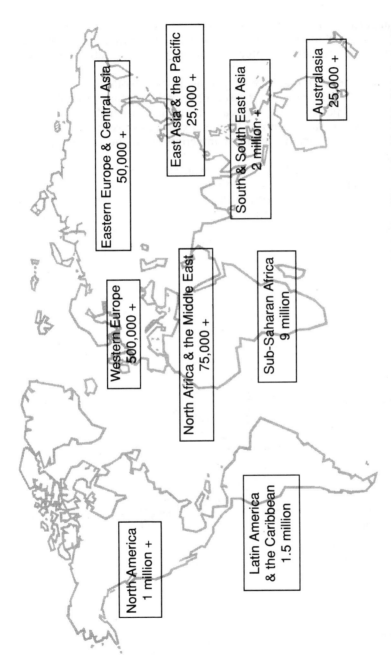

Fig. 1.2   Estimated global distribution of total adult HIV infections from late 1970s/early 1980s until mid-1994. Global total 16 million +

sexual partners of persons with AIDS or 'at risk' for AIDS, recipients of transfused blood or blood components, or children from families in which the mother was infected with HIV, the causative agent of AIDS.

Today, the vast majority of people in this world who become infected with HIV do so as a result of sexual exposure to HIV (Fig. 1.3), over 70 per cent of them as a result of heterosexual intercourse. In many developing countries, heterosexual transmission has always been the predominant means of infection since the outset of the epidemic.

The World Health Organization estimates that almost half of all newly infected adults are women (see Chapter 10). As infections in women rise, so do infections in the infants born to them[14]. By the end of 1993, there were at least 1 million infected infants in our world. Millions more are destined to become infected with or affected by HIV within the remaining years of this decade (see Chapter 11).

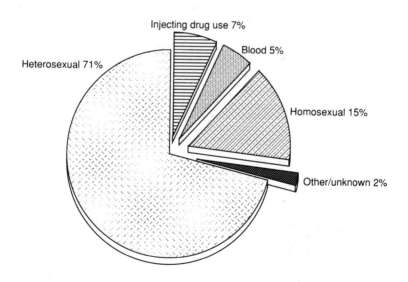

Fig. 1.3   Global proportion of cumulative adult HIV infections by mode of transmission 1992[13]

Conclusion

We already have the means to prevent infection, i.e. health education and behavioural change. However, the entire continuum of humanity remains at risk. In no country on this planet can it be said that this epidemic is under control. It continues as a volatile, unstable and escalating situation. The danger is compounded by the re-emergence, out of the shadows, of one of the great killers of the past – tuberculosis (see Chapter 7). The two, forming a dangerous liaison, and having been termed 'the cursed duet'[15], make the future for humankind somewhat more precarious than most had expected.

References

1. Centers for Disease Control (1981). Pneumocystis pneumonia. Los Angeles. *Morbidity and Mortality Weekly Report (MMWR)*, 5 June, **30**(21), 250–2.
2. Centers for Disease Control (1981). Kaposi's sarcoma and pneumocystis pneumonia among homosexual men. New York City and California. *Morbidity and Mortality Weekly Report (MMWR)*, 3 July, **30**(25), 305–8.
3. Centers for Disease Control (1981). Follow-up on Kaposi's sarcoma and pneumocystis pneumonia. *Morbidity and Mortality Weekly Report (MMWR)*, 28 August, **30**(33), 409–10.
4. Centers for Disease Control (1982). Persistent, generalized lymphadenopathy among homosexual males. *Morbidity and Mortality Weekly Report (MMWR)*, 21 May, **31**(19), 249–51.
5. Centers for Disease Control (1994). Update: Impact of the Expanded AIDS Surveillance Case Definition for Adolescents and Adults on Case Report – United States, 1993. *Morbidity and Mortality Weekly Report (MMWR)*, 11 March, **43**(9), 160–1, 167–70.
6. Centers for Disease Control (1992). Projections for the number of persons diagnosed with AIDS and the number of immunosuppressed HIV-infected persons, United States, 1992–1994. *Morbidity and Mortality Weekly Report (MMWR)* **41**(RR-18), 1–29.
7. Centers for Disease Control (1990). HIV prevalence estimates and AIDS case projections for the United States: Report based upon a workshop. *Morbidity and Mortality Weekly Report (MMWR)* **39**(RR-16), 1–31.
8. Dubois, R.M., Branthwaite, M.A., Mikhail, J.R. *et al.* (1981). Primary *Pneumocystis carinii* and cytomegalovirus infection. *Lancet*, 12 December, **ii**(8259), 1339.
9. PHLS Communicable Disease Surveillance Centre (1994). AIDS and HIV-1 infection in the United Kingdom: monthly report. *Communicable Disease Report* **4**(28), 131–4.
10. PHLS Communicable Disease Surveillance Centre (1993). The inci-

dence and prevalence of AIDS and other severe HIV disease in England and Wales for 1992–1997: Projections using data to the end of June 1992. *Communicable Disease Report*, June, **3**(Suppl. 1), S1–S17.

11. National Reports to the European Centre for the Epidemiological Monitoring of AIDS (1993). AIDS surveillance in Europe. *Quarterly Report*, 31 December, Report no. 40.
12. Mann, J., Tarantola, D.J., and Netter, T.W. (1992). *AIDS in the World: A Global Report*. Harvard University Press, Cambridge, MA.
13. World Health Organization Global Programme on AIDS (WHO/GPA) (1994). GPA publishes new HIV/AIDS data. *Global AIDS News – The Newsletter of the WHO/GPA*, **1**, 11–12.
14. WHO (1993). Press Release. WHO/69 (7 September). World Health Organization, Geneva.
15. Chretien, J. (1990). Tuberculosis and HIV. The cursed duet. *Bulletin of the International Union against Tuberculosis and Lung Disease* **65**(1), 25–8.

Further Reading

Gould, Peter (1993). *The Slow Plague: A Geography of the AIDS Pandemic*. Blackwell Publishers, Oxford (ISBN 1-55786-419-5).

Grmek, Mirko D. (1990). *History of AIDS: Emergence and Origin of a Modern Pandemic*. Princeton University Press, Oxford (ISBN 0-691-08552-8).

Mann, J., Tarantola, D.J., and Netter, T.W. (1992). *AIDS in the World: A Global Report*. Harvard University Press, Cambridge, MA (ISBN 0-674-01266-6).

Shilts, Randy (1987). *And The Band Played On: Politics, People and the AIDS Epidemic*. Viking (The Penguin Group), London (ISBN 0-670-82270-1).

2

The Biology of HIV – The Cause of AIDS

From the beginning of the epidemic, AIDS exhibited all the classic signs of an infectious disease and the only convincing explanation for its cause was the emergence of a new infectious agent. An infective aetiology was consistent with the geographical clustering of early cases and epidemiological proof of case-to-case contact[1, 2], the newness of the disease, the pattern of groups at risk, its occurrence, within the same time scale, in the diverse groups affected, and, finally, its exponential spread.

Various researchers independently discovered the causative agent of AIDS at approximately the same time (1983–4) and named the virus responsible: **LAV**, the 'lymphadenopathy-associated virus'[3]; **HTLV-III**, the 'human T-cell leukaemia (lymphotropic) virus, type III'[4]; and **ARV**, the AIDS-associated retrovirus'[5]. In May 1986, a subcommittee of the International Committee on the Taxonomy of Viruses proposed that the AIDS retroviruses be officially designated as the **'human immunodeficiency viruses'** (**HIV**). This has become the standard term for the viruses which can cause immunosuppression in humans and refers to two viruses: **HIV-1**, the predominant AIDS-causing virus in the world, and **HIV-2**, a biologically distinct second type of AIDS virus, identified in 1986 and generally restricted to West Africa, e.g. Guinea-Bissau, Cape Verde Islands, The Gambia, Senegal, Guinea, Burkina Faso and the Côte d'Ivoire (The Ivory Coast).

Characteristics of viruses

All viruses have certain characteristics which distinguish them from other microbes. These characteristics have to do with their composition, shape, method of reproduction, size, their viral antigenic characters and the host cell receptors to which they are attracted.

Composition (Fig. 2.1)

Genome   The core of the virus is composed of **nucleic acid**. The nucleic acid is *either* **DNA** (deoxyribonucleic acid) *or* **RNA** (ribonucleic acid); *never* both. This core is referred to as the **viral genome** and contains the genetic material (i.e. the complete gene complement) which the virus will use to survive and to reproduce.

Viruses are classified as being *either* **DNA viruses** *or* **RNA viruses**, depending on the composition of their genome.

Capsid   The genome is enclosed within and intimately attached to a protein outer shell, known as the **capsid**. The capsid is built from numerous smaller units **(capsomeres)** and serves to protect the delicate nucleic acid of the virus.

Envelope   Some viruses are enclosed in a **lipoprotein envelope** (or 'coat'), made up of fat and protein derived from material (nuclear and cytoplasmic membranes) from the cells they infect, which clings to them when they escape, by the process of **budding**.

Virion   The genome in the core surrounded by the capsid (and the envelope, if present) composes the complete infective viral particle

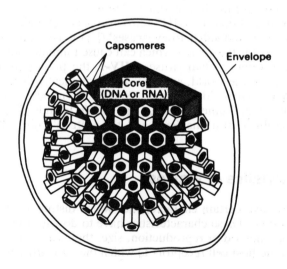

Fig. 2.1   The structure of a virus. (With acknowledgement to *Medical Microbiology*, Vol. 1, published by Churchill Livingstone.)

and is known as a **virion**. The virion is the **extracellular form of the virus** and can be found prior to the virus entering and parasitizing another cell. The virion serves as a transportation mechanism, carrying the viral genome to other cells targeted for infection.

Viruses are not classified as true cells as they do not contain a limiting plasma membrane, cytoplasm, ribosomes, mitochondria, enzymes to generate high energy bonds, or muramic acid in their outer coverings. However, because they contain nucleic acid (i.e. RNA or DNA), the fundamental property of life, they are able to reproduce, but *only inside another cell*, thus being intracellular parasites.

Shape

The capsid and genome of the virus are closely integrated to form a **nucleocapsid** of an exactly defined symmetry (i.e. **shape**). The capsids of different viruses have various shapes (symmetry). Some are **icosahedral** (cubical) in shape, some are **helical**, and still others are so **complex** that their symmetry has not yet been described. Viruses can be further classified according to their shape, i.e. they are either icosahedral, helical or complex.

Reproduction

When a virion enters a cell (the **host cell**) it loses its protein capsid (and lipoprotein envelope, if it has one). Because viruses lack the necessary cellular components needed for reproduction, they use the synthetic machinery in their genome to hijack the nucleus of the cell they have invaded. The viral nucleic acid infects the genetic material of the host cell, along with the cell's raw materials, energy-producing and metabolic systems. It then reprogrammes the nucleus of the host cell and commands it to produce more viruses: the infected host cell becomes a 'virus factory' . Several hundred new viruses can be produced in each infected host cell which then go on to infect other cells.

Size

Virions are extremely small, varying in diameter from 18 to 300 nanometres (a nanometre, or 'nm', is one-thousandth of a micrometre or one-millionth of a millimetre). There are hundreds of viruses which can infect man. They are usually classified according to their shape, size and the composition of their nucleic acid, i.e. they are either DNA viruses or RNA viruses.

Viral antigenic characters and host cell-surface receptors

Viruses have **antigenic characters** which usually reside in their surface structure. Various types of host cells (cells which the virion targets for invasion and infection) carry **cell-surface receptors** for these antigens, to which the virus can bind. The antigenic characters can be thought of as 'keys' and the host cell-surface receptors as 'locks'. Each virus which successfully invades man has a key for a certain lock, but not all locks. When a virion enters the human body, it searches for those host cells which have a lock its key will unlock. By using its key, the virus can open the lock and enter and infect the host cell.

The T-cell surface receptors (TCRs), i.e. the 'locks' on T lymphocytes have been characterized by the unique combination of glycoprotein adhesion molecules that are associated with each TCR and are classified by **CD** (cluster of differentiation) numbers. Different types of T lymphocytes are associated with different types of adhesion molecules, e.g. CD3, CD4, CD8, CD26, etc. The molecules of the **major histocompatibility complex (MCH)** (also known as the 'human leucocyte antigen', or **HLA genes**) are found on the surface of various cells and present antigen fragments to the TCR. Cell-surface receptors on B lymphocytes are mediated by **surface antibody molecules,** e.g. IgM, IgG and IgD. This will be discussed in more detail in Chapter 4.

Summary

Viruses are extremely small life forms, being composed of a piece of nucleic acid (either DNA or RNA, but not both), the viral genome, surrounded by a protein outer shell (the capsid) and sometimes, in addition, the capsid being surrounded by an envelope made up of fat and protein (lipoproteins). Viruses are of varying but exactly defined shapes and, in order to reproduce, must infect and take over the nucleus of a living cell. When viruses infect man, they search for host cells which contain specific surface receptors (e.g. CD4+ receptors on T lymphocytes) to which their antigenic characters can bind, and then invade and infect that cell. Different viruses have different antigenic characters and, as such, are attracted to different host cells. This attraction for specific host cells is known as **tropism.**

Human immunodeficiency viruses

Human immunodeficiency viruses belong to a group of viruses known as the **Retroviridae** (retroviruses). Retroviruses have an

RNA genome and a lipid-containing membrane surrounding their capsid. They also have a special viral enzyme, known as **reverse transcriptase,** which allows the virus to make a DNA copy of its RNA genetic material, facilitating its integration into the genetic material of the host cell. Once inserted into the nucleus of the host cell, it directs this cell to produce more RNA retroviruses. Reverse transcriptase facilitates the process of making DNA from RNA, and the presence of this enzyme is a unique feature of all retroviruses.

Although retroviruses were known to cause disease in some animals, it was not thought that they were involved in human disease. In 1980, a new retrovirus, associated with the aetiology of an aggressive, human, adult T-cell leukaemia, and named **human T-cell leukaemia virus (HTLV)**, was isolated by Robert Gallo[6]. In 1982 Gallo identified another similar, but distinct retrovirus from a patient with hairy cell leukaemia. This was named the **human T-cell leukaemia virus, type II (HTLV-II)**[7]. Human T-cell leukaemia viruses were especially (but not exclusively) attracted to T lymphocytes of the helper subgroup (CD4+ T lymphocytes), which became their targets. This attraction (tropism) for helper cells made them likely candidates for investigation into the aetiology of AIDS as it was known that patients with this disease had a decreased number of CD4+ T lymphocytes.

The possibility that a retrovirus of the HTLV group was involved in the aetiology of AIDS was first reported by Robert Gallo in February 1982[8]. This was followed by the discovery in 1983 of the **lymphadenopathy-associated virus (LAV)** by Françoise Barré-Sinoussi and Luc Montagnier at the Pasteur Institute in Paris, and Robert Gallo's discovery of a new type of **human T-cell leukaemia virus, type III (HTLV-III)** a year later. In 1984, Jay Levy in San Francisco also identified a virus which causes AIDS, which he named the **AIDS-associated retrovirus (ARV)**. All three of these viruses were shown to be associated with AIDS and it soon became clear that they were all different isolates of the same virus. However, they did not belong to the same genus of retroviruses as the HTLVs and, by 1986, they were all renamed **human immunodeficiency viruses (HIV)**.

Retroviruses

Retroviruses (family name: *Retroviridae*) are classified into genera and species. Most retroviruses are associated with disease in fish, reptiles, birds and mammals. The only known retroviruses which can cause disease in humans are **HTLV-I** and **HTLV-II** (oncoviruses, which are species of the retrovirus genus HTLV-BV) and **HIV-1** and **HIV-2** (which are species of the retrovirus genus *Lentivirus* – 'slow' viruses). HIV (and simian immunodeficiency viruses – SIV) are primate lentiviruses. Other species within the genus *Lentivirus* include immunodeficiency viruses associated with disease in horses (**EIAV**), cats (**FIV**), cows (**BIV**) and sheep (**Visna maedi**).

Retroviruses are associated with a wide variety of malignant, degenerative and immunologic diseases. These viruses are not easily transmitted and are very fragile, being easily inactivated by mild detergent, gentle heating, drying, or moderately high or low pH. In general, they can only be transmitted either vertically (from infected mother to her child, at or before parturition or in the immediate postnatal period) or by close physical contact involving the exchange of blood or semen. Infection with retroviruses is characterized by a long period of latency, during which time viral DNA is integrated into the host genome, thereby becoming a permanent infection.

Special characteristics of HIV-1

HIV-1 is 100–120 nm in diameter (Fig. 2.2) . It is icosahedral in shape and contains a helical nucleocapsid.

The HIV genome

The genome of HIV is composed of two identical strands of RNA which contain many genes which give directions (i.e. **encode**) to make either **structural** or **regulatory proteins** (Fig. 2.3). The proteins that make up various parts of the virus are referred to by their size as measured by the mass of protein in thousands of daltons (a unit of mass), or kilodaltons (kDa). For example, p17 refers to a protein with a mass, measured in kilodaltons, of between 17 and 18; gp120 refers to a glycoprotein (proteins linked to sugars) with a protein mass of 120 kilodaltons.

Genes encoding **structural proteins** include the *env* gene which encodes the glycoproteins gp41 and gp120 in the viral envelope, the *gag* gene which encodes the core proteins in the virus (p6, p9, p24, pl7), the and *pol* gene which encodes viral enzymes, i.e. reverse transcriptase (p66/p51), protease (p10) and integrase (p32).

Genes encoding for **early regulatory proteins**, important for viral replication, are *tat* (p14) and *rev* (p19), which, when switched on, increase viral replication, and *nef* (p27), which, when activated, may suppress HIV replication. Other genes which encode for **late regulatory proteins** include *vif* (p23) and, in HIV-1 only, *vpu* (p15). Another gene, *vpr* (p15) encodes for accessory proteins and is important for

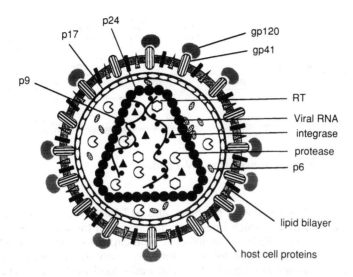

Fig. 2.2 Schematic representation of the HIV virion. (Adapted, with permission from Beatrice Hahn (1994). Viral genes and their products. In *Textbook of AIDS Medicine*, eds Broder, S., Merigan, T.C. Jr. and Bolognesi, D., Williams & Wilkins.)

efficient viral replication in the natural target cells. In addition, *vpx* (p16) is a special gene which encodes for accessory proteins, but only in HIV-2. It is not found in HIV-1.

The genomes of all retroviruses contain **long terminal repeat (LTR)** elements, generated during reverse transcription and only completely present in the DNA copy of the viral genome. LTRs do not encode for protein but are essential for the regulation of viral gene expression. The two strands of RNA are attached to molecules of the enzyme **reverse transcriptase**, which transcribes the viral RNA into DNA once the virus has entered a cell. Other enzymes are also found within the viral genome, including **integrase, protease** (also referred to as **proteinase**) and **ribonuclease**. Two other proteins are present in the genome: **p9**, which is a binding protein for the two strands of RNA, and **p6**, which plays a critical role in virion assembly and release.

Core proteins, glycoproteins and lipid bilayer

Surrounding the viral genome is a double protein coat (the **core proteins**). There are two core proteins: **p24** is the major capsid protein

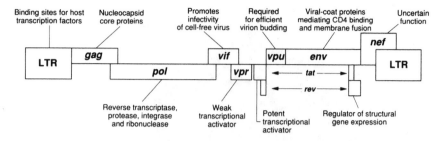

Fig. 2.3   Genetic structure of the HIV-1 genome

which surrounds the viral genome, and **p17** (also referred to as **p18**) is a matrix protein which lines and interacts with the inner surface of the lipid bilayer. These proteins (the viral capsid) are surrounded by a fatty membrane (**lipid bilayer**) with glycoprotein (proteins linked to sugars) structures attached to and embedded in it. The **gp120** is the external portion of the viral envelope and **gp41** spans the lipid bilayer and anchors the glycoprotein complex to the surface of the virion. The lipid bilayer, derived from human cells, and carrying host antigens, is the viral **envelope** (Fig. 2.2). This bilayer is studded with cellular proteins, including β_2-microglobulin and proteins of human origin, known as **class I** and **class II major histocompatibility complex** molecules. These proteins may help the virus to dock onto the host cell and further facilitate virus/cell fusion and core penetration.

Pathophysiology of HIV infection (Fig. 2.4)

The attack

Stage 1: Targeting for invasion   The outer glycoproteins, gp120, act as the antigenic 'keys' which are attracted to, and bind with, the special host cell receptors ('locks') – CD4. Host cells which contain the CD4+ surface receptors, and which are targeted for HIV infection, are[9]:

- CD4+ T lymphocytes ('T4' helper cells);
- CD4+ macrophages, monocytes and brain macrophages, i.e. microglia cells; and
- CD4+ recticulo-endothelial blood dendritic cells and related 'Langerhans cells' in the skin and mucous membranes.

There are most probably other cell-surface receptors for HIV

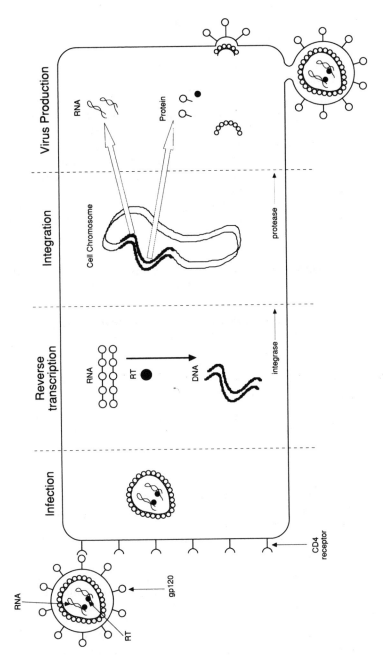

Fig. 2.4 Infection, integration and virus production in CD4 cell

which the virus can dock on to and this is currently the subject of intense research. In addition to the CD4+ cell-surface receptor, other 'secondary' or 'alternative' receptor(s) may be needed for viral penetration, e.g. CD26, cell-surface proteinase and galactosylcerebroside[9,10].

Stage 2: Cell invasion   The virus, once bound to the host cell CD4 receptors, gains entry into the cell in one of two ways. Cells constantly take in new materials by a process of **endocytosis**, i.e. the cell membrane folds inwards to form a tiny vesicle which carries the material, or in this case, the virus, inside the cell. Eventually the vesicle carrying the virus releases it into the cytoplasm of the host cell. Alternatively, once the gp120 of the virus is locked on to the CD4 receptor, the virus might simply **fuse** its surrounding membrane with the membrane of the cell and quickly enter the cytoplasm of the host cell. Membrane fusion is most likely the predominant mechanism involved in HIV entry.

Stage 3: Shedding the viral coats   Once inside the host cell, the viral structure disintegrates, releasing the RNA and the reverse transcriptase enzymes.

Stage 4: Making the master copy   Using the reverse transcriptase enzymes, the viral genome copies the two identical strands of RNA to DNA genetic material. The presence of the enzyme reverse transcriptase, and the ability of the viral genome to copy itself from RNA to DNA, is a fundamental characteristic of all retroviruses and distinguishes them from other viruses.

Stage 5: Entering the nucleus   The viral DNA then enters the nucleus of the host cell and becomes intimately integrated into the host cell's own DNA. The virus has thus become a permanent part of an infected person's own nucleic acid, i.e. establishing a permanent infection and becoming immortalized.

Stage 6: The calm before the storm   A period of calm (latency) now ensues and the virus, as it was, ceases to exist. However, the original infective virus has become a latent **provirus** which is sitting in the nucleus of the infected cell awaiting an external signal to start reproducing.

Stage 7: Viral replication   The cell is stimulated by chemical signals which may be the result of a new infection and would normally result in the cell reproducing itself. However, the nucleus is now reprogrammed by the provirus and, instead, reacts to these stimulating signals by manufacturing more virus. The proviral DNA is transcribed into RNA and new viral proteins are formed by cleavage of precursor proteins and the action of viral enzymes, e.g. protease (proteinase). New virions are constructed just beneath the cell membrane and the newly transcribed strands of identical RNA are inserted into the virion prior to release from the cell. The replication cycle is very inefficient, as possibly only 1 in 100 new virions are functional and infectious.

Stage 8: Cell exit As more and more viruses are manufactured within the infected cell, they eventually explode outwards through the cytoplasmic membrane of the host cell by a process known as **budding.** As they leave the infected cell, they surround themselves with protein, lipid and glycoprotein coats which they hijack from the cytoplasmic membranes of the host cell. Once released into the bloodstream, they start searching for new target cells which have the special CD4 'lock' and the cycle starts all over again.

Stage 9: Cell death The process of new viruses budding out of the original infected host cell may cause holes to be punched into the cell membrane of the host cell. Through these holes, essential cellular ingredients escape through the sieve-like membrane until the cell can no longer survive. Other cells in the immune system, and antibodies, may also destroy host cells that were damaged by the budding out of new viruses (an **autoimmune response**).

Summary

HIV has a special affinity for CD4+ T lymphocytes (T4 helper cells) and infects some but certainly not all of them. Those infected are turned into virus-producing cells and will eventually be destroyed. Viral replication increases when the infected CD4+ T-lymphocyte cell is activated. These cells are activated by infections (e.g. sexually transmitted diseases) or by the presence of substances containing non-infective antigen, such as the antigenic components of concentrated Factor VIII. Newly produced viruses are liberated by 'budding' out from the host cell and infect more helper cells, eventually leading to their destruction. The presence of HIV in some helper cells may also provoke an autoimmune response against non-infected helper cells, causing further destruction of these important cells[11]. HIV infection also induces a premature programmed cell death (**apoptosis**) in infected CD4+ T lymphocytes, which further depletes their numbers[12].

Once helper cells are depleted, B lymphocytes are inefficient as they require the 'help' of helper cells to produce specific antibody. Both the function and activities of cytotoxic CD8+ T lymphocytes (**killer cells**) are impaired[13], resulting in a decreased ability of the immune system to destroy neoplastic and virus-infected cells. Macrophages, having CD4+ cell-surface receptors, are also infected and destroyed[14], leading to a diminished phagocytic response and a decreased ability of the body to defend itself against extracellular pathogens, such as bacteria.

The origins of the virus

It may be that the exact origins of AIDS will never be completely elicited. There are, however, certain facts that have led to a more or less general agreement as to the source of this epidemic. It is plausible to conclude that HIV is a pathogen new to the human race, probably resulting from a non-pathogenic, subhuman primate retrovirus, which made a 'species jump' from African primates (monkeys) to humans. There is widespread evidence that many Old World primates, e.g. chimpanzees, mandrills, sooty mangabeys and African green monkeys, in sub-Saharan Africa have been infected with retroviruses similar to HIV for thousands of years[15], although they are non-pathogenic and do not cause disease in these animals. These viruses are referred to as **simian immunodeficiency viruses** (**SIV**). They have the same complex genomic structure as HIV, share 40–50 per cent homology (structural similarity) with HIV and infect T lymphocytes through the CD4+ cell-surface receptor, just as HIV does. It is probable that these retroviruses are the progenitor viruses from which HIV either mutated or recombined into the human population.

Humans may have been exposed to these viruses as a result of killing and butchering a monkey. In doing so, blood from an SIV-infected primate could have infected a human through non-intact skin on the hands. Once SIV had gained entry to the human body, it found it could thrive in what was, after all, simply a closely related primate species. This concept, i.e. a **zoonosis**, refers to a disease or infection of animals which may be transmitted to man under natural conditions. Several other infectious diseases have a zoonotic origin, e.g. rabies, brucellosis, Lassa fever and various tropical haemorrhagic fevers.

The 'species leap' probably occurred, from time to time, for many hundreds of years. However, HIV infection (and subsequent disease) remained episodic. Because of the rural (village) lifestyle, short life span and lack of sexual promiscuity in Africans at that time, the infection was not widely transmitted to other humans and remained localized to the village. Several factors conspired to change this episodic infection to first an epidemic, and then pandemic infection, including the migration of rural populations into cities, changes in sexual behaviour and increasing promiscuity, improved road, rail and air travel routes and international travel. In addition, increasing reliance on non-barrier forms of contraception, i.e. 'the pill', and injecting drug use also hastened the spread of HIV infection.

Cases of AIDS in sub-Saharan Africa became known at about the same time (1981) as American and European cases, although it is likely that human HIV infection existed in Africa long before the disease was recognized[16]. AIDS is now epidemic in most Central and East African countries (Zambia, Zaïre, Rwanda, Uganda and Tanzania). The current pandemic may have started in Africa and have spread simultaneously to the USA, Haiti and Europe. Certainly many Haitians lived in Zaïre from the early 1960s to the mid-1970s, and then moved to the United States, Europe, or returned to Haiti. It is likely that the spread of AIDS into the UK occurred via British tourists returning from American holidays. However the spread of AIDS into the rest of Europe was more likely a direct result of African links (Fig. 2.5). It then took less than ten years for HIV infection to spread to the most densely populated areas of the world, i.e. Latin America, the Caribbean, India and South-East Asia, where, currently, the pandemic is rapidly accelerating out of control.

HIV-1 and HIV-2

In 1985, serologic surveys in Dakar, Senegal (West Africa) identified antibody patterns in female sex workers which indicated infection with a virus closely related to HIV[17]. In 1986, a retrovirus, similar to but distinct from HIV was isolated from patients ill with an AIDS-like illness in Guinea-Bissau and the Cape Verde Islands in West Africa[18]. This was originally referred to as LAV-2 but has now been renamed **HIV-2**. Although similar to HIV-1, HIV-2 has a different sequence of nucleotides in its genome. In addition, HIV-1 has one gene (*vpu*) which is not found in HIV-2 and HIV-2 has a gene (*vpx*) which is not found in HIV-1, but is found in SIV[19]. Studies focused on the structural similarity (homology) of the viral genome of each virus suggest that they both evolved from SIV, but from different simian species, i.e. HIV-1 diverging from chimpanzee SIV and HIV-2 diverging from sooty mangabey SIV. These data confirm that the two viruses are distinct elements of the HIV family and cannot be considered 'strains' of the same virus[20].

Seroprevalence surveys have shown HIV-2 infection in most West African countries, the highest prevalence being in Guinea-Bissau, Côte d'Ivoire and Burkina Faso[21]. Some individuals are infected

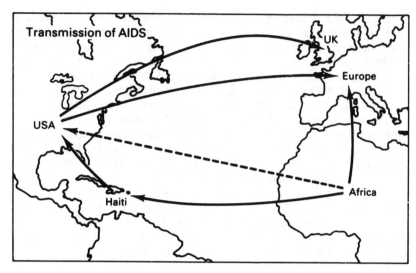

Fig. 2.5 The early spread of HIV-1

with both viruses and although HIV-1 was introduced much later than HIV-2, in some countries, e.g. Côte d'Ivoire, it is now present at higher levels than HIV-2. HIV-2 infection in Europe, Central or East Africa and North America is extremely rare and individuals who are infected are almost always West African immigrants or those who have had sexual contact (directly or indirectly) with West Africans.

Both viruses have the same method of transmission, i.e. close, intimate contact where blood or semen is exchanged, target the same cell-surface receptors (CD4) and, consequently, the same range of cells, i.e. CD4+ T lymphocytes (helper cells), monocytes, macrophages and microglia cells in the central nervous system.

HIV-2 is significantly less transmissible than HIV-1, both from mother to child (vertical transmission) and between sexual partners. HIV-2 infection, unlike HIV-1 infection, is frequently seen in older persons, confirming that it is spread less efficiently than HIV-1, i.e. it takes more exposures over a longer period of time to get infected with HIV-2. Following infection with HIV-2, the level of virus in the blood is much lower than in those infected with HIV-1. HIV-2 also seems less virulent than HIV-1 but still causes disease. Once infected with HIV-2, progression to end-stage disease, i.e. AIDS, is much slower than in HIV-1 infection[20].

HIV-1-O: A variant of HIV-1

A new variant of HIV-1 has recently been described in persons in, or originating from, West Central Africa (Cameroon, Gabon) and has been classified as '**subtype O**' (**HIV-1-O**)[22]. These variants were designated 'O' because genetic studies showed that they were 'outliers' from other known subtypes. HIV-1-O differs significantly from HIV-1 and HIV-2 in its proteins and nucleotide sequences. It is most likely an unusual infection, even in that part of Africa. However, some of the current HIV antibody tests will not detect HIV-1-O infection[23]. This could represent a potential risk to public health, particularly in relation to maintaining the safety of blood products[24]. It is probable that other variants of HIV may emerge and medical scientists all over the world are engaged in cooperative, active surveillance for the early detection of new variants, and to appropriately modify test kits so that HIV-1-O infection can be serologically identified[25].

References

1. Auerbach, D.M., Bennett, J.V., Brachman, P.J. and the CDC Task Force (1982). Epidemiologic aspects of the current outbreak of Kaposi's sarcoma and opportunistic infections. *New England Journal of Medicine*, 26 January, **306**(4), 248–52.
2. Gazzard, B.G., Farthing, C. *et al.* (1984). Clinical findings and serological evidence of HTLV-III infections in homosexual contacts of patients with AIDS and persistent generalised lymphadenopathy. *Lancet*, 1 September, **ii**(8401), 480–3.
3. Barre-Sinoussi, F., Chermann, J.C. *et al.* (1983). Isolation of a T-lymphotropic retrovirus from a patient at risk from acquired immune deficiency syndrome (AIDS). *Science*, 20 May, **220**(4599), 868–71.
4. Gallo, R.C., Salahuddin, S.Z. *et al.* (1984). Frequent detection and isolation of cytopathic retroviruses (HTLV-III) from patients with AIDS and at risk from AIDS. *Science*, 4 May, **224**(4648), 500–3.
5. Levy, J.A., Hoffman, A.D. *et al.* (1984). Isolation of lymphocytopathic retroviruses from San Francisco patients with AIDS. *Science*, 225, 840–2.
6. Poiesz, B.J., Ruscetti, F.W. *et al.* (1980). Detection and isolation of type-C retrovirus particles from fresh and cultured lymphocytes of a patient with cutaneous T-cell lymphoma. *Proceedings of the National Academy of Science USA*, **77**, 7415–19.
7. Kalyanaraman, V.S., Sarngaddharan, M.G. *et al.* (1982). A new subtype of human T-cell leukemia virus (HTLV-II) associated with a T-cell variant of hairy cell leukemia. *Science*, **218**, 571–3.

8. Gallo, R.C., Essex, M. and Gross, L. (1982). *Human T-cell Leukemia/Lymphoma Virus*. Cold Spring Harbor Press, New York.

9. Weiss, Robin A. (1994). The virus and its target cells. In *Textbook of AIDS Medicine*, eds Broder, S., Merigan, T.C. Jr. and Bolognesi, D., Williams & Wilkins, Baltimore, MD, pp. 15–20.

10. Dalgleish, A.G. (1993). Shooting the messenger. *Current AIDS Literature*, December **6**(12), 423.

11. Pantaleo, G., Graziosi, C. and Fauci, A.S. (1993). The immunopathogenesis of human immunodeficiency virus infection. *New England Journal of Medicine*, 4 February, **328**(5), 327–35.

12. Carson, D.A. and Ribeiro, J.M. (1993). Apoptosis and disease: Review article. *The Lancet*, 15 May, **341**(8855), 1251–4.

13. Buseyne, F. and Rivière, Y. (1993). HIV-specific CD8+ T-cell immune responses and viral replication. *AIDS*, **7**(Suppl. 2), S81–S85.

14. Fauci, A.S. and Rosenberg, Z.F. (1994). Immunopathogenesis. In *Textbook of AIDS Medicine*, eds Broder, S., Merigan, T.C. Jr. and Bolognesi, D., Williams & Wilkins, Baltimore, MD, pp. 55–76.

15. Essex, M. (1992). Origin of AIDS. In *AIDS: Etiology, Diagnosis, Treatment and Prevention*, 3rd edn, eds DeVita, V.T. Jr., Hellman, S. and Rosenberg, S.A., J.B. Lippincott, Philadelphia, pp. 3–12.

16. Grmek, Mirko D. (1990). *History of AIDS: Emergence and Origin of a Modern Pandemic*, Trans. Maulitz, R.C. and Duffin, J., Princeton University Press, Princeton, NJ, Chapter 15.

17. Barin, F., Mboup, S., Denis, F. *et al.* (1985). Serological evidence for virus related to simian T-lymphotropic retrovirus III in residents of West Africa. *Lancet* **ii**: 1387–9.

18. Clavel, F., Guétard, D., Brun-Vézinet, F. *et. al.* (1986). Isolation of a new human retrovirus from West African patients with AIDS. *Science* **233**, 343–6.

19. Kanki, P.J. (1992). Virologic and biologic features of HIV-2. In *AIDS and Other Manifestations of HIV Infection*, 2nd edn, ed. Wormser, G.P., Raven Press, New York, pp. 88–94.

20. Essex, M. and Kanki, P. (1994). Human immunodeficiency virus type 2 (HIV-2). In *Textbook of AIDS Medicine*, eds Broder, S., Merigan, T.C. Jr. and Bolognesi, D., Williams & Wilkins, Baltimore.

21. Brown, P. (1992). HIV-2: slower, still deadly. *WorldAIDS*, July, **22**, 10.

22. Gürtler, L.G., Hauser, P.H., Eberle, J. *et al.* (1994). A new subtype of human immunodeficiency virus type 1 (MVP-5180). *Journal of Virology* **68**, 1581–5.

23. Loussert-Ajaka, I., Ly, T.D., Chaix, M.L. *et al.* (1994). HIV-1/HIV-2 seronegativity in HIV-1 subtype O infected patients. *Lancet* **343**, 1393–4.

24. Dondero, T.J., Hu, D.J. and George, J.R. (1994). HIV-1 variants: yet another challenge to public health. *Lancet* **343**, 1376.

25. PHLS Communicable Disease Surveillance Centre (1994). HIV-1-O: a variant of HIV-1. *Communicable Disease Report Weekly*, 17 June, **4**(24), 109.

Further Reading

Grmek, Mirko D. (1990). *History of AIDS: Emergence and Origin of a Modern Pandemic*, trans. Maulitz, R.C. and Duffin, J., Princeton University Press, Princeton, NJ (ISBN 0-691-08552-8).

Hahn, B.H. (1994). Viral genes and their products. In *Textbook of AIDS Medicine*, eds Broder, S., Merigan, T.C. Jr. and Bolognesi, D., Williams & Wilkins, Baltimore, MD, (ISBN 0-683-01072-7).

3

HIV Transmission

The AIDS epidemic is a composite of many individual, though overlapping, smaller epidemics, each with its own dynamics and time course.

MMWR (1987) 36(49)

Now, well into the second decade of our experience with this disease, the known means of viral transmission are generally understood. HIV is a bloodborne virus and has been isolated from blood[1], semen[2], saliva[3], tears[4], breast milk[5] and cerebrospinal fluid[6].

Domains of exposure

HIV is transmitted through sexual contact and exposure to infected blood or blood components and, perinatally, from mother to neonate. Transmission potentials can be conveniently categorized into four major domains of possible exposure:

- Drug use
- Sexual transmission
- Vertical transmission
- Iatrogenic transmission

Drug use

Individuals who use injectable drugs account for the second largest group of individuals who have contracted HIV infection, both in the United States and in Western Europe. In the European Community (EC), by 1989, the incidence of new AIDS cases among injecting drug users had become equal to that occurring among homo/bisexual men[7]. In the United Kingdom, the known prevalence of HIV infection among injecting drug users remains low, being estimated at less than 2 per cent in most parts of the country. However, there are high prevalence areas in Scotland where, in Edinburgh and Dundee, approximately 25 per cent of drug injectors are thought to be infected and in England where, in London, approximately 8 per cent of drug injectors are probably infected[8].

HIV infection is transmitted by sharing blood-contaminated needles, syringes and injecting paraphernalia. However, drug users are, by and large, sexually active individuals, and may acquire HIV infection as a result of sexual exposure. Other, non-injectable drugs which often remove protective behavioural inhibitions may increase the risk of drug users to infection, as will trading or selling sex for drugs or money.

Smoking 'crack' cocaine is associated with increased risk of becoming infected with HIV[9]. Finally, the chaos in which many drug users live, e.g. homelessness, unemployment, etc., may make it difficult for them to incorporate harm reduction strategies into both their sexual and drug taking behaviour.

Sharing contaminated injecting equipment is the principal risk faced by injecting drug users. However, the risk of sexual exposure to HIV may be enhanced by the use of other, non-injectable drugs, e.g. 'crack' cocaine, various stimulants and alcohol which may alter protective behavioural restraints. Clearly the risk of sexual exposure is increased if drug users are exchanging sex for drugs or money.

Vertical transmission

AIDS in children was first reported in 1982[10,11]. The risk of an HIV-infected mother infecting her infant exists principally either in *utero* or during delivery (intrapartum). Postpartum risks exist from infectious breast milk, especially if the mother was postnatally infected (Fig. 3.1). It is not absolutely clear when most maternal–infant transmission takes place. This will be discussed in more detail in Chapter 11).

Sexual transmission

The majority of persons who have become infected with this virus have done so as a result of sexual exposure to HIV. Sexual behaviours which can efficiently facilitate HIV transmission can occur in both heterosexual and homosexual encounters and globally, the vast majority of persons infected sexually are as a result of heterosexual exposure (Fig. 3.2).

The chief route of HIV transmission is via sexual activity. Homosexual (and heterosexual) anal intercourse is an efficient means of transmission, due to the presence of both potentially infected semen

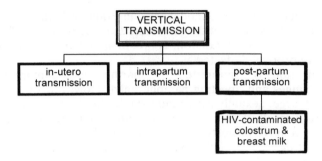

Fig. 3.1   Vertical transmission

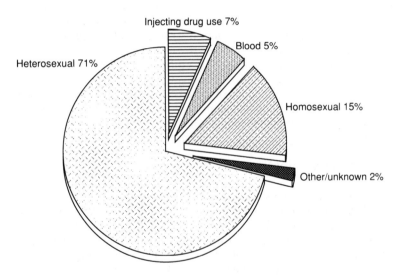

Fig. 3.2   Proportion of cumulative adult HIV infections by mode of transmission[12]

and small amounts of blood, which are common in penetrative rectal intercourse. In Europe and the United States, homosexual or bisexual men constitute the largest group of individuals who have contracted HIV infection. This is due to the propensity for anal sex and the multiplicity of sexual partners often associated with this group. Heterosexual vaginal intercourse is also an efficient means of virus transmission, due to both potentially infected semen and vaginal and cervical secretions containing infected lymphocytes. In sub-Saharan Africa, the Caribbean, and South-East Asia, AIDS is principally a heterosexually spread disease and is a significant exposure domain in North-East Asia, Latin America, the southeastern Mediterranean and Western Europe[12]. The principal sexual behaviours which are associated with sexually transmitting HIV are receptive anal intercourse and insertive and receptive vaginal intercourse. In addition, although a lesser risk, receptive oral intercourse (fellatio) is a risk if the male insertive partner is infected with HIV[13,14].

Iatrogenic transmission

Iatrogenesis refers to the creation of additional problems or complications resulting from treatment or care. HIV transmission has been documented following exposure as a result of the items listed in Fig. 3.3. I will return to the conundrum of the HIV-infected health care worker in Chapter 13. The number of individuals becoming infected via iatrogenic exposure will continue to decline in the industrialized world as the epidemic continues but, although they currently account for only a small percentage of those who have become infected, they continue to haunt the public perception of risk completely out of proportion to the actual risk.

Blood and blood products

HIV has been transmitted following transfusion of whole human blood, blood components and the administration of concentrated Factor VIII, manufactured from pooled plasma and used in the treatment of haemophilia. The routine screening of donor blood for the presence of HIV antibodies (indicating infection) and the self-exclusion of donors who, on the known means of transmission, may have been exposed to HIV, will substantially decrease (but not

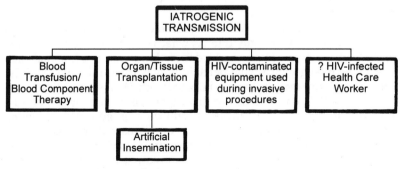

Fig. 3.3 Iatrogenic transmission

totally eliminate) infection from this source. By 1992, transmission through blood or blood components accounted for 2–3 per cent of HIV infections in North America and Western Europe. However, in the southeastern Mediterranean, 18 per cent of infections were acquired through blood transfusions or blood component therapy, as were 10 per cent of infections in North-east Asia. Rates of infection through this mode varied between 4 and 6 per cent in sub-Saharan Africa, the Caribbean and South-East Asia[12].

Organ transplants and artificial insemination by donor semen

Donor organs (kidneys, corneas, hearts, etc.) are a potential risk and individuals whose previous behaviour has put them at risk of acquiring HIV infection are advised not to donate organs or to carry 'donor cards'. The routine screening of donors for HIV infection will diminish this risk substantially. However, the risk will not disappear completely as the donor may have only recently become infected and serological tests for HIV infection will be negative[15]. Cases have been reported of recipients of artificial insemination of donor semen acquiring HIV infection[16]. This risk will decrease with screening of donors, the voluntary self-exclusion of donors who may have been exposed to HIV, and the exclusive use of cryopreserved donor semen, stored for 3–6 months and not used until the donor has been retested for anti-HIV. The use of fresh semen in artificial insemination programmes will remain a potential risk and is not recommended.

Transmission categories

In both the UK and the USA, most cases of AIDS (80 per cent in the UK and 60 per cent in the USA) have occurred in men with homosexual or bisexual orientation. This transmission group is often referred to as the '**first wave**' of the epidemic and it is important to remember that because of the long incubation period of AIDS, the current cases of gay men with AIDS only reflects what was happening 10–15 years ago. There is now convincing evidence that many homosexual men started changing their sexual behaviour as early as mid-1987 and the numbers of gay men becoming infected with HIV started to decline at that time[17]. Whether or not this change in behaviour can be sustained is not certain. In Europe, recent data on gonorrhoea among homosexual men from London, Leeds and Amsterdam seem to indicate that high risk sexual practices have once again increased[18,19].

The '**second wave**' of the epidemic involves individuals who use injectable drugs. In both Europe and the USA, this transmission group is accounting for an ever increasing number of individuals with HIV disease, and they comprise the second largest exposure category[12]. It is important to remember that individuals who use injectable drugs are generally sexually active (both heterosexually and homosexually) and it is usually impossible to ascertain exactly how they became infected. However, it is acknowledged that sharing blood-contaminated injecting equipment is a more efficient means of viral transmission than sexual intercourse.

Finally, the '**third wave**' of the epidemic involves men and women who have become infected with HIV as a result of heterosexual exposure. As more women become infected, more perinatally infected infants will be born. During the 1990s, individuals from the second and third waves of the epidemic will come to dominate the numbers of patients/clients requiring nursing care as a result of symptomatic HIV infection.

Transmission categories are different, dynamic and evolving in the various parts of the world affected by this pandemic and have been described by the World Health Organization (WHO). They describe three categories of countries:

WHO pattern I countries In Europe and North America, HIV began to spread extensively during the latter half of the 1970s, principally among homosexual and bisexual men. Later, drug users would enter the epidemic, and by the end of the 1980s an escalating number of heterosexual men and women would become infected.

WHO pattern II countries In other parts of the world, notably sub-Saharan Africa and, increasingly, Latin America and the Caribbean, HIV also started to spread during the latter half of the 1970s, principally among heterosexual men and women. Transmission from HIV-contaminated blood transfusions and unsterile medical equipment (needles, syringes, etc.) also accounted for significant numbers of new infections. Illicit drug use was an uncommon means of HIV transmission in these countries.

WHO pattern III countries In Eastern Europe, the Middle East, North Africa and most countries in Asia and the Pacific, HIV slowly began to spread during the 1980s, initially from imported blood or blood products, or contact with individuals from pattern I or pattern II countries. Commercial sex workers would become infected by the end of the 1980s, as would significant numbers of injecting drug users.

Risk factors

Male-to-male (via anal intercourse or, more rarely, from fellatio) and **male-to-female** (via vaginal or anal intercourse) are the two most efficient means of sexually transmitting HIV. **Female-to-male** and **passive male-to-active male** (during anal/oral intercourse) transmission is less efficient because the concentration of virus (i.e. the number of 'infectious particles per million' or ppm) is generally higher in semen than in vaginal or cervical secretions. However, an increased number of white cells in cervical or vaginal secretions (as seen in chronic pelvic inflammatory diseases, e.g. sexually transmitted diseases) or the presence of even small amounts of blood will enhance the effectiveness of female-to-male (or passive male-to-active male during anal intercourse) viral transmission. **Female-to-female** transmission is reported from time to time but must be extremely rare[20].

Other factors involved in the probability of efficient sexual transmission of HIV include:

Type of sexual activity   Penetrative vaginal and anal intercourse, sexual intercourse during the menstrual cycle and the number of times an individual has unprotected penetrative intercourse with an infected partner all increase the likelihood of viral transmission. Passive (i.e. receptive) vaginal and anal intercourse are significantly associated with a higher risk of HIV acquisition than active (i.e. insertive) intercourse. Receptive oral–genital sex has now been conclusively associated with HIV transmission, although the risk is probably less than one-sixth the risk of receptive anal sex for men who have sex with men[21,22]. Incidents in which HIV has been transmitted from an infected woman to a man via oral intercourse have been reported[23,24]. Although active anal–oral sex ('rimming') is not linked to HIV transmission, it may be associated with the transmission of an infectious agent which, in combination with a deteriorating immune response secondary to HIV infection, may cause Kaposi's sarcoma[25,26]. Deep, passionate kissing ('French kissing') has also not conclusively been shown to be associated with HIV transmission.

Male-to-female transmission   Available evidence strongly suggests that male-to-female transmission is more efficient than female-to-male transmission [27,28]. Increased risk factors associated with HIV acquisition in women include the presence of a sexually transmitted disease in the woman, anal sex, and symptomatic HIV disease in the woman's male partner[27].

Disease stage of the index case (i.e. the infected partner) It is probable that an individual is most infectious, from a sexual transmission point of view, shortly after becoming infected and then after a long period of time when they become unwell as a result of that infection. Infectiousness in the index case may be associated with a positive HIV culture and/or the presence of p24 antigen and a declining CD4+ T-lymphocyte count (< 400 mm^3)[27,29].

Viral variants There is significant genetic diversity among different strains of both HIV-1 and HIV-2 and an HIV-infected individual is host to many different strains of the virus, which are continually evolving. Biological variants in different viral strains are likely to be more infectious and virulent than are other strains[30,31].

Presence of other sexually transmitted diseases (STDs) Not only do other concurrent STDs recruit additional white cells and macrophages to the sexual field, but they may also alter the protective mucosa of the vagina, rectum or urethra, increasing the probability of HIV transmission. This is especially true of ulcerative STDs, e.g. genital herpes, chancroid and primary syphilis. Consequently, the presence of an STD increases the risk of becoming infected with HIV, or, if already infected, transmitting HIV to a non-infected partner[31,32]. The presence of non-ulcerative STDs, e.g. gonorrhoea, is also associated with increased risk of HIV acquisition or transmission[33].

Viral load The amount of virus to which an individual is exposed is significant. Being exposed to a large amount of virus not only increases the risk of ultimately being infected but may also lead to an accelerated progression into fully expressed AIDS.

Lack of male circumcision If the male is uncircumcised, there is a greater probability of viral acquisition than in circumcised men[34,35].

Bleeding during sex Any open lesions, however small, which result from trauma during sexual activity, may cause bleeding which would increase the likelihood of both transmission and acquisition of HIV.

Number of sexual partners A direct relationship exists between the number of different sexual partners and the probability of contracting HIV infection during unprotected, penetrative sexual activity.

Conclusion

Although homosexual men were particularly vulnerable to this infection during the early years of the epidemic, AIDS and other manifestations of HIV infection are not exclusive to this group of individuals. All sexually active individuals can be infected, if exposed to the virus under the right circumstances. Nurses have both a unique responsibility and opportunity to assist in the health education efforts, aimed at primary prevention, currently being implemented by the health services. The role of the nurse in patient education, as related to HIV infection, is discussed in Chapter 17.

References

1. Gallo, R.C., Salahuddin, S.Z., Popovic, M. *et al.* (1984). Frequent detection and isolation of cytopathic retroviruses (HTLV-III) from patients with AIDS and at risk for AIDS. *Science* **224**, 500–3.
2. Zagury, D., Bernard, J., Leibowitch, J. *et al.* (1984). HTLV-III in cells cultured from semen of two patients with AIDS. *Science* **226**, 449.
3. Groopman, J.E., Salahuddin, S.Z., Sarngadharan, M.G. *et al.* (1984). HTLV-III in saliva of people with AIDS-related complex and healthy homosexual men at risk for AIDS. *Science* **226**, 447–9.
4. Fujikawa, L.S., Palestine, A.G., Nussenblatt, R.B. *et al.* (1985). Isolation of human T-lymphotropic virus type III from the tears of a patient with the acquired immune deficiency syndrome. *Lancet*, 7 September, ii(8454), 529–30.
5. Thirty, L., Sprecher-Goldberger, S., Jonckheer, T. *et al.* (1985). Isolation of AIDS virus from cell-free breast milk of three healthy virus carriers. *Lancet*, 19 October, ii(8460), 891–2.
6. Levy, J.A., Hollander, H., Shimabukura, J. *et al.* (1985). Isolation of AIDS-associated retroviruses from cerebrospinal fluid and brain of patients with neurological symptoms. *Lancet*, 14 September, ii(8455), 586–8.
7. Downs, A. (1990). *Europe: WHO Predictions to 1991.* Abstracts, VI International Conference on AIDS, San Francisco, USA.
8. Department of Health (1993). *AIDS and Drug Misuse Update: Report by the Advisory Council on the Misuse of Drugs.* HMSO, London.
9. Chaisson, M.A., Stoneburner, R.L., Hildebrandt, D.S. *et al.* (1991). Heterosexual transmission of HIV-1 associated with the use of smokable freebase cocaine (crack). *AIDS* **5**, 1121–6.
10. Centers for Disease Control (1982). Unexplained immunodeficiency and opportunistic infections in infants – New York, New Jersey, California. *Morbidity and Mortality Weekly Report (MMWR)* **31**, 665–7.
11. Oleske, J., Minnefor, A., Cooper, R. *et al.* (1983). Immune deficiency in children. *Journal of the American Medical Association* **249**, 2345–9.
12. Mann, Jonathan, Tarantola, Daniel J. and Netter, Thomas W. (eds) (1992). *AIDS in the World: A Global Report.* Harvard University Press, London.
13. Murray, A.B., Greenhouse, P.R., Nelson, W.L., Norman, J.E., Jeffries, D.J. and Anderson, J. (1991). Coincident acquisition of

Neisseria gonorrhoeae and HIV from fellatio. *Lancet* **338**, 830.
14. Lifson, A.R., O'Malley, P.M., Hessol, N.A. *et al.* (1990). HIV seroconversion in two homosexual men after receptive oral intercourse with ejaculation; implications for counseling concerning safe sexual practices, *American Journal of Public Health* **80**, 1509–11.
15. Simonds, R.J., Holmberg, S.D., Hurwitz, F.L. *et al.* (1992). Transmission of human immunodeficiency virus type 1 from a seronegative organ and tissue donor. *New England Journal of Medicine* **326**, 726–32.
16. Chaisson, M.A., Stoneburner, R.L. and Joseph, S.C. (1990). Human immunodeficiency virus transmission through artificial insemination. *Journal of Acquired Immunodeficiency Syndromes* **3**, 69–72.
17. Centers for Disease Control (1990). Update: acquired immunodeficiency syndrome – United States, 1989, *Morbidity and Mortality Weekly Report (MMWR)* **39**, 81–6.
18. Waugh, Michael A. (1991). Resurgent gonorrhoea in homosexual men. *Lancet* **337**, 375.
19. Van Den Hoek, J.A.R., Van Griesven, G.J.P., and Coutinho, R.A. (1990). Increase in unsafe homosexual behavior. *Lancet* **336**, 179–80.
20. Edwards, A. and Thin, R.N. (1990). Sexually transmitted diseases in lesbians. *International Journal of STD and AIDS*, May, **1**(3), 178–81.
21. Koopman, J.S., Simon, C.P., Jacquez, J.A. *et al.* (1992). HIV transmission probabilities for oral and anal sex by stage of infection. *Conference Abstracts*, Abstract PoC 4101, Eighth International Conference on AIDS, Amsterdam, The Netherlands, 19–24 July.
22. Samuel, M.C., Mohr, M.S., Speed, T.P. *et al.* (1992). Infectivity of HIV by anal and oral intercourse among gay men: estimates from a prospective study in San Francisco. *Conference Abstracts*, Abstract PoC 4104, Eighth International Conference on AIDS, Amsterdam, The Netherlands, 19–24 July.
23. Quarto, M., Germinario, C., Troiano, T. *et al.* (1990). HIV transmission by fellatio. *European Journal of Epidemiology* **6**, 339–40.
24. Spitzer, P.G. and Weiner, N.J. (1989). Transmission of HIV infection from a woman to a man by oral sex. *New England Journal of Medicine* **320**, 251.
25. Beral, V., Peterman, T.A., Berkelman, R.L. *et al.* (1990). Kaposi's sarcoma among persons with AIDS: a sexually transmitted infection? *Lancet* **335**, 123–8.
26. Peterman, T.A., Jaffe, H.W. and Beral, V. (1993). Epidemiologic clues to the etiology of Kaposi's sarcoma. *AIDS* **7**(5), 605–11.
27. European Study Group (1992). Comparison of female to male and male to female transmission of HIV in 563 stable couples. *British Medical Journal* **304**, 809–13.
28. Haverkos, H.W. and Battjes, R.J. (1992). Female-to-male transmission of HIV. *Journal of the American Medical Association* **268**, 1855.
29. Seage, G., Mayer, K., Horsburgh, C.R. (1991). The relationship between immunologic status and risk of HIV infection among partners of HIV infected men. *Conference Abstracts*, Abstract M.C. 3016, Seventh International Conference on AIDS, Florence, Italy, 16–21 June.

30. Wolinsky, S.M., Wike, C.M., Korber, B.T. *et al.* (1992). Selective transmission of human immunodeficiency virus type-1 variants from mothers to infants. *Science (Washington, D.C.)* **255**, 1134–7.
31. Holmberg, S.D., Horsburgh, C.R., Ward, J.W. *et al.* (1989). Biologic factors in the sexual transmission of human immunodeficiency virus. *Journal of Infectious Diseases* **160**, 116–25.
32. Alexander, N.J. (1990). Sexual transmission of human immunodeficiency virus: Virus entry into the male and female genital tract. *Fertility & Sterility* **54**, 1–8.
33. Sestak, P., Schechter, M.T., Carib, K.J. *et al.* (1991). Is gonorrhea a cofactor in HIV transmission in gay men? *Conference Abstracts*, Abstract M.C. 3004, Seventh International Conference on AIDS, Florence, Italy, 16–21 June.
34. Cameron, D.W., Simonsen, J.N., D/Costa, L.J. *et al.* (1989). Female-to-male transmission of human immunodeficiency virus type 1: Risk factors for seroconversion in men. *Lancet* **2**. 403.
35. Bongaarts, J., Reining, P., Way, P. *et al.* (1989). The relationship between male circumcision and HIV infection in African populations. *AIDS*, 1 June, **3**, 373–7.

4

Understanding Immunology

An understanding of normal immune mechanisms is necessary in order to appreciate fully the immune dysfunction seen during the course of HIV infection. Immunity has evolved in man over the centuries and affords essential protection against infectious diseases, without which survival would be impossible. **Immunology** is the study of systems, organs, cells and molecules which are involved in the **recognition** and **destruction** of foreign ('non-self') materials which enter the human body, e.g. infectious micro-organisms, proteins, etc. and their responses to, and interreactions with, each other. Immune responses can be divided into **innate** ('natural' or 'non-specific') and **acquired** ('adaptive') mechanisms.

Innate immunity

There are many natural, non-specific mechanisms available to everyone, which we employ to protect ourselves against infection; these are non-specific in that they are used to protect against a wide range of potential pathogens (micro-organisms which cause disease) which we recognize as foreign. Innate mechanisms have no **memory** (an essential feature of acquired immunity) and, consequently, they are not enhanced as a result of previous exposure to the invading material.

Innate immunity is geared towards either the prevention of pathogenic invasion or containment and eventual resolution should invasion occur. It encompasses mechanical and chemical barriers, normal bacterial flora and humoral and cell-mediated mechanisms.

Prevention of invasion

A variety of **mechanical barriers** and **surface secretions** protect us against invasion by pathogenic micro-organisms. These barriers include:

Intact skin A healthy, intact skin provides a good barrier against infection by pathogens. It is an effective barrier because the outer, horny layer of the skin is principally made of keratin, which most micro-organisms cannot digest and, consequently, protects the living cells of the epidermis from pathogens and toxins. In addition, the dry nature of the skin, covered by a film of salt (pH 5.5) from drying perspiration is either bacteriostatic (inhibitory to growth) or bacteriocidal (killing bacteria) to many micro-organisms.

A variety of substances and secretions further enhance the protective action of the skin in preventing infection, including the fatty acids in sweat and sebaceous secretions, and lactic acid, both of which are bactericidal and fungicidal. Other skin surface secretions, which have important antimicrobial activity, include secretions from sebaceous glands (triglycerides, wax alcohols) and sweat glands (amino acids, ammonia, uric acid) and substances produced as a result of ongoing skin cornification (steroids and complex polypeptides).

It is unusual, however, for skin to be perfectly intact (especially the skin on the hands of nurses) as all of us have small or microscopic abrasions or lesions. In addition, sweat glands, hair follicles, etc. provide an entry for many potential pathogens, such as *Staphylococcus aureus*.

Mucous membranes and ciliated cells   External openings of the body are guarded by mucous membranes. For example, the mouth, nose, urethra, vagina and rectum are all lined with mucous membranes. These membranes secrete sticky mucus so that when pathogens enter the body by one of these routes, they are impinged on these sticky, mucous surfaces. Many of these membranes are associated with cells which have hair-like processes, known as **cilia**, which are then able to waft pathogens away from deeper structures, eventually assisting in expelling them from the body, e.g. 'the mucus–cilia escalator' in the respiratory tract. Additional protection is afforded by **antiviral** (mucopolysaccharides) and **antibacterial substances** (IgA antibody) in nasal secretions and saliva and antibacterial **lysozyme** in tears and in mucous secretions of the respiratory, alimentary and genito-urinary tracts.

pH changes   Various substances and secretions in different parts of the body determine its acid, alkaline or neutral basis. On a pH scale, 7 is neutral; above it alkalinity increases and below it acidity increases. Some areas of the body have a pH which is often hostile to many pathogens. For example, the pH of the skin and vagina is acid and pathogens which require an alkaline medium to reproduce would not be successful in establishing infection in this environment. The pH changes in the gastro-intestinal tract, where ingested food is first mixed with alkaline saliva in the mouth, is then swallowed into the acid environment of the stomach, and eventually passes into the alkaline environment of the duodenum, can be either bacteriostatic or bacteriocidal for many pathogens.

Washing and flushing actions   The washing action of tears, flowing away from the eye, and the flushing action of urine are both effective mechanisms employed in preventing pathogenic invasion.

Resident bacterial population

The normal bacterial flora of the body provides good protection by two mechanisms. First, their growth results in the production of substances, e.g. bacteriocins and lactic acid, which have antimicrobial activity. Second, by competing with potential pathogens for essential nutrients, the growth of normal bacterial flora protects by excluding the growth of other, harmful micro-organisms. This is an important consideration in antimicrobial therapy, where antibiotics may destroy normal gut flora, allowing other, antibiotic-resistant pathogens to establish infection. It is important to remember that **commensals**, i.e. those bacteria which make up the normal flora, are both beneficial and harmless in those areas in which they are normally present, but may cause illness if they are transported to other areas of the body where they do not normally reside. For example, *Escherichia coli*, a common gut commensal, is also a frequent cause of genito-urinary tract infection, gaining access to the genito-urinary tract via a urinary catheter.

Containment of invading pathogens

Effective as these non-specific mechanisms are, pathogenic invasion does occur from time to time. The body still has some fairly sophisticated, innate mechanisms available to deal with these pathogens, which, if successful, contain them, limit the damage they may cause and eventually, destroy them. These innate devices include both **humoral** and **cell-mediated** mechanisms (not to be confused with humoral and cell-mediated mechanisms in acquired immunity).

Humoral innate mechanisms

Humoral refers to those antimicrobial substances in the tissues and body fluids. They include lysozymes, basic polypeptides, acute phase proteins, interferon and complement enzymes.

Lysozyme   This enzyme is found in most tissue fluids (except cerebrospinal fluid, sweat and urine). It attacks the sugars making up part of the cell wall on Gram-positive (and some Gram-negative) bacteria, causing their lysis (dissolution).

Basic polypeptides   These are antibacterial basic proteins which also attack the micro-organism's cell surface. They are derived from tissues and blood cells. Important basic polypeptides include spermine and spermidine, which can kill *Mycobacteria tuberculosis* and some staphylococci, and arginine, protamine and histone.

Acute phase proteins   During the acute phase of infection, macrophages (mononuclear phagocytic cells found in tissues and serous cavities such as the pleura and peritoneum) release small protein messenger molecules (**cytokines**) known as **interleukin-1 (IL-1)**. IL-1 is an endogenous pyrogen and is responsible for the rise in temperature seen in acute infection. Its role is to stimulate the liver to release acute phase proteins, such as **C-reactive protein**, which binds to the cell walls of some micro-organisms and activates the **classical complement pathway**. Other acute phase proteins include fibrinogen and serum amyloid A protein. These protein molecules are greatly increased during acute infection and help to contain the spread of the infecting micro-organism and facilitate further immune responses.

Interferon   Interferons are cytokines which have a powerful, broad-spectrum, antiviral effect. There are two types of interferon: type 1 interferons consist of alpha-interferon (**INFα**) and beta-interferon (**INFβ**), both of which are part of innate immunity; type 2 interferon is gamma-interferon (**INFγ**), synthesized by T lymphocytes in acquired immunity. There are over a dozen types of INFα, produced by white blood cells (leucocytes). INFβ (of which there is only one type) is manufactured by fibroblasts (but probably can be produced by many other cells in the body).

Once cells are infected with viruses, they secrete interferons into the extracellular fluid, where they bind onto specific surface receptors of uninfected neighbouring cells. The 'interferon-treated cell' then makes a variety of enzymes which are toxic to the virus, inhibiting further viral replication and destroying viral nucleic acid. This results in a chain of uninfected cells being thrown around the virus-infected cell, isolating it and containing the infection.

Complement   There are approximately twenty different serum complement enzymes which can be sequentially activated along two different pathways, known as the **classical** (because it was the first described) and **alternative** pathways (Fig. 4.1).

The **classical pathway** is activated by **immunoglobulins** (antibodies), either attached to cell surfaces or by the formation of

immune complexes, especially IgM or IgG complexes. A complex is formed by the attachment of an antibody to an antigen. Both C-reactive protein (an acute phase protein discussed above) and protein A (a cell wall protein found in many strains of *Staphylococcus aureus*) can also activate the classical pathway.

The **alternative pathway** is activated by some immune complexes composed of IgA and IgE, but principally by **activators** found in the cell walls of many bacteria, viruses, yeasts and some tumours. Both pathways converge via C3 onto a final **lytic** pathway.

Inactive complement enzymes are thus triggered into action in a

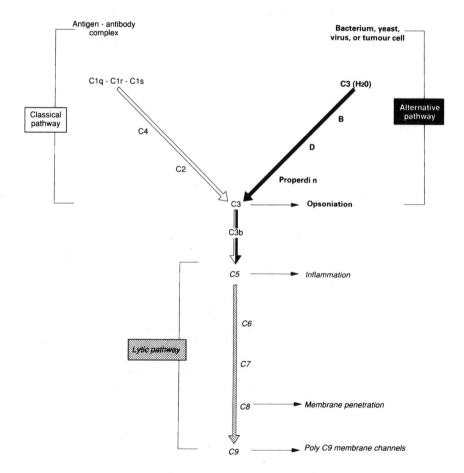

Fig. 4.1 Complement and its activation

sequential cascade, the end result being the formation of **active complement** (C3b, C5 and C8, C9) which results in important protective consequences. First, **C3b** attaches to specific receptors on phagocytic cells (**opsonization**), switching them on and promoting enhanced **phagocytosis**. Second, **C5** releases peptides which induce **inflammation**, destroying immune complexes. Inflammation is generally a protective mechanism, which results in an increase in local blood supply to the area under attack. This **hyperaemia** is the cause of the classic signs of inflammation (heat, redness, swelling and pain). With this increased blood supply come cells which are able to engage in phagocytosis.

Third, **C8** and **C9** (**membrane attack complex**) causes cell wall damage and **lysis** to many pathogens, such as malaria parasites, trypanosomes and (with the help of lysozymes), some Gram-negative bacteria.

The net result of activating the complement network is, in summary, opsonization, cell wall lysis, enhanced phagocytosis and destruction of immune complexes by inflammation.

Cell-mediated innate mechanisms

Phagocytosis

This is a scavenging function of **phagocytes**, cells which engulf (phagocytosis) and digest micro-organisms which enter the tissue fluids or bloodstream. There is a wide variety of cells which are phagocytic, but the principal 'professional' phagocytes are **neutrophils** and **macrophages** (Table 4.1).

Macrophages ('big eaters') are long-lived phagocytic cells which are strategically sited throughout the body where they are likely to encounter invading micro-organisms, e.g. in the lungs, liver, spleen sinusoids, lymph node medullary sinuses and kidney glomerulosis. They act as sentries and are usually the first phagocytic cells which invading micro-organisms encounter. Their function is somewhat different from that of neutrophils. Although they are capable of cell killing, in general, when they have attacked and ingested foreign material, they secrete several soluble substances, e.g. lysozymes, cytokines (IL-1, INFα, INFβ), complement components and coagulation factors (to name but a few!). These substances summon the real killers to the scene of the battle, the **neutrophils**.

Macrophages are activated by a variety of stimuli, and can be up-regulated from a **resting** state to higher degrees of activation, where they function as **activated** and **hyperactivated** macrophages[1]. Resting macrophages travel around the body, but basically do not do anything until they are stimulated by encounters with invading

Table 4.1 Phagocytes

Polymorphonuclear (PMN) phagocytes
Neutrophils
Eosinophils

Monocyte/macrophage series (mononuclear phagocytes)
Blood monocytes
 Promonocytes
Macrophages
 Alveolar macrophages
 Splenic macrophages
 Lymph node macrophages
 Brain microglial cells
 Liver Kupffer cells
 Kidney mesangial phagocytes
 Synovial A cells

---

micro-organisms. Once activated, they engage in scavenging and phagocytosis. If hyperactivated, they are capable of killing tumour cells.

Neutrophils, often referred to as PMNs, are the chief 'killer phagocytes'. They are short-lived cells which migrate into tissues when stimulated by the presence of invading micro-organisms and engulf foreign material, destroying it, and then, they themselves dying. **Eosinophils** are reserved for the extracellular killing of giant invaders, e.g. multicellular parasites.

Cell killing in phagocytosis is achieved by three phases. First, during the **attachment phase**, the invading micro-organism (antigen) is recognized as foreign and firm contact is made between the phagocyte and the micro-organism. In *The Doctor's Dilemma* (George Bernard Shaw), a famous line reads 'The phagocytes won't eat the microbes unless the microbes are nicely buttered for them.' The 'butter' which coats the antigen are special molecules known as **opsonins**, which become attached to the surface of the antigen. There are two types of opsonins: **antibodies** (IgM, IgG) and certain **complement fragments** (e.g. C3b). Phagocytes have specialized receptors (Fc receptors for antibodies and C3b receptors) which will latch on to the opsonins, securing the attachment.

The second phase is the **ingestion phase**, during which the antigen is engulfed into the cytoplasm of the phagocytes and enclosed within a pocket (**phagosome**).

The final phase is the **digestion phase**. Within the cytoplasm of the phagocytes are numerous compartments of potentially toxic molecules, known as either **lysosomes** (in macrophages) or **granules** (in PMNs). These molecules are compartmentalized so that they do not kill the phagocytic cell. However, the lysosomes fuse with the phagosome and the ingested material is killed and digested.

Natural killer cells
Natural killing refers to the process in which cells which have been **infected with viruses** are destroyed by an extracellular killing mechanism. Natural killer (NK) cells look like large granular lymphocytes, although they are of uncertain origin. They are sometimes referred to as 'null lymphocytes' (non-T, non-B). It is likely that a variety of cells can carry out natural killing. NK cells are activated by **interferons**, which stimulate the production of more NK cells and increase their killing speed. In addition to detecting and killing cells infected with viruses, NK cells can detect those cells undergoing neoplastic change and destroy them, thus protecting us against **cancers**. They are an important part of our normal tumour surveillance systems. NK cells kill by first binding to their targets, then discharging a toxin (Ca-dependent endonuclease) into the target cell which acts on the cellular DNA and programmes the target cell for self-destruction, i.e. **programmed cell death** (apoptosis).

Other determinants of innate immunity

Other determinants of innate immunity which influence the ability of the individual to withstand infectious disease include:

- **Nutrition**   A well nourished individual is better able to deal with an infectious process than people who suffer from malnutrition (see Chapter 15).
- **Age**   The very young and the very old are less able to ward off infectious diseases.
- **Individual differences**   Heredity is important in determining resistance to different infectious diseases.
- **Species**   Man is immune to many of the diseases that affect animals and vice versa.
- **Race**   Some races are either more susceptible or more resistant to certain infections than other races.
- **Hormonal factors**   Increased susceptibility to infections is seen in various endocrine diseases, e.g. diabetes mellitus and hypothyroidism.

All of these factors, associated with innate immunity, offer good protection against infectious diseases. However, by themselves, they are not adequate for survival in the hostile environment in which man finds himself. We need much more specific protection and this is afforded by the specific immune response of **acquired immunity**.

Acquired immunity – the specific immune response

During the first few months of life, the infant begins to acquire protection against specific pathogens. This type of immunity, known as **acquired immunity**, allows the child to mount a **specific immune response** towards each pathogen the child encounters as it progresses through those first, vulnerable months and years. For the first 3 months of its life, the child is protected by the natural, passive immunity conferred by the mother. During this time, antibodies from the mother pass to the child while it is still in the uterus. However, these antibodies are short-lived and, by the end of 3 months, the child must begin to acquire its own immunity.

Acquired immunity involves two different but interrelated processes; **cell-mediated immunity** and **humoral immunity**.

Antigens

Before discussing the two arms of acquired immunity, it might be useful to review the characteristics of **antigens**, the substances which provoke the specific immune response in both systems. Antigens are foreign material, such as bacteria, viruses, foreign tissue cells or proteins, etc., and are recognized by the body as different, alien and 'not self'. The first requirement, then, of an antigen is that it must be foreign. Another requirement is that, in general, antigens, unless they are going to be attached to a special 'carrier molecule', have to be large (having a molecular weight > 5000). An antigen is usually composed of several antigenic determinants, or **epitopes** (Fig. 4.2). These epitopes must be topographical, i.e. appear on the surface of the antigen in order for them to be recognized and interact with the special receptors on lymphocytes.

Antigen receptors

The ability of the immune system to recognize antigens as foreign and bind on to them is contingent upon the antigen making contact with the **lymphocyte cell-surface receptors**. The genes of the antigen cell-surface receptors on lymphocytes have the ability to combine in potentially unlimited arrangements, providing an

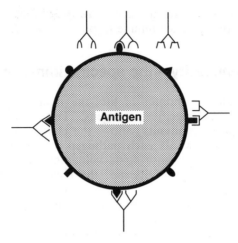

Fig. 4.2   Antigen

infinite number of cell-surface receptors which recognize specific antigens. The cell-surface receptors associated with B lymphocytes will be discussed in association with a description of humoral immunity and the cell-surface receptors associated with T lymphocytes will be described in the section outlining cell-mediated responses.

Humoral immunity

The active agents of acquired immunity are the lymphocytes, of which there are two distinct types: **B lymphocytes** and **T lymphocytes**. Both originate from **stem cells**, which are manufactured in the bone marrow. Some of these stem cells, destined to become B lymphocytes (B cells), are known as B-cell precursors. The remaining stem cells, destined to become T lymphocytes, are T-cell precursors. The B-cell precursors migrate back to the bone marrow, where they are 'processed' into B lymphocytes. They are known as B lymphocytes because they were first identified in the hindgut of a bird, an area known as the 'bursa of Fabricius'. Although humans do not have this special tissue, it is thought that they have similar areas (**bursa equivalent areas**), such as the foetal liver and the bone marrow, which 'process' or train B-cell precursors in such a way that when they develop into fully mature B lymphocytes, they respond in a specific manner to pathogens. The manner in which they respond is known as **humoral immunity**. B lymphocytes account for about

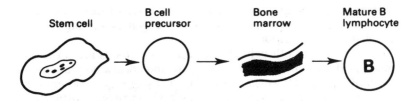

Fig. 4.3 The maturation of a B lymphocyte

30 per cent of all lymphocytes (the remaining 70 per cent being T lymphocytes). Figure 4.3 illustrates the development of a mature B lymphocyte.

Humoral immunity is activated as follows: following digestion by phagocytic cells, an antigen is eventually presented to the B lymphocytes in lymphatic tissue (e.g. spleen, liver, bone marrow and lymph nodes). The **antigen cell-surface receptor** on B lymphocytes is mediated by **surface antibodies**, typically IgM, IgC and IgD. Following the capture of the antigen by the cell-surface receptor, a series of events (explained below), culminates in the secretion of additional antibody which is the specific antibody for that particular antigen.

The presence of this antigen stimulates the B cell to proliferate and change into **plasma cells** and **memory cells**. Plasma cells have a specific function which is to secrete a protein substance known as **antibody**. Another name for antibody is **immunoglobulin**, sometimes abbreviated as **Ig**; the terms antibody and immunoglobulin are synonymous. The rate of 'antibody secretion is impressive, in the order of 2000 antibody molecules per second for each plasma cell. This goes on for several days until the plasma cell dies (4–5 days).

Immunoglobulins (antibodies)

Immunoglobulins are glycoproteins that bind specifically to the antigen which provoked its formation, e.g. measles virus antibody will be produced in response to an encounter by a B lymphocyte with the measles virus (the antigen). When the two molecules are bound together, this combination of 'antibody bound to antigen' is known as an **immune complex** (Fig. 4.4).

All antibodies have a four chain structure, being made up of two identical **light chains** and two identical **heavy chains** (Fig. 4.5). The chains are made out of polypeptides which are bound to each other by disulphide bonds. The light chains are identified by the Greek letters

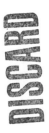

lambda (λ) and **kappa** (κ). There are five types of heavy chains and they are also identified by Greek letters, i.e. **gamma** (γ), **alpha** (α), **mu** (μ), **delta** (δ) and **epsilon** (ε).

Some parts of both light chains and heavy chains are made up of amino acid combinations that never vary and are always the same (the **constant region**). However, the amino acid sequence in other parts of both light and heavy chains in the antibody changes constantly, i.e.

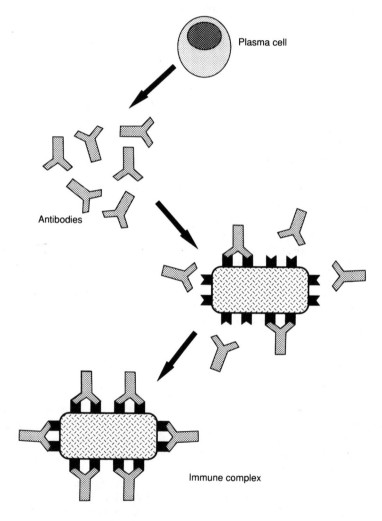

Fig. 4.4 Immune complex

the amino acid sequence differs from molecule to molecule. This part of the antibody fragment is known as the **hypervariable region**.

In the laboratory, antibody molecules can be split into three large pieces by a protein-digesting enzyme (papain). Two of these pieces are exactly the same and contain the **antibody binding site**. They are known as the **Fab fragment**. The Fab fragment consists of the entire

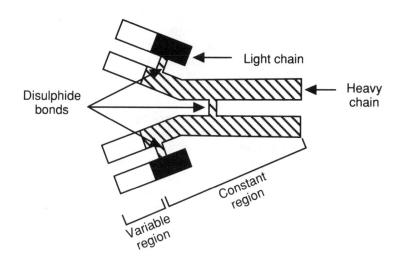

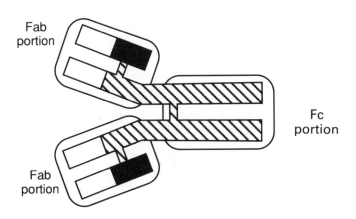

Fig. 4.5 Structure of an antibody

light chain and almost half of the heavy chain (linked together by the disulphide bonds). The hypervariable region of the antibody is in the Fab fragment and this is where the specific lock is made to bind onto a specific antigen. The locks (i.e. the complete antibody repertoire) in the hypervariable region are made as a result of constant antibody gene rearrangement during the growth and development of B lymphocytes, long before exposure to antigens with the corresponding epitopes. This results in a vast number (thousands) of combinations of molecules which will recognize similar combinations of amino acid molecules on the surface of the thousands of different antigens it may meet throughout the course of our existence.

The remaining fragment of the antibody is known as the **Fc fragment** and is important in determining essential characteristics of the antibody (e.g. whether it can or cannot cross the placenta and enter the foetal circulation). The Fc fragment also binds to certain antigens, e.g. bacteria, and **activates the complement system**. In addition, by Fc binding, the antigen becomes 'buttered' (as in G.B. Shaw, above), the Fc fragment of certain types of immunoglobulins acting as **opsonins**, sticking to the antigen and attracting phagocytes.

Antibodies are very diverse and provide **different** and **specific** binding sites to the thousands of different antigenic shapes that they can potentially encounter throughout life. They protect the individual in several ways: first, the antibody attacks the antigen's cell wall, weakening and eventually destroying it; this is known as **lysis**. More importantly, when the antibody 'coats' or attaches itself to an antigen, the formation of immune complexes activates **complement**. As discussed previously, complement has two important functions: it initiates a **local inflammatory reaction** at the invasion site, which increases the local blood supply, and second, by-products of inflammation chemically attract neutrophils, monocytes and macrophages to the area under attack. This chemical attraction of phagocytic cells to the invasion site is known as **chemotaxis**. Some antigens are destroyed by direct cell wall damage when coated by complement.

We can see that it is critically important for plasma cells to secrete antibody. There are two important points to remember: first, the antibody produced is **specific** to that particular antigen, for example if the antigen was the chickenpox virus, then the antibody produced would bind only to the chickenpox virus; it would not bind to the measles virus. Second, antibody is **formed in a sequential manner**, something like: antibody 1, antibody 2, antibody 3, etc. Hence, soon after invasion, antibody 1 is formed, then, approximately 3–4 weeks later, antibody 2 is formed, and so on. If we took a sample of blood at week three of the infection, we might find the first antibody (antibody number 1) still there, but disappearing, and the second antibody (antibody number 2) just appearing. A special characteristic of antibody 1 is that it is a short-lived molecule. It will disappear within a month but antibody 2 will stay in the serum for years, or for life. This is important, as the presence of antibody 1 is a diagnostic marker of acute infection while antibody 2 is a marker of previous exposure. However, all the antibodies will be antibodies to that specific antigen (e.g. the chickenpox virus); they will simply be different classes of the antibody. In reality, these immunoglobulins are not referred to as numbers 1, 2, 3, etc., but rather according to their **class name**. B lymphocytes are capable of making five major classes (or **isotypes**) of antibodies which are named after the Greek letter that designates the heavy chains of the antibody molecule, i.e. gamma (γ), alpha (α), mu (μ), delta (δ) and epsilon (ϵ).

Consequently, the working names for these different classes of immunoglobulins are **IgM, IgG, IgA, IgD** and **IgE** (the 'Ig' stands for immunoglobulin). A few points about the different classes of immunoglobulins:

IgM This is a large immunoglobulin (macroglobulin) which appears early in the course of an infectious disease and disappears as the patient recovers. Hence it is a marker of acute infection. Because this antibody appears early after initial infection, IgM is mainly confined to the bloodstream and accounts for about 10 per cent of the total amount of immunoglobulins. As IgM is highly efficient at binding and agglutinating micro-organisms, it plays an important role as the first line of defence in bacteraemia (bacterial infection of the blood).

IgG (gamma globulin) This small antibody accounts for 70 per cent of all the immunoglobulin formed and appears after IgM, during the secondary response to infection. Because of its small size, IgG diffuses more easily than other antibodies out of the bloodstream and into the tissue fluids of the body, where it is the principal antibody responsible for neutralizing bacterial toxins, binding to micro-organisms, activating complement and promoting phagocytosis. It also readily crosses the placenta and maternal IgG provides the principal means of defence against infection for the first few months of a baby's life. Because it appears after IgM and remains in the body for long periods of time (years, or a lifetime), its presence is not an indication of acute infection, but rather of previous exposure.

IgA IgA accounts for up to 13 per cent of the total amount of immunoglobulin formed, but accounts for over 90 per cent of the immunoglobulin found on mucosal surfaces (e.g. nose, mouth) and protects the body by blocking and neutralizing antigens that enter by these routes (mucosal 'paint'). It is found in high levels in many secretions (tears, sweat, saliva, urine, gut secretions, secretions in the lungs, etc.). This immunoglobulin does not cross the placenta. However, it is present in large quantities in colostrum and breast milk, protecting the infant from infection via breast feeding.

IgD accounts for less than 1 per cent of the total amount of circulating immunoglobulins and not much is known for certain about its specific function. However, it is found residing on the surface of B lymphocytes, along with IgM and they both most likely operate as mutually interacting antigen receptors, controlling further lymphocyte activation and suppression[2].

IgE This antibody accounts for only about 0.002 per cent of immunoglobulin formed. It binds to the surface membranes of 'mast cells' and basophils, causing these cells to release vasoactive substances, such as histamine, heparin and serotonin, which are responsible for the common signs and symptoms of acute allergic reactions. Mast cells are 'fixed' in tissues, such as the lungs, whereas basophils are circulating mast cells. As elevated levels of IgE are found during parasitic infections, IgE may be important in protecting against this type of infection[3].

Killer cells

Different from 'natural killer (NK) cells', killer cells are able to kill a whole variety of micro-organisms as long as they are first attached to the Fc fragment of antibody. This process is known as **antibody-dependent cell-mediated cytotoxicity**. It works because, like phagocytes, the killer cells have a special **Fc receptor** that recognizes antigen bound to antibody, i.e. immune complexes.

Memory cells

When provoked by the presence of an antigen, both T cells and B cells produce **memory cells**, clones of the stimulated parent cell. Should the individual encounter the same antigen any time in the future, the cascade of events which constitute a specific immune response will be accelerated. This is because memory cells 'remember' the characteristics of each specific antigen and respond quickly.

Summary

Humoral immunity is the process whereby B lymphocytes, provoked by the presence of an antigen, proliferate and undergo change, some changing into memory cells, but most changing into plasma cells. Plasma cells have just one function – to secrete specific antibody which can combine with the antigen, forming immune complexes, activating the complement system and, by different methods, eventually destroying the invading pathogen.

Humoral responses are directly linked to the other arm of acquired immunity – cell-mediated responses, by cytokines secreted by one type of activated T lymphocyte, the Th2 CD4+ helper cell.

Cell-mediated immunity

The other process involved in acquired immunity is that of **cell-mediated immunity**. This involves the T lymphocytes which are derived from the same stem cells as B lymphocytes, but which migrate to the **thymus gland** for processing, rather than to bone marrow and other bursa equivalent areas (Fig. 4.6). In the thymus gland, these T-cell precursors are 'processed' to react differently when they encounter antigens. Mature T lymphocytes account for about 70 per cent of the total number of lymphocytes.

T-cell antigen receptors

As discussed in Chapter 2, the **cell-surface receptors** on T lymphocytes (**TCR**) have been characterized by the unique glycoprotein combination of their adhesion molecules, which are classified by **CD** (cluster of differentiation) numbers. The complex of glycoproteins on TCRs includes: **CD3**, which is present on all TCRs and has a constant structure, having an important role in conveying the antigen

| Stem cell | T cell precursor | Thymus gland | Mature T lymphocyte |

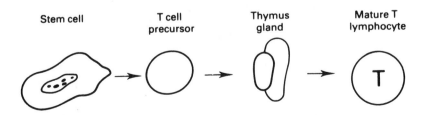

Fig. 4.6 The maturation of a T lymphocyte

recognition signal received by the TCR to the inside of the T cell, i.e. **signal transduction** [2,4]; **CD4** which binds to **exogenous** antigen fragments (e.g. from bacteria) presented by MHC Class II molecules; **CD8** which binds to **endogenous** antigen fragments (e.g. from viruses) presented by MHC Class I molecules (NB CD4 and CD8 are mutually exclusive molecules)[4].

Cell-mediated response

The invading antigen is engulfed by a phagocytic cell. Once it has been ingested, bits of the antigen are embedded in special molecules known as **MHC molecules** (discussed below). The complex of the antigen bound to MHC molecules is carried to the surface of the phagocytic cell (becoming topographical) and presented by the phagocytic cell (now known as an **antigen presenting cell**, or **APC**) to the T lymphocyte. This **antigenic presentation** stimulates the T cell to change (differentiate) into two major subsets: **helper cells (Th CD4+)** and **cytotoxic (killer) cells (Tc CD8+)**.

In addition to antigenic presentation, another important stimulation necessary for T-cell activation is the secretion, by APCs, of the cytokine interleukin-1 (IL-1). IL-1 binds to T-cell receptors, regulates their activation and stimulates the production of other cytokines (discussed below). **Memory cells** are also formed but the specific immune response to this invasion will now be the responsibility of these quite remarkable helper and killer cells.

Helper cells (Th CD4+)

Helper cells function by giving help in the form of chemical assistance. The chemical assistance arrives in the form of **cytokines**, soluble proteins which interact with specific cell-surface receptors. Helper cells control and modulate the development of the immune response and their main function is to produce cytokines. Two types of helper cells are formed when the T cell has been stimulated by APCs: helper cells 1 (**Th1**) and helper cells 2 (**Th2**). These two types of helper cells are distinguished by the cytokines they produce. One type of helper cell can become predominant, switching off the other type. For example, if a Th1 response is the strongest response, there will be a down-regulation of the Th2 response. This is important to remember when we come to discussing the pathogenesis of HIV infection.

Th1 cells produce interleukin-2 (IL-2) and gamma-interferon (IFN-γ). Consequently, Th1 cells activate macrophages and promote cytotoxic (killer) cell responses, i.e. they promote an effective cell-mediated response.

Th2 cells produce interleukins 4, 5, 6 and 10 (IL-4, IL-5, IL-6 and IL-10). These interleukins further stimulate the plasma cells to secrete antibody and, consequently, they augment the humoral response (Fig. 4.7).

Th1→Th2 switch

It is important that the right subset of Th cell is **switched on** during infection. If the infecting antigen is an **extracellular** invader, e.g. bacteria, then a **Th2 response** is best, as it will be humoral defences, i.e. antibodies, which neutralize this threat. However, if the antigen is an **intracellular** attacker, e.g. a virus or intracellular bacterium, then a **Th1 response** is needed as it is killer cells,

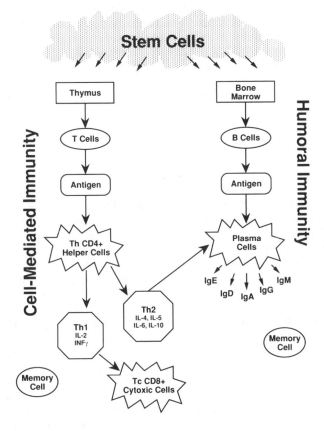

Fig. 4.7 Acquired immunity

not antibodies, which can destroy cells infected with viruses. Unfortunately, in HIV infection, cytokine mis-signalling produces a **Th1→Th2 switch**, promoting antibody production but depressing killer cell activity[5]. A tremendous amount of research is currently focused on how to re-programme helper cell activity back to an effective Th1 response which would activate the killer cells needed to destroy HIV-infected cells and, incidentally, cells infected with the tubercle bacilli[6].

Cytotoxic (killer) cells (Tc CD8+)

These small subsets of activated T cells recognize and destroy virus-infected cells. They can also detect and destroy cells showing neoplastic change (malignant) and foreign (histoincompatible) cells, e.g. tissue and organ transplants. An extremely important function of Tc killer cells is their ability to find and destroy cells infected with intracellular bacteria, e.g. *Mycobacterium tuberculosis*.

An effective Tc CD8+ killer cell response is able to suppress HIV replication in infected Th CD4+ helper cells and helps maintain a low viral load *in vivo*, allowing a long asymptomatic period of infection[7].

Major histocompatibility complex (MHC)

The molecules of the MHC (also known as the 'human leucocyte antigen', or **HLA genes**) are found on the surface of various cells and present antigen fragments to the CD4+ or CD8+ adhesion molecules in the T-lymphocyte receptors. This interaction is essential in initiating a cell-mediated response. There are two types of MHC molecules: **MHC Class I molecules** bind peptides produced from **endogenously** produced proteins (e.g. viral proteins) and present them to CD8+ T-cell receptors. **Exogenous** antigens (e.g. foreign material, bacteria, etc.) taken into a cell by endocytosis, are processed within that cell and the resultant peptides presented by **MHC Class II molecules** to CD4+ T-cell receptors. Although B lymphocytes can respond to soluble antigen, T cells rarely do so and recognize antigen only when it is embedded within the MHC, i.e. a 'complex of antigen + MHC molecules'. Phagocytic cells, which capture antigen, process the antigen so that it is combined with MHC molecules before it is presented to the T cell. These cells, e.g. Langerhans' cells, monocytes, macrophages, follicular dendritic cells, etc., consequently are also known as **antigen-presenting cells (APCs)**.

Cytokines

Cytokines are soluble protein molecules which act as 'cell-to-cell messengers', much like hormones. These molecules are made by cells of the immune system, e.g. monocytes, lymphocytes, NK cells, macrophages, etc., when they are stimulated to do so. They are secreted in small amounts but are very powerful. Their principal function is to act, via special **cytokine receptors**, on cells of the immune system and stimulate or inhibit the development and growth of immune system cells and amplify or depress the immune response. In the past, a variety of other names was given to cytokines, depending on their cell of origin, e.g. **lymphokines**, **monokines**, **interleukins** and **interferons**, etc.

These messenger molecules are now known collectively as **cytokines** ('molecules which move between cells'). Another characteristic of cytokines is that they have multiple effects on growth and differentiation of a variety of cell types, often overlapping and sometimes mutually synergistic or antagonistic. They have potentially harmful as well as beneficial effects in disease. Table 4.2 describes the activities of some of the better known cytokines.

Table 4.2 Cytokines and their function

Cytokine	Function
Interleukins (IL)	
IL-1 (α & β)	Activates lymphocytes, promotes the release of acute phase proteins from the liver, induces fever and inflammation
IL-2	Made by Th1 CD4+T cells (and Tc CD8+ cells); powerful growth factor for and activator of T cells, including those cells producing it
IL-4	Produced by T cells (Th2 CD4+) and is a powerful growth factor for B lymphocytes, especially promoting IgG and IgE production from plasma cells
IL-6	Produced by T cells (Th2 CD4+) and stimulates B cells to differentiate into plasma cells
IL-10	Produced by T cells (Th2 CD4+) and inhibits the production of IFNγ, inhibits antigen presentation and macrophage production of other cytokines[8]
IL-3, IL-5, IL-7, IL-8, IL-9	Other interleukins fully described in reference text[4]
Interferons (IFN)	
IFNα, IFNβ	Antiviral activity, regulate other immune system cells, activate NK cells

Table 4.2   *continued*

Cytokine	Function
IFNγ	Immunoregulation, secreted by Th1 cells, activates Tc CD8+ killer cells and macrophages, some antiviral activity
Colony stimulating factors (CSF)	
GM-CSF, G-CSF	Stimulates growth of granulocytes, macrophages, neutrophils
M-CSF	Stimulates monocyte and macrophage development and activity
EPO	Produced by the kidneys and regulates red blood corpuscle (erythrocyte) growth
Tumour necrosis factors (TNF)	
TNFα, TNFβ	Acts on the blood supply to tumours to shrink them, mediates inflammation and healing, promotes release of acute phase proteins, has antiviral and antiparasitic activity, activates phagocytes If produced in excess or inappropriately, can cause vascular shock, induces wasting (cachexia) in illnesses such as HIV disease and TB
Other cytokines	
TGFβ	'Transforming growth factors' inhibit the activities of other cytokines
Chemotactic factors	Attract phagocytic cells to site of infection or tissue damage

Immune dysfunction

Survival is impossible without a well-functioning immune system. However, immune dysfunction is clinically well recognized. Some children are born with a **primary immune dysfunction**, such as severe combined immunodeficiency (SCID) or DiGeorge syndrome. In these conditions, fatal flaws in the immune system render the child unable to mount a specific immune response to invading pathogens. The child will die of infectious diseases that take the opportunity of establishing themselves in a host who is unable to defend himself effectively – hence these infections are referred to as **opportunistic infections**.

Most individuals, however, are born with an effective and fully functional immune system. As life progresses, events and incidents can occur which may depress the immune system, either temporarily or permanently. These are the immunodeficiencies, which are secondary to another cause or condition, i.e. **secondary immunodeficiency**. Secondary immunodeficiencies can be caused by the following:

Drugs Administration of corticosteroids, immunosuppressants, and most anti-cancer drugs will depress the immune system. During this period, the patient is at increased risk of opportunistic infections, a fact well known to nurses as evidenced by their careful monitoring of patients while on this type of treatment.

Malignant conditions Hodgkin's disease, leukaemia and other malignancies can cause a severe immunodeficiency.

Protein depletion conditions Antibodies are made up of protein molecules. Any condition in which there is an inadequate supply of protein in the body leads to an immunodeficient state. This can be seen in conditions such as the nephrotic syndrome in which there is a renal loss of protein (especially IgG), and in starvation, where inadequate protein renders the individual (often a child) prone to common infections, such as measles, which may then be rapidly fatal.

Radiation Radiation can depress the bone marrow, affecting its ability to produce the stem cells which eventually become fully mature lymphocytes. Any type of radiation can be harmful, including ultraviolet radiation from the sun (or sun-tanning lamps).

Stress Both the nervous system and the endocrine system (which interact with each other) have a powerful influence on the immune response. The blood supply to lymphatic tissue is innervated by the **sympathetic nervous system** (the 'fright, fight, flight' system), which is activated during periods of stress. Lymphocytes have receptors for many hormones released from various endocrine glands as a result of sympathetic nervous system stimulation. These include **steroids**, **thyroxine** and **catecholamines** (adrenaline and noradrenaline). In addition, **enkephalins**, **endorphins** and other neurotransmitters and neuropeptides are released as a result of active nervous system stimulation. These substances are released during times of stress, depressing the immune response and reducing the ability of patients to recover from infections[8].

Other conditions Ageing, debilitation, various infectious diseases, diseases such as sarcoidosis, leprosy, and miliary TB can all cause immunodeficiency, resulting in the individual becoming vulnerable to opportunistic disease.

Summary

Various immunological mechanisms protect us from infectious diseases. **Innate** mechanisms, associated with **non-specific**, or **natural immunity**, provide protection against invasion of disease-causing micro-organisms and also help contain those pathogens which have breached this first line of defence. A more **specific immune response** complements these innate mechanisms and is provided by factors and processes associated with **acquired**, or **adaptive immunity**. These allow for the production of a specific immune response (both **humoral** and **cell-mediated**) to specific invading micro-organisms. Unlike innate mechanisms, acquired immunity is associated with **memory**, which allows a faster response on re-presentation of the same pathogen. The immune system is an interrelated 'dynamic', with its own **chemical mediators** to facilitate effective and appropriate responses and, as importantly, its own **inhibitors**, to slow down the immune response once the invader is removed. Because of the dynamic nature and close interdependence in this system, damage to any one element will result in wide-reaching detrimental effects throughout the whole system. This has never been more clearly exemplified than in HIV disease, where infection, and then injury, to CD4+ T lymphocytes results in such catastrophic, global damage to the entire immune system, allowing the onset of life-threatening opportunistic events, i.e. **AIDS**.

References

1. Klein, Jan (1990). *Immunology*. Blackwell Scientific, Oxford.
2. Roitt, I. (1994). *Essential Immunology*, 8th edn. Blackwell Scientific, Oxford.
3. Kirkwood, E. and Lewis, C. (1989). *Understanding Medical Immunology*, 2nd edn. John Wiley & Sons, Chichester.
4. Weir, D.M. and Stewart, J. (1993.) *Immunology*, 7th edn. Churchill Livingstone, London.
5. Clerici, M. and Shearer, G.M. (1993). A Th1→Th2 switch is a critical step in the etiology of HIV infection. *Immunology Today* **14**(3), 107–11.
6. Standford, J.L., Onyebujoh, P.C., Rook, G.A.W. *et al.* (1993). Old plague, new plague, and a treatment for both? *AIDS* **7**(9), 1275–7.
7. Buseyne, F. and Rivière, Y. (1993). HIV-specific CD8+ T-cell immune responses and viral replication. *AIDS* **7**(Suppl. 2), S81–S85.
8. Roitt, I., Brostoff, J. and Male, D. (1993). *Immunology*, 3rd edn. Mosby, London.

Further reading

Kirkwood, E. and Lewis, C. (1989). *Understanding Medical Immunology*, 2nd edn. John Wiley & Sons, Chichester (ISBN 0-471-91577-7).

Klein, Jan (1990). *Immunology*. Blackwell Scientific, Oxford. (ISBN 0-86542-151-X).

Playfair, J.H.L. (1992). *Immunology at a Glance*, 5th edn. Blackwell Scientific, Oxford (ISBN 0-632-03315-0).

Roitt, I. (1994). *Essential Immunology*, 8th edn. Blackwell Scientific, Oxford (ISBN 0-632-03313-4).

Roitt, I., Brostoff, J. and Male, D. (1993). *Immunology*, 3rd edn. Mosby, London (ISBN 0-397-44765-5).

Scientific American (September 1993) **269**(3), 20–108 (Special Issue: Life, Death and The Immune System).

Weir, D.M. and Stewart, J. (1993). *Immunology*, 7th edn. Churchill Livingstone, London. (ISBN 0-443-04660-3).

5

Pathways of Destruction in HIV Disease

AIDS is the end stage of a long process beginning with primary HIV infection. Most scientific opinion agrees that the cause of AIDS is infection with the human immunodeficiency virus (HIV), although there are a few scientists who do not believe this to be true[1]. The exact way by which HIV causes the relentless, progressive and profound immunosuppression seen in HIV disease is only now just beginning to be understood. However, there are several straightforward facts which help to explain the **immunopathogenesis** (i.e. the cellular events leading to disease) of HIV infection.

Immunopathogenesis of HIV infection

HIV is unique in using the **CD4 cell-surface receptor** on T lymphocytes ('helper' cells) as a docking site for attachment, and then infection of this cell[2]. No other virus does this. Infection of CD4+ T cells results in a step-by-step depletion of these important cells over time, continuously increasing the severity of the developing immunosuppression[3]. This depletion of CD4+ T cells is the fundamental abnormality in HIV infection. HIV, all by itself, is sufficient to cause AIDS, although co-factors, e.g. other micro-organisms such as cytomegalovirus, *Mycoplasma penetrans*, etc., may impact adversely on the rate of progression to AIDS following infection, and may also exacerbate disease late in the course of HIV infection[4].

The concept of 'HIV disease'

During the course of infection, HIV exists as a mixture of **active** and **inactive** virus in different cells throughout the body. Cells with inactive virus (**latently infected cells**) can be activated in the future and start to produce more virus. Cells infected with virus which is active and replicating are generating new viruses (**virus-producing cells**)[5].

There are always some cells infected with virus which is active and replicating, budding out and seeking other CD4+ T cells to infect. Consequently, following infection, there is never a period of microbiological latency; the virus is always working, replicating, infecting and destroying more and more cells[6]. Although there are usually long periods of **clinical latency**, i.e. intervals where individuals are **asymptomatic**, the gradual deterioration of the immune system, taking place day by day, month by month, year by year, has led to the use of the concept of '**HIV disease**' as a model in HIV pathogenesis. By definition, HIV disease begins on the day of infection and continues until the patient dies. This allows for a more rational staging system, which is described in the next chapter, and moves away from the imprecise language (e.g. HIV+, ARC, AIDS, AIDS-related, etc.) used in the earlier years of the epidemic.

The natural history of HIV disease

Following primary infection, the virus quickly starts to replicate and there is an early burst of viraemia, i.e. a high level of virus in the blood (Fig. 5.1), with the virus rapidly spreading widely throughout the body. Initially, there is a good immune response with the production of HIV-specific neutralizing antibodies and a strong cell-mediated CD8+ cytotoxic killer-cell effect[7]. However, many viruses escape immune surveillance and destruction by frequently **mutating**, keeping 'one step ahead' of the immune defences. In addition, the virus causes cells in the immune system to send out the wrong signals. These signals are in the form of **cytokines**, produced and secreted by the two types of CD4+ T cells (helper cells), as discussed in the previous chapter. Helper cells belonging to the subset known as **Th2 cells** (helping humoral immunity) send out cytokine messages to plasma cells, instructing them to secrete more antibody. Unfortunately, the correct message would be that sent out by **Th1 cells** (helping cell-mediated immunity), which activates cytotoxic killer cells, tailor-made to destroy those cells which are infected with viruses. The dominant activity of the Th2 helper cells suppresses Th1 helper cell responses. This switch from Th1 to Th2 activity is a fatal immune system error and the resulting immune response is inadequate in destroying or containing the infection[8].

The virus in the blood will start to be filtered by the **follicular dendritic cells (FDC)** in the lymph nodes, reducing both the viral load and replication in the peripheral blood, but infecting more helper cells in the **reticulo-endothelial system**, e.g. in the spleen, adenoid glands, tonsils and lymph nodes (the sites where most helper cells reside)[9,10].

This early burst of viraemia is associated with a rapid depletion of helper cells and, during this period, between 50 and 70 per cent of infected persons will develop an acute (mononucleosis) glandular fever-like syndrome, which is known as **acute HIV syndrome**[11]. The development of significant illness during this acute syndrome, i.e. signs and symptoms lasting > 14 days, is associated with a more rapid progression to end-stage disease (AIDS) as compared with individuals who experience more short-lived illness as a result of primary infection[12]. As the patient recovers, the plasma viraemia declines and the helper cell count recovers somewhat.

The infected person will then generally experience many years (median 10 years) of **clinical latency**, during which time they are usually asymptomatic (often unaware that they are infected with HIV). However, during this period of clinical latency, there continues to be a persistent and progressive loss of helper cells. In time, a critical depletion of helper cells (< 500 cells/mm³) will accelerate viral replication. The inevitable outcome of a further deterioration of the immune system, and a rising level of viral activity, is clinically apparent disease. The types of disease seen during end-stage disease

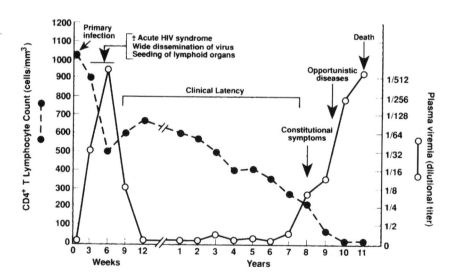

Fig. 5.1 The typical course of HIV infection. (Reprinted, with permission, from Fauci, A.S. (1993). Immunopathogenesis of HIV infection. *Journal of Acquired Immune Deficiency Syndromes*, 6(6).)

are discussed in more detail in the next chapter and include severe and persistent constitutional signs and symptoms (diarrhoea, night sweats, weight loss, skin conditions, etc.) and/or AIDS-defining opportunistic infections and neoplasms.

Mechanisms of HIV cell killing

Although the mechanisms HIV uses to kill CD4+ T cells is not completely understood, medical scientists have identified several phenomena to explain the probable means by which HIV kills cells in the immune system (Fig. 5.2):

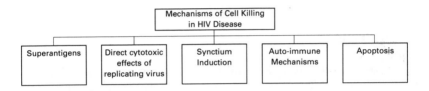

Fig. 5.2 Mechanisms of cell killing in HIV disease

Viral replication

HIV replicating in CD4+ T cells is one cause of cell death. The infected cell dies as a result of attack by CD8+ T cells (cytotoxic killer cells) which detect that they are infected with a virus. In addition, the production of new virions inside the host cell will eventually cause that cell to die as a result of the damage caused by tiny holes punched out of its cell wall by budding virions.

Syncytium induction

Some (but not all) types of HIV will cause the formation of **syncytia**, a mass of merged cells. Syncytia develop after a single cell becomes infected with a **syncytium inducing (SI)** form of HIV. This cell then produces viral proteins, including gp120, which the host cell (i.e. the infected cell) displays on its cell surface. Because CD4+ T cells have a high affinity for gp120, a mass of uninfected helper cells bind to the infected cell. The original cell is destroyed and the uninfected cells bound to it in the syncytium are killed by a so-called 'innocent bystander' effect. SI forms of HIV are more cytotoxic than **non-syncytium inducing (NSI)** forms of HIV. Individuals are infected with a mixture of both forms.

Autoimmune mechanisms

Free viral gp120 (i.e. extra fragments of HIV envelope glycoprotein, which is not attached to the intact virion) is found freely circulating in the plasma following HIV infection and will bind to uninfected CD4+ T cells. Although the CD4+ T cell is not infected, it will appear to be so by the killer cells of the immune system because it has this extra fragment of gp120 attached to its cell surface, and it will be destroyed.

Apoptosis

Apoptosis (pronounced: ap"o-to'sis) refers to **programmed cell death** (suicide), a normal phenomenon which occurs in the thymus gland to eliminate abnormal (autoreactive) T cells which would otherwise attack the body's own tissue, causing autoimmune disease. HIV infection primes T lymphocytes (even those not infected with HIV) to commit cellular suicide when they are stimulated by foreign proteins, rather than dividing as they should[13]. This untimely and inappropriate induction of apoptosis not only affects helper cells, but also appears to involve uninfected CD8+ cytotoxic killer cells[4]. These are the cells, which, when functioning effectively, kill those very cells which are infected with viruses!

Superantigens

Superantigens are special antigens which react and bind with all T lymphocytes which have a particular T cell receptor ('Vβ **subset**') and stimulate a much larger number of cells than do conventional antigens[14]. Proteins made by HIV during its replication cycle, acting as a superantigen, can bind to and stimulate the whole Vβ subset population of T cells. Following superantigen exposure, the stimulated cells undergo expansion and are then either killed or made impotent (**anergic**)[15].

Other immune system abnormalities in HIV disease

Directly, or indirectly, HIV causes widespread havoc throughout the immune system. In addition to the progressive loss of helper cells, many of the remaining helper cells become impaired, unable to function effectively. In addition, B lymphocytes also become defective, developing into a state of chronic stimulation (polyclonal activation) and secrete large amounts of non-specific antibody (hypergammaglobulinaemia), especially IgG and IgA. Natural killer cells also become dysfunctional[16]. There is an inappropriate secretion of a whole range of cytokines, e.g. tumour necrosis factor, which may enhance HIV replication. Many immune system abnormalities can be monitored by physicians to determine the rate of progression to end-stage disease. These markers include elevated levels of neopterin and β_2-microglobulin. Finally, a progressive anaemia is a common feature of HIV disease. Upwards of 10–20 per cent of patients are anaemic when they are first diagnosed as being infected with HIV and, as the infection progresses, 70–80 per cent of all patients will become anaemic[17]. A falling haemocrit and haemoglobin level is another useful laboratory marker of disease progression.

Summary

Following infection, a variety of complex interactions take place between HIV and the host cells it targets for infection. One important cause of the progressive destruction of helper cells is that brought about by the virus causing immune system 'mis-signalling'. This activates a Th2, rather than an effective Th1 helper cell response, giving the virus valuable 'break-away' time to spread throughout the body, especially to the lymph nodes, seeding infection. **Direct cell killing** occurs through the cytolytic effect of the virus, infecting and replicating in cells, and **indirect cell killing** occurs by syncytium induction, autoimmune mechanisms, inappropriate apoptosis and the activities of superantigens manufactured by the virus. It is likely that other mechanisms of cell killing are involved in the immunopathogenesis of HIV disease and this is an area of intense scientific scrutiny.

It can be appreciated that perhaps the most devastating immunological defect in patients with AIDS is the absolute reduction in helper (T4) cells. Without the 'help' of these cells, the entire, intricate pattern of the immune system is defective. It is thus easy to understand why patients with AIDS present with opportunistic infections and neoplastic conditions. It is this new understanding of these defects of acquired immunity which is pointing the way for many researchers as they quickly move forward in investigating the treatment of this catastrophic condition.

Long-term non-progressors and long-term survivors

Some individuals who become infected with HIV survive in good health long past the usual incubation period, and these persons are known as **long-term survivors**. They do, however, show evidence of gradual immune system deterioration. In addition, it has recently been recognized that some other individuals who become infected with HIV, do not show any immune system deterioration, i.e. 12 years following documented infection, they still have normal and stable CD4+ T-cell counts (and have a strong cytoxic CD8+ killer cell response). They remain in good health and are referred to as **long-term, non-progressors**.

References

1. Duesberg, P. (1993) HIV and the aetiology of AIDS. *Lancet*, 10 April, **341**(8850), 957–8.
2. Weiss, Robin A. (1994). The virus and its target cells. In *Textbook of AIDS Medicine*, eds Broder, S., Merigan, T.C. Jr. and Bolognesi, D., Williams & Wilkins, Baltimore, MD, pp. 15–20.
3. Giorgi, J.V. and Detels, R. (1989). T cell subset alterations in HIV-infected homosexual men: NIAID Multicenter AIDS Cohort Study. *Clinical Immunology and Immunopathology* **52**, 10–18.
4. Weiss, Robin A. (1993). How does HIV cause AIDS? *Science*, 28 May, **260**(5112), 1273–9.
5. Temin, Howard M. and Bolognesi, Dani P. (1993). Where has HIV been hiding? *Nature*, 25 March, **362**, 292–3.
6. Fauci, Anthony S. (1993). Immunopathogenesis of HIV infection. *Journal of Acquired Immune Deficiency Syndromes* **6**(6), 655–62.
7. Ada, Gordon (1994). An immunologist's view of HIV infection. In *Textbook of AIDS Medicine*, eds Broder, S., Merigan, T.C. Jr. and Bolognesi, D., Williams & Wilkins, Baltimore, MD, pp. 77–87.
8. Clerici, Mario and Shearer, Gene M. (1993). A Th1→Th2 switch is a critical step in the etiology of HIV infection. *Immunology Today* **14**(3), 107–11.
9. Pantaleo, G., Graziosi, C., Demarest, J.F. *et al.* (1993). HIV infection is active and progressive in lymphoid tissue during the clinically latent stage of disease. *Nature*, 25 March, **362**, 355-8.
10. Embretson, J., Zupancic, M., Ribas, J.L. *et al.* (1993). Massive covert infection of helper T lymphocytes and macrophages by HIV during the incubation period of AIDS. *Nature*, 25 March, **362**, 359–62.

11. Pantaleo, G., Graziosi, C. and Fauci, A. (1993). The immuno-pathogenesis of human immunodeficiency virus infection. *New England Journal of Medicine*, 4 February, **328**(5), 327–35.
12. Pederson, C., Orskov, L.B., Jensen, B.L. *et al.* (1989). Clinical course of primary HIV infection. *British Medical Journal*, 15 July, **299**(6692), 154–7.
13. Greene, Warner C. (1993). AIDS and the immune system. *Scientific American*, September, **269**(3), 99–105.
14. Roitt, Ivan (1994). *Essential Immunology*, 8th edn. Blackwell Scientific, Oxford.
15. Fauci, Anthony S. and Rosenberg, Zelda F. (1994). Immuno-pathogenesis. In *Textbook of AIDS Medicine*, eds Broder, S., Merigan, T.C. Jr. and Bolognesi, D., Williams & Wilkins, Baltimore, MD, pp. 55–75.
16. Rosenberg, Zelda F. and Fauci, Anthony S. (1992). Immuno-pathogenesis of HIV infection. In *AIDS: Etiology, Diagnosis, Treatment, and Prevention*, 3rd edn, eds DeVita, V.T., Hellman, S. and Rosenberg, S.A., J.B. Lippincott & Co, Philadelphia, pp. 61–76.
17. Doweiko, John P. and Groopman, Jerome E. (1994). Hematological consequences of HIV infection. In *Textbook of AIDS Medicine*, eds Broder, S., Merigan, T.C. Jr. and Bolognesi, D., Williams & Wilkins, Baltimore, MD, pp. 617–28.

6

The Clinical Consequences of HIV Infection

> A succession of disasters came on him so swiftly and with such
> unexpected violence that it is hard to say when exactly I recognised
> that my friend was in deep trouble.
>
> *Brideshead Revisited*, Evelyn Waugh

The shape of HIV disease

In August 1987, the Centers for Disease Control (CDC) in Atlanta
published their latest surveillance case definition of AIDS[1]. This
was then revised at the end of 1992[2]. The current CDC Classification System for HIV Infection and the Expanded Surveillance Case
Definition for AIDS Among Adolescents and Adults is reproduced
in Appendix 1.

It is probable that most individuals infected with HIV will
eventually develop some form of ill health as a result of infection.
HIV infection is a dynamic process incorporating various phases,
which are illustrated in Fig. 6.1.

Phase A: Acute primary HIV infection

As previously mentioned in Chapter 5, some (but not all) individuals
develop an acute 'glandular fever-like illness' 2–6 weeks after primary
or initial infection with HIV. This is a result of an immunological
response to rapid and widespread dissemination of HIV following
primary infection. This acute illness is characterized by lethargy and
malaise, headache, fever, joint pains (arthralgias), tenderness and
pain in the muscles (myalgias), diarrhoea and a maculopapular rash.
Individuals may also develop a variety of self-limiting, neurological
manifestations of acute HIV infection, for example, atypical, aseptic meningitis and acute encephalitis. These are discussed in more
detail in Chapter 8. Some individuals develop generalized, swollen
lymph glands (lymphadenopathy) in response to acute HIV infection,

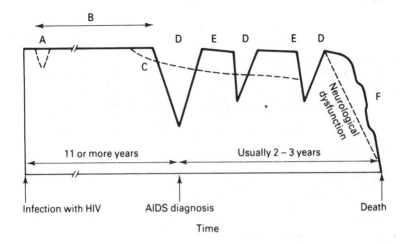

Fig. 6.1 Clinical dynamics of HIV disease

which resolve in several weeks[3]. Towards the end of this acute illness, the infected individual will start to produce antibodies to HIV (i.e. seroconversion).

This acute reaction to HIV infection, often referred to as **Acute HIV syndrome**, may go unrecognized in many individuals. However, the following typical immune system abnormalities can be detected in everyone following primary HIV infection:

- High plasma viraemia
- Depressed T-helper (T4) cell number and function
- Raised immunoglobulin levels
- Leucopenia (white blood cells $< 5.0 \times 10^9$/l)
- (Differential count, i.e. percentage of different types of white blood cells, is usually normal in the early or asymptomatic stages).

Phase B: Antibody positive phase

Following seroconversion, the infected individual becomes antibody positive and may remain asymptomatic for many years prior to developing clinical illness as a result of infection. This phase of infection can be subdivided into two subphases.

Phase B-1: Asymptomatic HIV infection

Many individuals infected with HIV remain clinically asymptomatic (at least in the first 11–12 year period). However, several laboratory abnormalities characteristic of overt disease may be found in these individuals (Table 6.1, see p. 78). As infection progresses, **leucopenia** may become more serious and a reduction in lymphocytes (**lymphocytopenia**) can develop. A reduction in thrombocytes (**thrombocytopenia**) may also be seen but is not usually associated with bleeding unless aggravated by a drug reaction, for example trimethoprim-sulphamethoxazole (Septrin®)[4].

Individuals who are asymptomatically infected with HIV remain infected, probably for life, and remain infectious. It is not known if HIV antibody positive individuals are infectious throughout the course of their infection. It may be that they are infectious (or more infectious) at different stages of the infection and non-infectious (or less infectious) at other stages. Infectivity may relate to the presence of HIV antigens in the blood.

It is currently not known how many individuals who are asymptomatically infected with HIV will eventually become ill. It is generally thought that the majority will develop symptomatic disease within a 10–15 year period. In the face of no other advances in medical treatment and no changes in the pathogenicity of the virus, they will eventually die as a consequence of their disease. Considering the vast numbers of individuals now asymptomatically infected with this virus all over the world, the magnitude of the epidemic becomes more sinister as the years go by. The chilling possibility of an entire generation of young people becoming ill, either with AIDS or with HIV-related neurological dysfunction, leaves little doubt that we are potentially facing the most serious threat to the public health in our human experience.

Phase B-2: Persistent generalized lymphadenopathy (PGL)

Many individuals infected with HIV develop a persistent generalized lymphadenopathy (known as PGL or LAS – lymphadenopathy syndrome). PGL is defined as palpable lymph node enlargement (more than 1 cm) at two or more extra-inguinal sites, persisting for more than 3 months in the absence of an identifiable cause other than HIV infection. Axillary and cervical lymph nodes are commonly involved in this condition. Herpes (varicella) zoster commonly occurs in patients with PGL and may be a poor prognostic sign[5]. PGL can persist in some individuals for many years without any progression to clinical illness and it may be that this lymphadenopathy represents, in some individuals at any rate, a successful containment of the infection. The presence of PGL in and of itself does not affect the patient's clinical prognosis and is now considered to be compatible with asymptomatic HIV disease[6]. Consequently, this diagnostic term is generally reserved for those individuals in which lymphadenopathy is the principal manifestation of infection and is included in group 'A' of the current CDC classification system for HIV infection[2].

Phase C: Early symptomatic disease

Many individuals develop a variety of indicators of ill health due to HIV infection without developing major opportunistic infections or secondary cancers. These constitutional symptoms and signs are a manifestation of **early symptomatic disease** (sometimes referred to as the AIDS-related complex – ARC) and are represented in group 'B' in the current CDC classification system for HIV infection[2]. Symptomatic conditions in an HIV-infected adolescent or adult that are included in this group are discussed in further detail later in this chapter.

Individuals with HIV disease at this stage usually appear chronically ill or even cachectic and may display a variety of minor opportunistic infections such as oral candidiasis (thrush) and skin conditions, for example, seborrhoeic dermatitis. Seborrhoeic dermatitis presents as a red, scaly rash which commonly affects the face and scalp, although the entire body may be affected. This condition can occur in individuals with no prior history of skin disease and may be extremely serious. Some individuals also present with white, elevated lesions on the side of their tongue, known as hairy leucoplakia. Hairy leucoplakia is almost exclusively seen in patients with HIV infection and is thought to be caused by a virus (e.g. Epstein–Barr virus or human papilloma virus).

Hairy leucoplakia and oral candidiasis are important prognostic indicators and are seen as harbingers of AIDS-defining illnesses in persons infected with HIV[7]. In addition, persons with early symptomatic HIV disease are prone to a variety of bacterial, fungal and viral infections. *Tinea cruris* (a fungal skin disease of surfaces of contact in the scrotal, crural and genital areas) and *Tinea pedis* (athlete's foot) are frequently seen. Many individuals may also have enlarged spleens (splenomegaly) and most will have serological evidence of past exposure to various viruses, for example cytomegalovirus (CMV), Epstein–Barr virus (EBV), herpes simplex and hepatitis B virus.

Herpes simplex infection may reactivate in patients during this phase of HIV disease and healing may be prolonged. Herpes zoster (shingles) infection may also be seen at this stage. Genital warts (*condyloma acuminata*) and molluscum contagiosum, presenting as large, multiple molluscum situated in the face, are sometimes seen in patients with early symptomatic disease and both conditions are relatively unresponsive to conventional treatment. Testicular atrophy and malabsorptive diarrhoea may also be seen. During this stage, many patients will develop unusually thick and elongated eyelashes[4].

Oral candidiasis   Candidiasis can be treated with topical antifungal preparations (e.g. clotrimazole, nystatin or natamycin oral suspension) or, if these fail, with systemic imidazole antifungal drugs, such as ketoconazole, fluconazole or itraconazole. First line treatment is often **ketoconazole**. It is effective, the cheapest systemic drug available and side-effects are rare. However, absorption is variable, depending on gastric acidity. Acid beverages, e.g. Coca-Cola® (pH = 2.5), may be used to improve the absorption of ketoconazole if acid production is reduced, as is common in patients with HIV disease, or in patients who have to take anti-ulcer medications. **Fluconazole** is more expensive but better absorbed and has fewer side-effects. All of these drugs are very effective but resistance can occur, resulting in a serious clinical management problem.

Oral hairy leucoplakia   Antifungal drugs are usually given to reduce or eliminate superinfection with *Candida* and **acyclovir** (Zovirax®) or **ganciclovir** may be of some benefit. The antiviral agent **desciclovir** is often effective[8].

Tinea cruris/pedis   These can be treated with topical antifungal preparations such as 2 per cent miconazole cream (Daktarin®) or 1 per cent clotrimazole cream (Canesten®), or with oral griseofulvin, 125 mg 4 times daily.

Seborrhoeic dermatitis   Treatment depends on location and severity. Tars are used to depress the proliferation of cells and have antipruritic and antiseptic properties. Salicylic acid is frequently combined with tars for its keratolytic action, i.e. it helps remove scales, allowing the tars access to the underlying diseased areas. Seborrhoeic dermatitis of the body can be treated with a combination of tars and salicylic acid, for example Gelcosal®. Seborrhoeic dermatitis of the scalp can be treated with a similar preparation, for example Ionil T®. Topical steroids also reduce epidermal cell turnover and low-dose (0.5 per cent) hydrocortisone cream can be used sparingly to treat small areas, such as the scalp and flexures. Aqueous creams are used and bath emollients (e.g. Aveeno Colloidal®, Balneum®, Alpha Keri®) may be useful. Quinoderm Cream® (potassium hydroxyquinoline sulphate 0.5 per cent with benzoyl peroxide 10 per cent) is effective for facial folliculitis.

Herpes zoster   Acyclovir (Zovirax) is effective and is generally prescribed as 800 mg orally, 5 times a day (at 4-hourly intervals) for 7 days.

Herpes simplex   Acyclovir (Zovirax) is used and is generally prescribed as 200 mg orally, 5 times a day (at 4-hourly intervals) for 5 days. Long-term, low-dose acyclovir prophylaxis may be required. Acyclovir-resistant lesions usually respond to foscarnet (Foscavir®) or ganciclovir (Cymevene®).

Diarrhoea   Antidiarrhoeals, for example loperamide hydrochloride (Imodium®), diphenoxylate hydrochloride with atropine sulphate (Lomotil®) or codeine phosphate may be useful. If diarrhoea is severe, an oral fluid and electrolyte replacement preparation, such as Rehidrat® may be beneficial.

Malnutrition/cachexia   The patient should be assessed by a dietitian and appropriate diet, dietary supplements and nutritional interventions implemented. This is discussed in greater detail in Chapter 15.

HIV infection   A variety of antiretroviral drugs may be prescribed and these are discussed in detail in Chapter 19.

Most patients with early symptomatic disease will, in time (e.g. within 3–4 years), progress to fully expressed AIDS.

Phase D: Late symptomatic disease, i.e. AIDS

The diagnosis of AIDS is made when Phase D first occurs. Patients are admitted to hospital for a variety of opportunistic infections associated with this syndrome. They are called 'opportunistic' as they are infections caused by pathogens which the body, in health, contains quite easily. However, in late HIV disease, these pathogens have taken the 'opportunity' of a depressed immune system to establish clinical illness. Although it is possible for a patient to be admitted with just one infectious disease, patients with AIDS more commonly present with a host of infections. We will look at each individually, remembering then that they frequently occur together in various combinations (Table 6.1).

Table 6.1   Opportunistic pathogens seen in HIV infection

Protozoal infections
Pneumocystis carinii
Toxoplasma gondii
Cryptosporidium species
Giardia lamblia
Entamoeba histolytica
Isospora species

Bacterial infections
Mycobacterium tuberculosis
Mycobacterium avium-intracellulare
Mycobacterium kansasii/xenopi
Salmonella typhimurium
Shigella flexneri
Legionella species
Listeria monocytogenes
Nocardia species
Pyogenic bacteria, e.g. *Haemophilus, Streptococcus*
(including *Pneumococcus*)

Fungal infections
Candida albicans
Cryptococcus neoformans
Aspergillus species
Coccidioides immitis
Tinea species

Viral infections
Cytomegalovirus
Herpes simplex
Herpes zoster
Epstein–Barr virus
Papovaviruses (JC/SV-40)

Pneumocystis carinii pneumonia (PCP)

PCP (also referred to as 'pneumocystosis') is not only the main presenting disease seen in AIDS, it is by far the most frequent cause of death in persons with AIDS. The organism was first described in 1909 as a multiflagellate protozoan and was first recognized as a human pathogen during the Second World War when it caused a fatal pneumonia in severely malnourished refugee children. *Pneumocystis carinii* is now thought to be more closely related to fungi and yeasts, rather than being a protozoan, i.e. a 'protist'[9,10]. It is part of the normal flora of most adults, rarely causing disease unless the immune system becomes compromised[11]. In the United States, the first case in an adult of pneumonia caused by *P. carinii* was observed in 1954. Until the present epidemic of AIDS, PCP was only seen in patients whose immune system had been depressed either by a known primary or secondary cause, for example congenital immunodeficiency disorders, or in patients receiving chemotherapy for cancer or immunosuppressant drugs following transplant surgery. It is a relatively important point for the nurse to note that PCP only occurs in immunocompromised individuals; hence hospital personnel and other patients, who are not immunocompromised, are not at risk of acquiring this infection.

Patients usually develop symptoms insidiously, often giving a 3–4 week history of cough, dyspnoea, chest pain, fever and chills. Tachypnoea (rapid respirations) and cyanosis are usually present when the patient is seen in hospital. Patients frequently complain of not being able to take a deep breath. Some patients have a more fulminate course with a much shorter history. The patient may be in acute respiratory failure and in extreme distress.

The diagnosis of PCP is difficult. All the usual causes of pneumonia will need to be excluded and sputum will need to be obtained for routine culture and sensitivity. Chest X-rays usually show alveolar and interstitial infiltrates in both the right and left lung fields (bilateral). These changes, however, may be so mild as to be interpreted as normal in many patients[12]. Abnormalities of arterial blood gases (associated with hypoxaemia) are common. The diagnosis of PCP is generally made as a result of bronchoalveolar lavage of subsegmental bronchi, or transbronchial biopsy, both distressing procedures in patients with an already established respiratory impairment. Biopsy can also help to diagnose coexisting pulmonary infection with mycobacterium, CMV or *Cryptococcus neoformans*.

Nursing staff must wear protective clothing (a water-repellent, long-sleeved gown), disposable rubber latex or good quality plastic gloves, an effective, high filtration mask or a particulate respirator and eye protection when assisting with bronchoscopy.

A 'dedicated' bronchoscope is not necessary. Following bronchoscopy, the bronchoscope is thoroughly cleaned and then immersed in 2 per cent glutaraldehyde for 1 hour (preferably 2 hours). This is adequate disinfection and it can then be used for any other patient without fear of transmitting HIV and, more importantly, *Mycobacterium* tuberculosis and environmental mycobacteria, which are commonly associated with HIV disease[13]. Mycobacterial diseases and associated infection control precautions are discussed more fully in Chapter 7.

Patients with PCP frequently have a dry, non-productive cough. The protocol for sputum induction consists of having the patient fast the night before. To avoid contamination of the sputum specimen with oral debris, patients are asked to brush the buccal mucosa, tongue and gums with a wet toothbrush and rinse their mouths thoroughly with water. Sputum is then induced by inhalation of 20–30 ml of 3 per cent saline through an ultrasonic nebulizer. Gentle chest percussion to aid expectoration is used when necessary and two sputum specimens are then taken promptly to the laboratory. Examination of sputum obtained in this manner can detect evidence of *Pneumocystis carinii* infection in over 95 per cent of patients, consequently sparing them from bronchoscopy[14]. Prior to sputum induction, chest X-rays are needed to rule out pleural effusions. Sputum induction is contraindicated in a patient with a pleural effusion, as forceful coughing could fatally worsen the effusion[15].

Treatment

Once PCP has been diagnosed, treatment is initiated with either pentamidine isethionate or trimethoprim-sulphamethoxazole (Bactrim®, Septrin®).

Pentamidine isethionate   This drug is administered intravenously or intramuscularly in a dose of 3 or 4 mg/kg, once daily for at least 21 days.

Almost half of all patients receiving pentamidine experience side-effects ranging from nephrotoxicity (with elevated creatinine levels), hypoglycaemia (and sometimes hyperglycaemia), sterile abscesses at the injection site, disorders of blood clotting (e.g. thrombocytopenia), skin rashes and pruritus (severe itching), tachycardia and hypotension. The most frequent major adverse reaction to pentamidine is neutropenia (< 1000 polymorphonuclear leucocytes/μL) and the most frequent minor reactions are hyponatremia (salt depletion), abnormal liver function and azotemia (excess urea and other nitrogenous compounds in the blood)[16].

The abscesses at the injection site may become secondarily infected, providing yet another focus of infection for this immunocompromised patient, and can be so painful that the patient may refuse further injections. Intramuscular injections into a wasted, catabolic patient present nursing care problems and although using alternative sites is helpful, the formation of abscesses, or the bleeding disorders sometimes caused by this drug, may preclude it being used intramuscularly. For these reasons, intravenous administration of pentamidine is often preferred. Pentamidine, diluted in at least 250 ml of 5 per cent dextrose/water, is given slowly (over 1–2 hours), once daily, under close supervision, as this route of administration has been associated with intractable hypotension.

For patients receiving pentamidine therapy urine specimens should be tested and blood glucose levels measured daily. Arterial blood pressure should be taken and recorded 4-hourly, unless unstable, when it should be taken more frequently. During intravenous administrations of pentamidine, the blood pressure should be taken every 15 minutes.

Aerosolized pentamidine The use of aerosolized pentamidine is also successful in both treating patients with PCP and as a prophylactic measure. Ultrasonic or jet nebulizers (Respirgard II®, Acorn system 22 Miser®) are used to deliver appropriate size particles of pentamidine (2–4 μm) into the alveoli. Pentamidine isethionate (600 mg) is dissolved in 6 ml of sterile water and shaken until all the solute is dissolved. The solution is stable for 48 hours at 20°C. Using a 10 ml syringe, all the drug from the vial is withdrawn and injected into the drug chamber of the nebulizer system. The patient is treated in a sitting position and then lying on each side (to increase upper lobe distribution of the drug). The psi gas flow rate is determined by the nebulizer used but 6 l/min is usual.

Aerosolized pentamidine should be administered in a room with good external ventilation and nursing personnel must wear effective, high filtration masks or particulate respirators while caring for patients during this treatment[17]. The use of aerosolized pentamidine avoids many of the grave systemic side-effects of this drug. Side-effects of aerosolized pentamidine include cough and bronchospasm which can be treated with ipratropium bromide (Atrovent®). Aerosolized pentamidine therapy can be used on an outpatient basis and at home[18]. This form of treatment requires the use of a special nebulizer as shown in Fig. 6.2[19].

Extrapulmonary pneumocystosis and pulmonary breakthrough infection with *P. carinii* can occur while clients are on prophylactic aerosolized pentamidine[20]. A nursing assessment for clients on such therapy must incorporate a high index of suspicion for developing infections, and the patient's temperature should be taken on each visit.

Trimethoprim-sulphamethoxazole Also known as 'co-trimoxazole', this drug is given in high doses (e.g. 20 mg trimethoprim/100 mg

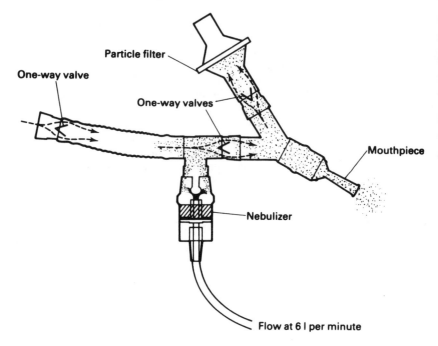

Fig. 6.2   Diagram of a nebulizer and delivery system for pentamidine aerosol

sulphamethoxazole/kg) either orally or intravenously, in divided doses, every 8 hours, again for at least 21 days. Although generally this drug is associated with fewer side-effects than pentamidine, a high percentage of patients with AIDS (up to 80 per cent) develop a drug fever, rash and significant leucopenia when treated with this compound. Side-effects may be controlled by the administration of antihistamines, and/or by giving trimethoprim separately and reducing the dose of sulphonamide. Co-trimoxazole for intravenous use is diluted 1/25 in either 0.9 per cent sodium chloride or 5 per cent dextrose and is infused slowly (over 1½ hours) and care should be taken **not to mistake intramuscular preparations for intravenous use**. When given orally, nausea, vomiting and diarrhoea are not uncommon.

It is usual for the medical staff to prescribe folinic acid (calcium folinate) 15 mg 2–3 times weekly in an attempt to prevent the bone marrow depression due to high dose trimethoprim-sulphamethoxazole therapy; this may be given orally or intravenously.

Other drugs Other drugs used in the treatment of PCP include diaminodiphenylsulphone (dapsone) with or without trimethoprim, DFMO (alpha-difluromethylornithine) (also known as Elflornithine), trimetrexate with leucovorin, the combination of clindamycin and primaquin or sulfadoxine and pyrimethamine (Fansidar®).

All of these drugs have serious side-effects and patients must be carefully observed for these, especially in the second week of therapy. The most common side-effects include haematological abnormalities, nephrotoxicity and severe skin rashes.

Improvement, if it is to be seen, usually occurs within 5–10 days. Although perhaps as many as 90 per cent of patients with AIDS who present with PCP can be successfully treated with the above drugs, they will eventually return to hospital with another episode, more difficult to treat. The long-term survival rate in patients who have AIDS and present with PCP is poor; the median cumulative survival is approximately 35 weeks. The quality of life is also poor, with many patients (up to 40 per cent) spending more than half the time, from date of diagnosis until death, in hospital.

Other causes of pneumonia in HIV disease

The somewhat aggressive investigations required to diagnose PCP are needed not only because the drugs used to treat this pneumonia are relatively toxic, hence the physician wants to be sure of treating *P. carinii*, but also because several other opportunistic pathogens, some of which are treatable, are also known to cause pneumonia in patients with HIV disease. These include mycobacteria (i.e. *M. tuberculosis* and environmental mycobacteria, such as *M. avium-intracellulare*), bacteria (e.g. *Streptococcus pneumoniae, Haemophilus influenzae, Pseudomonas aeruginosa*), viruses (e.g. CMV and herpes simplex), protozoa (e.g. *Toxoplasma gondii*) and fungi (*Aspergillus* and *Cryptococcus*). Most patients with Kaposi's sarcoma (KS) develop lung disease but it is usually asymptomatic. In some patients, KS may cause severe pulmonary symptoms (e.g. haemoptysis, dyspnoea, cough) which may be unresponsive to treatment. Both lymphoid interstitial pneumonia and alveolar proteinosis are sometimes seen in patients with HIV disease.

Mycobacterial infections are treated with antituberculosis drugs, which are described in more detail in Chapter 7. Bacterial infections are treated with the appropriate antibiotics as indicated by culture and sensitivity, and other therapies are available for some of the varied agents which can cause pneumonia in the patient with HIV disease. Bronchoalveolar lavage allows the physician to culture many of these opportunists and transbronchial biopsy (or open lung biopsy) can demonstrate pulmonary involvement of Kaposi's sarcoma.

Toxoplasmosis

Toxoplasmosis is caused by a small, intracellular protozoan parasite, *Toxoplasma gondii*. It exists as three forms (all potentially infectious to man) and is found in felines (cats) and some mammals. Humans become infected when exposed to the parasite in cat faeces (e.g. litter trays or when gardening) or by eating undercooked, infected beef, lamb or pork. Although humans frequently become asymptomatically infected, it is only when the immune system fails to keep this parasite in check that it is able to cause clinical illness. In patients with HIV disease, *T. gondii* can cause a variety of clinical disorders, but the most common illness seen related to infection with this agent is **toxoplasma encephalitis**.

Patients with toxoplasma encephalitis frequently present with neurological signs such as confusion, headache, vertigo and seizures. The patient often has an elevated temperature and is lethargic. The various signs and symptoms may resemble those seen in space-occupying lesions of the brain or those following stroke. The patient is seriously ill and can deteriorate with alarming speed.

Although encephalitis is by far the most frequent manifestation of toxoplasmosis in patients with HIV disease, **pneumonia** and/or **myocarditis** can also occur.

In toxoplasma encephalitis, X-rays, CT scans, lumbar punctures and serological blood tests are usually abnormal, but changes seen are non-specific and the diagnosis is made by brain biopsy.

Once diagnosed, treatment is initiated with pyrimethamine and sulphadiazine. Folinic acid (calcium folinate) is often concurrently prescribed to prevent the serious consequences of depressed folate metabolism associated with pyrimethamine, for example leucopenia, thrombocytopenia and anaemia.

Intravenous clindamycin, with or without sulphadiazine or pyrimethamine, may also be used. Other drugs used include piritrexin, Dapsone and trimetrexate. Newer macrolide antibiotics (e.g. azithromycin, roxithromycin, clarithromycin) may also be used in the future. Corticosteroids and anticonvulsants may also be prescribed.

As it is impossible to eradicate *T. gondii* completely, treatment with these powerful drugs may have to continue for the remaining length of the patient's life.

Cryptosporidiosis

The intracellular protozoan parasite *Cryptosporidium* has been recognized only in the last 10 years as a potential human pathogen, causing a self-limited diarrhoea in animal workers (e.g. veterinarians and slaughterhouse workers). It is spread by a faecal–oral route and, in the immunodeficient individual, attacks the intestines (principally the small intestines), causing abdominal cramps, fever, nausea and vomiting and a profuse diarrhoea. In HIV disease this can be a catastrophic complication – diarrhoea can range from three to four bowel movements a day, to patients passing large amounts (10–12 litres/day) of watery diarrhoea, becoming hypotensive and showing signs and symptoms of electrolyte imbalance. This wasting, weakening disease attacks not only the small bowel, but also the patient's self-esteem, causing psychological havoc.

The diagnosis is made by using special techniques of staining smears of stool specimens or by biopsy of the gastro-intestinal mucosa.

At the present time there is no specific therapy which is curative for this infection. Anti-retroviral drugs, such as zidovudine, are often associated with clinical improvement, remission of symptoms and, in some patients, clearance of *Cryptosporidium*[21].

Supportive treatment includes antidiarrhoeals, such as loperamide hydrochloride (Imodium) and diphenoxylate hydrochloride with atropine sulphate (Lomotil), rehydration, electrolyte replacement, and nutritional support.

Diarrhoea

Diarrhoea is seen in most patients with HIV disease and only in some is *Cryptosporidium* the cause. Other causes include amoebiasis (caused by the protozoon *Entamoeba histolytica*) and giardiasis (caused by another protozoon, *Giardia lamblia*). These are not uncommon enteric infections in homosexual men and the diarrhoea seen is generally less than that seen in cryptosporidiosis. Amoebiasis is treated with oral metronidazole (Flagyl®) and di-iodohydroxyquin, and giardiasis is treated with atabrine or metronidazole.

Other opportunists associated with diarrhoea in patients with HIV disease include *Shigella, Isospora belli, Helicobacter pylori (Campylobacter), Microsporidia, Salmonella, Strongyloides stercoralis*, CMV and *Mycobacterium avium-intracellulare*. Kaposi's sarcoma may be an additional cause. Diarrhoea caused by isoporiasis is treated with co-trimoxazole (Septrin, Bactrim) and metronidazole (e.g. Flagyl) is sometimes used to treat idiopathic diarrhoea.

Diarrhoea is perhaps one of the most distressing complications of HIV disease, and often one of the most difficult to treat.

Mycobacterial infections

There are several mycobacterial diseases associated with HIV disease and these are discussed in detail in the following chapter.

Cryptococcal infection

Infection caused by the fungus *Cryptococcus neoformans* var. *neoformans* is a ubiquitous organism in nature, found in soil and the excreta of pigeons and other birds. It mainly causes a subacute meningitis or a meningoencephalitis in immunocompromised individuals. It can affect other areas in the body (e.g. lungs, bone and the genito-urinary system) and prior to the current epidemic of AIDS was seen mainly in individuals with Hodgkin's disease.

Patients with AIDS may present with a slowly developing meningitis, complaining of headache, mild pyrexia and sometimes blurred vision. Other neurological signs and symptoms associated with meningitis (e.g. positive Kernig's sign, confusion, changes in level of consciousness) may develop, and the patient may become nauseated and start vomiting.

Cryptococcal meningitis is diagnosed by finding the fungus in cerebrospinal fluid, sputum, urine and blood cultures.

Treatment
Drugs used for treating this severe infection include amphotericin B, 5–flucytosine and fluconazole.

Amphotericin B (Fungizone®)   This is a major drug used to treat systemic fungal infections and is active against most fungi and yeasts. As it is frequently used for many of the systemic mycoses in patients with HIV disease, it is covered in detail here.

Amphotericin B is a fungicidal and fungistatic antibiotic and is given intravenously for systemic disease. It is given in an initial dose of 0.25 mg/kg daily, increasing to 0.5 mg/kg daily to 1 mg/kg daily. The maximum daily dose is 1.5 mg/kg a day or on alternate days. Amphotericin B for intravenous infusion is available from the pharmacy as a dry powder in a 50 mg vial. The vial must be kept refrigerated and protected from light. It is reconstituted with large volumes of 5 per cent dextrose/water (**never** normal saline, which can precipitate the drug) and is infused promptly after reconstitution via a central line over a 6 hour period. It is essential that the 5 per cent dextrose infusion is issued by the pharmacy and has a specific pH of greater than 4.2. Each container of 5 per cent dextrose must be checked for its pH and the infusion container must be protected from light (the use of aluminium foil is convenient and effective) once the amphotericin has been added.

Amphotericin B is a toxic drug and side-effects are common. Some patients experience chills, fever, headache, anorexia, nausea and occasionally vomiting, particularly with the initial infusion. Paracetamol (acetaminophen USP) and an antihistamine (e.g. chlorpheniramine maleate) may be prescribed concurrently with the infusion to lessen the incidence of these side-effects. Further side-effects include epigastric cramps, diarrhoea, haemorrhagic gastroenteritis with melaena, peripheral neuropathies, maculopapular rash, transient vertigo, tinnitus, hearing loss, blurred vision, diplopia, anaemia and convulsions.

Rarely, anaphylactoid reactions, hypertension or hypotension, ventricular fibrillation and cardiac arrest can occur. Acute hepatic failure has also been encountered. Chemical thrombophlebitis may occur; adding 25 mg of hydrocortisone to the infusion may lessen the incidence. The concomitant administration of heparin has not been shown to be helpful. Serum potassium levels must be monitored frequently as hypokalaemia is common and occasionally is dramatic and dangerous. If hypokalaemia is detected, oral potassium supplements are usually adequate; if intravenous potassium is required, it is **not** added to the amphotericin B 5 per cent dextrose solution. This drug is nephrotoxic and blood tests for renal function (e.g. blood urea nitrogen, serum creatinine) must be determined before and periodically during treatment. Patients must be monitored closely during therapy and vital signs are taken and recorded every 30 minutes during the infusion and for 1 hour after the infusion has been completed. Corticosteroids may enhance the potassium depletion caused by amphotericin B. This potassium depletion may enhance the effects of curariform muscle relaxants and increase the toxicity of digitalis glycosides. It interacts with cyclosporin, increasing the risk of nephrotoxicity.

It is possible to administer amphotericin B via an intrathecal injection. The usual technique employed for intrathecal injection is to first painstakingly dissolve 50 mg of amphotericin B in 10 ml of sterile water for injection. The total volume should then be diluted in a 250 ml bottle of 5 per cent dextrose/water from which 10 ml has been removed. From 0.5 ml (0.1 mg) to 5.0 ml (1.0 mg) is then drawn into a 10 ml syringe, further diluted to 10 ml with CSF and injected **slowly** (over at least 2 minutes). A lumbar, cisternal, or ventricular (by an Ommaya reservoir) site may be used.

Flucytosine (Alcobon®)   This is available from the pharmacy in a ready prepared 250 ml infusion (and administration set) containing 10 mg/ml. It is also available as 500 mg tablets. The usual dose by mouth or by intravenous infusion is 200 mg/kg daily in four divided doses. The dose is reduced in the presence of renal impairment. It is frequently given with amphotericin B for its synergistic effect on this drug. Flucytosine can cause nausea, vomiting, diarrhoea, rashes, thrombocytopenia and leucopenia. Weekly blood counts are necessary during prolonged treatment.

Fluconazole (Diflucan®)   This is a novel triazole antifungal drug and may hopefully replace both amphotericin and flucytosine in the treatment of cryptococcal meningitis. It can be given either orally or intravenously; both routes are equally effective and it has a wide margin of safety and few side-effects. It is given in a single dose of 400 mg on the first day, followed by a single daily dose of 200 mg. Intravenous fluconazole is supplied in either 25 ml or 100 ml bottles (each containing 2 mg. of fluconazole per ml). It is infused at a maximum rate of 200 mg/h as a continuous infusion. Therapy with fluconazole usually continues for 10–12 weeks after CSF cultures become negative. For prophylaxis, the patient is continued on 100–200 mg daily.

Viral infections – herpesviruses

Patients with AIDS are particularly prone to infection with, or re-activation of, various herpesviruses, the most significant being cytomegaloviruses (CMV), herpes simplex viruses, varicella-zoster virus, and Epstein–Barr virus.

Cytomegalovirus infection
As children and young adults, most of us will have been exposed to **cytomegaloviruses** (CMV), a common, airborne spread group of viruses ('salivary gland viruses'). CMV infection may also occur congenitally, postnatally, and can be acquired following blood transfusion ('post-perfusion syndrome').

Infection with CMV produces variable results. Most infants infected show no clinical disease, but congenitally acquired CMV infection may cause abortion, stillbirth, postnatal death, or severe central nervous system damage. In children and adults who acquire this infection, most are asymptomatic, and a few may develop a mononucleosis or hepatitis. CMV are ubiquitous and 60–90 per cent of adults will have been exposed to this virus group and will have developed antibodies. When infected with CMV, individuals will excrete this virus in urine, saliva, cervical secretions, semen, faeces and breast milk for several months. Eventually, the process of cell-mediated immunity contains the infection, the individual developing a **latent infection** and, in most cases, never being aware that he or she had been infected in the first place. Like other latent infections normally contained by the immune system, in HIV disease, CMV infection becomes re-activated as cell-mediated immunity is destroyed by HIV.

Most patients with HIV disease will have re-activated CMV infection and usually are viraemic (i.e. have virus in their blood). In the constellation of opportunistic infections seen in patients with HIV disease, it is often difficult to establish just what the clinical consequences of re-activated CMV infection are. However, as it may cause ulcerations of the gastro-intestinal tract, it may be implicated as yet another cause of diarrhoea seen in these patients. CMV can cause a terminal pneumonitis and sometimes also causes a retinochoroiditis which may lead to blindness.

Effective treatment for CMV infection has been unsatisfactory. New drugs currently being used are **ganciclovir** and **foscarnet** (Foscavir®). Ganciclovir 2.5–5 mg/kg is given intravenously every 8 hours for 14–21 days. Oral ganciclovir is now in final trials and should be available for clinical use. Patients with CMV pneumonitis and encephalitis do not respond well to ganciclovir, and in CMV retinopathy it only seems to delay the progression of disease. Maintenance treatment (usually daily injections via a central line) are usually necessary and these can be self-administered or administered by community nurses at home. Foscarnet 0.05–0.16 mg/kg per minute is administered by a continuous intravenous infusion for 14–21 days, and is useful in ganciclovir-resistant infections.

The major side-effect of foscarnet therapy is nephrotoxicity, and clients on this medication must be kept well hydrated. As ganciclovir (but not foscarnet) may cause severe neutropenia, it is often not pre-scribed for individuals who are taking zidovudine (Retrovir® – AZT). Clearly this may reduce its usefulness, as most individuals who are at this stage of HIV disease will already be on zidovudine therapy. If zidovudine and ganciclovir are being prescribed together, weekly white blood cell counts are usually done and nurses must be alert to developing pyogenic infections.

Herpes simplex virus infection
Many adults (including a large proportion of homosexual men) have

been exposed to **herpes simplex** and consequently harbour these latent viruses. During HIV disease, these viruses are frequently re-activated and may cause severe perineal or facial lesions. They will usually respond to treatment with the antiviral drug, **acyclovir**. Acyclovir-resistant lesions are usually treated with foscarnet or vidarabine.

Other viral infections
Many other latent viruses can be re-activated in AIDS and they include:

Varicella-zoster virus   This causes herpes zoster (shingles) and is generally seen in patients with early symptomatic HIV disease. Its occurrence may be prognostic of progression to fully expressed AIDS. These lesions respond to acyclovir, although oral acyclovir may have to be continued indefinitely to prevent relapse. This virus may also cause chickenpox (varicella) in non-immune individuals.

Epstein-Barr virus   This may cause fever, lassitude and lymphadenopathy in patients with HIV disease. There is no specific treatment available for illness associated with this virus.

Candidal species infection

Infection with **candidal species fungi** in healthy adults is now often considered to be a harbinger of AIDS. Most patients with HIV disease have oral candidiasis ('thrush'), often affecting the oesophagus and rectum. Disseminated candidiasis can occur, but it is usually associated with indwelling catheters or prolonged treatment with antibiotics. Although sometimes responsive to treatment with nystatin or clotrimazole, candidiasis is frequently resistant to these agents. In such cases, fluconazole (Diflucan®) is usually effective. Fluconazole is given orally as a single daily dose of 200 mg on the first day, followed by 100 mg daily. Candidal oesophagitis is serious and may cause perforation and haemorrhage. Treatment with the above agents has to be continued for the remainder of the patient's life because, if discontinued, relapse is invariable.

Other opportunistic pathogens in AIDS

Although the opportunistic conditions we have discussed are the ones most frequently seen as a manifestation of immunodeficiency in patients with HIV disease, and serve to define this disease, they are by no means the only potential pathogens which take the opportunity to establish clinical disease in the absence of immune competence.

Other opportunists which may be encountered include:

Isospora belli   This coccidian protozoan may cause severe diarrhoea.

Histoplasma capsulatum   This causes **histoplasmosis**, a progressive, disseminating fungal disease involving lungs, spleen, liver and the gastro-intestinal tract.

Coccidioides immitis   This causes **coccidioidomycosis**, another disseminated fungal disease involving many organs in the body, including the brain. *Coccidioides immitis* may also be involved in causing meningitis.

Nocardia asteroides   This causes **nocardiosis**, a disseminating disease associated with metastatic brain abscesses. It also causes skin or subcutaneous abscesses and pulmonary lesions.

Listeria monocytogenes   This causes **listeriosis**, meningitis being its most frequent clinical presentation.

Papova viruses   JC virus and SV-40 virus have been implicated in causing a severe, progressive, demyelinating disease in patients with AIDS, known as **progressive multifocal leucoencephalopathy (PML)**. This is a rare but serious infection of the central nervous system for which there is no effective therapy at present.

Salmonella   These Gram-negative bacteria commonly cause an enteritis from which septicaemia (**salmonellosis**) frequently develops in patients with AIDS. Drugs used to treat this condition include ampicillin, amoxicillin or chloramphenicol. The septicaemia is recurrent and often unresponsive to treatment.

Shigella   These are also Gram-negative bacteria and, like *Salmonella*, belong to a family of bacteria known as *Enterobacteriaceae*. *Shigella* cause enteritis, dysentery and, like *Salmonella*, can cause a persistent bacteraemia in patients with HIV disease. Drugs used to treat this condition include ampicillin, tetracycline and co-trimoxazole.

All patients with HIV disease will develop opportunistic infection at some time during the course of their illness. Even though most are initially treatable, eventually they become more difficult, if not impossible, to treat and eventually, after incapacitating illness, cause death in patients with AIDS.

The other remaining, major, opportunistic disease seen in AIDS is Kaposi's sarcoma.

Kaposi's sarcoma

Prior to the current epidemic of AIDS, Kaposi's sarcoma (KS) was a relatively unusual, vascular tumour, first described by a Hungarian dermatologist, Moriz Kaposi, in 1872. In the United States and in Western Europe, Kaposi's sarcoma was mainly seen in elderly men, especially those of Italian or Eastern European Jewish ancestry, and was relatively benign in its clinical course. Patients presented with discoloured patches, plaques or nodular skin lesions, brown, red or blue in colour, usually confined to lower extremities (especially the ankles and soles of the feet). These lesions are the result of a multicentric tumour arising from local hyperplasia of a cell of the vascular endothelium. Often, as the patients were in the age group 60–79 years, no specific treatment was indicated. This type of indolent, non-aggressive, non-invasive Kaposi's sarcoma has become known as **classic** Kaposi's sarcoma.

Another form of Kaposi's sarcoma was known to exist in Equatorial Africa, where it was more common. Four different types of Kaposi's sarcoma have been described in Africa, one of which is similar to classic Kaposi's sarcoma, the remaining three being more aggressive, rapidly progressive neoplastic conditions, affecting young African men, often fatal within a year. This African form of Kaposi's sarcoma is sometimes referred to as **endemic** Kaposi's sarcoma.

Prior to 1981, a type of Kaposi's sarcoma similar to the African endemic form was observed in renal patients following kidney transplant and iatrogenic immunosuppression. This too was aggressive, but responded well to discontinuation of immunosuppression therapy and restoration of the patient to immune competence.

With the advent of AIDS in 1981, an aggressive form of Kaposi's sarcoma, similar to African endemic Kaposi's sarcoma, was seen in young, previously healthy male homosexuals. This AIDS-associated Kaposi's sarcoma has become known as **epidemic** Kaposi's sarcoma and patients usually present with asymptomatic, pigmented skin lesions which may be on any part of the body. Lesions can usually be identified in the mouth, especially on the hard palate, and many will also have lymph node enlargement. The initial lesions are often multifocal at time of diagnosis, often involving visceral organs (e.g. lungs, liver, spleen, gastro-intestinal tract), and rapidly disseminate, usually in an orderly fashion.

The average life expectancy of patients with AIDS who have Kaposi's sarcoma is about 16 months, only a quarter of all patients surviving for 2 years or more.

Treatment
Treatment does not improve survival, nor the rate of the appearance of new lesions. However, it is useful for palliation and various treatment modalities can be effectively used.

Local irradiation therapy   Skin and oral lesions are often radiosensitive and doses under 20 Gy are used.

Interlesional chemotherapy   Small cutaneous lesions are sometimes treated for cosmetic purposes with interlesional injections of 0.01 mg of vinblastine in 0.1 ml of sterile water, using a tuberculin syringe. This has to be frequently repeated and a hyperpigmented area frequently remains following treatment.

Systemic chemotherapy   Various anti-cancer drugs have been tried and the following have been found to be the most useful. **Vinblastine** (given intravenously, once weekly in doses of 4–10 mg). This regime is associated with minimal toxicity and approximately 40 per cent of patients treated may show objective improvement. **VP-16 (epidophyllotoxin)** (given intravenously for 3 days every 3–4 weeks in doses of 150 mg/m^2 of body surface). Most patients will experience side-effects, especially leucopenia and alopecia; however, up to 75 per cent may show objective improvement.

One of the dangers of anti-cancer chemotherapy is the risk of further depressing the immune system and rendering the patient more prone to opportunistic infection. The use of VP-16 is not only associated with the highest objective response rate, but is also associated with the lowest rate of occurrence of opportunistic infection (seen in only 12 per cent of patients treated, as opposed to 25 per cent of patients treated with vinblastine).

Immune modulators   It seemed clear from the beginning of the epidemic that curative treatment for epidemic Kaposi's sarcoma would be available only if immune competence was restored, and various immune modulators have been used in combination with anti-cancer chemotherapy. **Alpha-interferons** have been widely used to stimulate the immune system in patients with HIV disease and may be useful in treating epidemic Kaposi's sarcoma. However, this has not been shown to restore immune competence. Intravenous administration has been shown to be associated with the fewest side-effects, which commonly include fever, malaise, headache, and transient, mild confusion. Alpha-interferon is often combined with zidovudine (Retrovir – AZT) as they exhibit synergistic activity in this disease.

Other tumours in AIDS

Although Kaposi's sarcoma is by far the most common malignancy seen in AIDS, **undifferentiated lymphomas** (non-Hodgkin's lymphomas), affecting various sites including the central nervous system, bone marrow and gastro-intestinal tract, may be seen. An increased incidence of other tumours may also be encountered. It may be that the various viruses present in patients with HIV disease are potentially oncogenic and once the immune system has broken down, may become involved in the pathogenesis of the various tumours seen.

Phase E: Periods of remission

Treatment of the opportunistic diseases encountered in AIDS will produce periods of remission and relative good health. This phase of HIV disease can be considerably prolonged if the patient is commenced on zidovudine therapy. However, neurological dysfunction either from CNS opportunistic disease secondary to HIV infection, or from the direct action of HIV on nervous tissues (e.g. dementia) may seriously limit the relative health of patients with HIV disease who are in remission. Periods of remission alternate with new opportunistic diseases (i.e. Phase D) and, eventually, patients proceed to Phase F.

Phase F: Terminal phase of illness

Patients eventually develop terminal, opportunistic illnesses from which they will die. Pneumonia caused by *Pneumocystis carinii is* the most common cause of death in patients with late, symptomatic HIV disease. In this phase, patients are frequently blind (due to CMV retinitis), bed-bound and incontinent, dementing and grossly malnourished and wasted. They may be extremely frightened and only nursing care of the highest quality is able to make a critical impact on the physical and psychological condition of these young patients who find themselves wide awake in their own worst nightmare.

Classification system for HIV infection

In 1986, the Centers for Disease Control (CDC) outlined a system which classified the manifestations of HIV infection into four mutually exclusive groups, designated by Roman numerals I–IV (Table

6.2)[22]. Classification in a particular group is not explicitly intended to have prognostic significance, nor to designate severity of illness. However, classification in the four principal groups, I–IV, is hierarchical in that persons classified in a particular group should not be reclassified in a preceding group if clinical findings resolve, since clinical improvements may not accurately reflect changes in the severity of the underlying disease. Although the CDC revised their classification system in 1993[2], the revised system has not been widely accepted in Europe and the 1986 classification system, as described in Table 6.2, continues to be widely used in the United Kingdom.

Group I This refers to the acute sero-conversion illness described in **Phase A**.

Group II This refers to asymptomatic HIV infection, as described in **Phase B-1**.

Group III This refers to PGL, as described in **Phase B-2**.

Group IV Other HIV diseases: the clinical manifestations of patients in this group may be designated by assignment to one or more subgroups (A–E) listed below. AIDS-defining illnesses are listed in Table 6.3 and discussed further in Appendix 1.

>   **Subgroup A** This refers to patients previously classified as having the AIDS-related complex (ARC), i.e. **Phase C**.

>   **Subgroup B** This refers to patients who develop neurological manifestations of HIV infection, i.e. **Phase D**.

Table 6.2 Summary of classification system for HIV infection

Group I	Acute primary infection
Group II	Asymptomatic infection
Group III	Persistent generalized lymphadenopathy
Group IV	Other diseases
Subgroup A	Constitutional disease
Subgroup B	Neurological disease
Subgroup C	Secondary infectious diseases
Category C-1	Specified secondary infectious diseases listed in the CDC surveillance definition for AIDS*
Category C-2	Other specified secondary infectious diseases*
Subgroup D	Secondary cancers*
Subgroup E	Other conditions

*See Table 6.3 and Appendix 1.

Table 6.3   AIDS indicator diseases[1,2]

Without laboratory evidence regarding HIV infection
If laboratory tests for HIV were not performed, or gave inconclusive results, and the patient had no other cause of immunodeficiency (see Appendix 1), then any disease listed in **Section 1** indicates AIDS if diagnosed by a definitive method.

Section 1
1   Candidiasis of the oesophagus, trachea, bronchi, or lungs
2   Cryptococcosis, extrapulmonary
3   Cryptosporidiosis with diarrhoea persisting > 1 month
4   Cytomegalovirus disease including retinitis with loss of vision and of any organ other than liver, spleen or lymph nodes in a patient > 1 month of age
5   Herpes simplex virus infection causing a mucocutaneous ulcer that persists longer than 1 month; or bronchitis, pneumonitis, or oesophagitis for any duration affecting a patient > 1 month of age
6   Kaposi's sarcoma affecting a patient < 60 years of age
7   Lymphoma of the brain (primary) affecting a patient < 60 years of age
8   Lymphoid interstitial pneumonia and/or pulmonary lymphoid hyperplasia (LIP/PLH complex) affecting a child < 13 years of age
9   *Mycobacterium avium* complex or *M. kansasii* disease, disseminated (at a site other than or in addition to lungs, skin, or cervical or hilar lymph nodes)
10   *Pneumocystis carinii* pneumonia
11   Progressive multifocal leucoencephalopathy
12   Toxoplasmosis of the brain affecting a patient > 1 month of age

With laboratory evidence for HIV infection
Regardless of the presence of other causes of immunodeficiency, any disease listed above or below indicates a diagnosis of AIDS in the presence of laboratory evidence for HIV infection

Section 1
13   Bacterial infections, multiple or recurrent (any combination within a 2-year period) of the following types affecting a child < 13 years of age: septicaemia, pneumonia, meningitis, bone or joint infection, or abscess of any internal organ or body cavity (excluding otitis media or superficial skin or mucosal abscesses), caused by *Haemophilus, Streptococcus* (including *Pneumococcus*), or other pyogenic bacteria
14   Coccidioidomycosis, disseminated (at a site other than or in addition to lungs or cervical or hilar lymph nodes)
15   HIV encephalopathy (AIDS dementia complex)
16   Isosporiasis with diarrhoea persisting > 1 month
17   Kaposi's sarcoma at any age
18   Lymphoma of the brain (primary) at any age
19   Other non-Hodgkin's lymphoma of B cell or unknown immunologic phenotype (see Appendix 1)

Table 6.3 *continued*

20 *Salmonella* (non-typhoid) septicaemia, recurrent
21 HIV wasting syndrome (emaciation, 'slim disease')
22 Any disseminated mycobacteria disease caused by mycobacteria other than *M. tuberculosis*
23 Tuberculosis; extrapulmonary disease caused by *M. tuberculosis*
24 Pulmonary tuberculosis*
25 Recurrent pneumonia (2 or more episodes within 1 year)*
26 Invasive cervical cancer*

*Diagnostic criteria as of January 1993[2].

Subgroup C   This is defined as the diagnosis of an infectious disease associated with HIV infection and/or at least moderately indicative of a defect in cell-mediated immunity. Patients in this subgroup are divided further into two categories:

> **Category C-1** includes patients with symptomatic or invasive disease due to one of the specified secondary infectious diseases listed in the surveillance definition of AIDS (Appendix 1), i.e. **Phase D**.

> **Category C-2** includes patients with symptomatic or invasive disease due to one of six specified secondary infectious diseases: oral hairy leucoplakia, multidermatomal herpes zoster, recurrent *Salmonella* bacteraemia, nocardiosis, tuberculosis, or oral candidiasis, i.e. can be either **Phase C** or **Phase D**.

Subgroup D   This is defined as the diagnosis of one or more kinds of cancer known to be associated with HIV infection, as listed in the surveillance definition of AIDS (Appendix 1), i.e. **Phase D**.

Subgroup E   This is defined as the presence of other clinical findings or diseases, not classifiable above, that may be attributed to HIV infection and/or may be indicative of a defect in cell-mediated immunity. Included are patients with adult, chronic lymphoid interstitial pneumonitis. Also included are those patients whose signs or symptoms could be attributed either to HIV infection or to another coexisting disease not classified elsewhere, and patients with other clinical illnesses, the course or management of which may be complicated or altered by HIV infection. Examples include patients with constitutional symptoms not meeting the criteria for subgroup IV-A; patients with infectious diseases not listed in subgroup IV-C; and patients with neoplasms not listed in subgroup D.

This classification system is meant to provide a means of grouping patients infected with HIV according to the clinical expression of disease. It defines a limited number of specified clinical presentations.

CDC 1993 Revised HIV Classification System for HIV Infection and Expanded Surveillance Case Definition for AIDS Among Adolescents and Adults

Background

The aetiologic agent of acquired immunodeficiency syndrome (AIDS) is a retrovirus designated human immunodeficiency virus (HIV). The CD4+ T lymphocyte is the primary target for HIV infection because of the affinity of the virus for the CD4 surface marker. The CD4+ T lymphocyte coordinates a number of important immunologic functions, and a loss of these functions results in progressive impairment of the immune responses. Studies of the natural history of HIV infection have documented a wide spectrum of disease manifestations, ranging from asymptomatic infection to life-threatening conditions characterized by severe immunodeficiency, serious opportunistic infections, and cancers. Other studies have shown a strong association between the development of life-threatening opportunistic illnesses and the absolute number (per microlitre of blood) or percentage of CD4+ T lymphocytes. As the number of CD4+ T lymphocytes decreases, the risk and severity of opportunistic illnesses increase.

The classification system for HIV infection among adolescents and adults has been revised to include the CD4+ T lymphocyte count as a marker for HIV-related immunosuppression. This revision establishes mutually exclusive subgroups for which the spectrum of clinical conditions is integrated with the CD4+ T lymphocytes count. The objectives of these changes are to simplify the classification of HIV infection, and to reflect more accurately HIV-related morbidity.

The revised CDC classification system for HIV-infected adolescents and adults categorizes persons on the basis of clinical conditions associated with HIV infection and CD4+ T lymphocyte counts. The system is based on three ranges of CD4+ T lymphocyte counts and three clinical categories and is represented by a matrix of nine mutually exclusive categories (Table 6.4). This system replaces the classification system published in 1986, which included only clinical disease criteria and which was developed before the widespread use of CD4+ T-cell testing.

Table 6.4 1993 revised classification system for HIV infection and expanded AIDS surveillance case definition for adolescents and adults (bold type, i.e. **A3**, **B3**, and **C1-3** indicates an AIDS diagnosis)

CD4+ T-cell categories	Clinical categories		
	(A) Asymptomatic, acute (primary) HIV or PGL	(B) Symptomatic, not (A) or (C) conditions	(C) AIDS-indicator conditions
(1) > 500/µl	A1	B1	**C1**
(2) 200–499/µl	A2	B2	**C2**
(3) < 200/µl AIDS-indicator T-cell count	**A3**	**B3**	**C3**

CD4+ T lymphocyte categories

The three CD4+ T-lymphocyte categories are defined as follows:

Category 1: > 500 cells/µl
Category 2: 200–499 cells/µl
Category 3: < 200 cells/µl

Clinical categories

The three clinical categories are defined as follows:

Category A This consists of one or more of the conditions listed below in an adolescent (13 years of age or over) or adult with documented HIV infection. Conditions listed in Categories B and C must not have occurred.

- Asymptomatic HIV infection
- Persistent generalized lymphadenopathy (PGL)
- Acute (primary) HIV infection with accompanying illness or history of acute HIV infection.

Category B This consists of symptomatic conditions in an HIV-infected adolescent or adult that are not included among conditions listed in clinical Category C and that meet at least one of the following criteria:

- The conditions are attributed to HIV infection or are indicative of a defect in cell-mediated immunity.
- The conditions are considered by physicians to have a clinical course or to require management that is complicated by HIV infection.

Examples of conditions in clinical Category B include but are not limited to:

- Bacillary angiomatosis
- Candidiasis, oropharyngeal (thrush)
- Candidiasis, vulvovaginal; persistent, frequent, or poorly responsive to therapy
- Cervical dysplasia (moderate or severe)/cervical carcinoma *in situ*
- Constitutional symptoms, such as fever (38.5 C) or diarrhoea lasting > 1 month
- Hairy leukoplakia, oral
- Herpes zoster (shingles), involving at least two distinct episodes or more than one dermatome
- Idiopathic thrombocytopenic purpura
- Listeriosis
- Pelvic inflammatory disease, particularly if complicated by tubo-ovarian abscess
- Peripheral neuropathy.

Note: For classification purposes, Category B conditions take precedence over those in Category A. For example, someone previously treated for oral or persistent vaginal candidiasis (and who has not developed a Category C disease) but who is now asymptomatic, should be classified in clinical Category B.

Category C   This includes the twenty-three clinical conditions listed in the 1987 CDC AIDS Surveillance Case Definition (Table 6.3 and Appendix 1) plus the following:

- pulmonary tuberculosis (TB)
- recurrent pneumonia
- invasive cervical cancer.

Note: For classification purposes, once a Category C condition has occurred, the person will remain in Category C.

The above three conditions were added to the previous 1987 surveillance case definition for the following reasons:

Pulmonary tuberculosis (TB)

Throughout the world, pulmonary TB is the most common type of TB in persons with HIV infection. The addition of pulmonary TB to the list of AIDS-indicator diseases is based on the strong epidemiological link between HIV infection and the development of TB. Longer courses of anti-TB chemotherapy and prophylaxis are recommended for HIV-infected patients.

Recurrent pneumonia

With the exception of conditions included in the 1987 AIDS Surveillance Case Definition, pneumonia, with or without a bacteriologic diagnosis, is the leading cause of HIV-related morbidity and death. Persons with HIV-related immunosuppression are at an increased risk of bacterial pneumonia. Recurrent episodes of pneumonia (two or more episodes within a 1 year period) are required for AIDS case reporting because pneumonia is a relatively common diagnosis and multiple episodes of pneumonia are more strongly associated with immunosuppression than are single episodes.

Invasive cervical cancer

Invasive cervical cancer is a more appropriate AIDS-indicator disease than is either cervical dysplasia or carcinoma *in situ* because these latter cervical lesions are common and frequently do not progress to invasive disease. Invasive cervical cancer is preventable by the proper recognition and treatment of cervical dysplasia. The addition of invasive cervical cancer to the list of AIDS-indicator diseases emphasizes the importance of integrating gynaecologic care into medical services for HIV-infected women.

Conclusion

The revised CDC HIV Classification System provides uniform and simple criteria for categorizing conditions among adolescents and adults with HIV infection and should facilitate efforts to evaluate current and future health care and referral needs for persons with HIV infection. The addition of a measure of severe immunosuppression, as defined by a CD4+ T-lymphocyte count of < 200 cells/μl or a CD4+ percentage of < 14, reflects the standard of immunologic monitoring for HIV-infected persons and will enable AIDS surveillance data to more accurately represent those who are recognized as being immunosuppressed, who are in greatest need of close medical follow-up, and who are at greatest risk for the full spectrum of severe HIV-related morbidity. The addition of three clinical conditions (pulmonary TB, recurrent pneumonia and invasive cervical cancer) to the AIDS surveillance criteria reflect the documented or potential importance of these diseases in the HIV pandemic. Two of these conditions (pulmonary TB and cervical cancer) are preventable if appropriate screening tests are linked with proper follow-up.

Although the 1993 revised classification system and expanded surveillance case definition for AIDS is being used in the USA, a European working group has decided not to adopt it in Europe[23]. The rationale for this decision includes: CD4+ T-lymphocyte typing is not sufficiently standardized or widely available in Europe; the negative impact an AIDS diagnosis, based solely on CD4+ counts might have on some HIV-1 infected persons; biases that would be introduced to epidemiological surveillance based solely on CD4+ counts; and finally, unlike the USA, access to medical care and social benefits within Europe do not depend upon a person meeting the case definition for AIDS. However, the three new indicator diseases, i.e. recurrent pneumonia, pulmonary tuberculosis and invasive cervical carcinoma, are being included in the list of the twenty-six AIDS-defining illnesses (Table 6.3). In addition, developed countries are using CD4+ cell counts for classification of HIV infection but not for defining AIDS[24].

WHO Clinical Staging System for HIV Infection and Disease

In 1990, the World Health Organization drafted a staging system for HIV infection and disease. This is reproduced in Appendix 2.

ICL syndrome – AIDS without HIV infection

In recent years, several reports have been published of persons who had an unexplained, severe immunosuppression, associated with a low CD4+ T-lymphocyte count, without evidence of HIV-1 or HIV-2 infection[25,26]. These persons differ from patients with AIDS in several ways: they are usually older, they do not have a progressive decline in CD4+ T lymphocytes and most lack risk factors usually associated with HIV infection. This condition has been defined by the Centers for Disease Control[27] and is referred to as **idiopathic CD4+ T**

lymphocytopenia (or **ICL syndrome**). 'Idiopathic' refers to any disease in which the cause is unknown. The clinical case definition for ICL syndrome includes:

- a depressed number of circulating CD4+ T lymphocytes (< 300 cells/mm³ or < 20 per cent of total T cells) on more than one occasion;
- no laboratory evidence of HIV-1 or HIV-2 infection;
- the absence of any defined immunodeficiency or therapy associated with depressed levels of CD4+ T cells[27].

In addition, there is no evidence in these patients that a transmissible agent is involved[28,29] or that this rare condition is epidemic[30]. None of the sexual partners of patients with ICL show any evidence of immunosuppression and cases of ICL are not increasing. It has probably always existed and its cause is presumably heterogeneous, i.e. there are many different causes. The existence of this rare condition cannot logically be associated with a hypothesis that HIV is not the cause of AIDS.

Summary

Fully expressed AIDS is an acquired immunodeficiency state in which individuals develop one or more opportunistic infections, usually due to latent, potential pathogens which are ubiquitous in nature and which, were it not for the underlying immune deficiency, would not be dangerous. The most common opportunistic infection seen is pneumonia, caused by the fungi, *Pneumocystis carinii*. The depressed immune state also involves a breakdown in the normal tumour surveillance carried out by activated natural killer cells and opportunistic cancers may be seen, chiefly Kaposi's sarcoma.

Treatment for either opportunistic infectious diseases or cancers is not curative as the principal defect is in the immune system and, until a way can be found to restore the competence of this system, AIDS will continue to be a fatal disease.

References

1. Centers for Disease Control and Prevention (1987). Revision of the CDC Surveillance Case Definition for Acquired Immunodeficiency Syndrome. *Morbidity and Mortality Weekly Report (MMWR)*, 14 August, **36**, 1S.
2. Centers for Disease Control and Prevention (1992). 1993 Revised Classification System for HIV Infection and Expanded Surveillance Case Definition for AIDS Among Adolescents and Adults. *Morbidity and*

Mortality Weekly Report (MMWR), 18 December, **RR-17**, 1–19.
3. Tindall, B. and Cooper, D.A. (1991). Editorial review: Primary HIV infection: host responses and intervention strategies. *AIDS*, 1 January, **5**, 1–14.
4. Mildvan, D. and Solomon, S.L. (1987). The spectrum of disease due to human immunodeficiency virus infection. In *Current Topics in AIDS*, Vol. 1, eds Gottlieb, M., Jeffries, D., Mildvan, D. *et al.*, John Wiley & Sons, Chichester, p. 35.
5. Weber, J. and Pinching, A. (1986). The clinical management of AIDS and HTLV-III Infection. In *The Management of AIDS Patients*, eds Miller, D., Weber, J. and Green, J., Macmillan, London, p. 11.
6. Volberding, Paul A. (1992). Clinical spectrum of HIV disease. In *AIDS: Etiology, Diagnosis, Treatment and Prevention*, 3rd edn. J.B. Lippincott, Philadelphia, p. 128.
7. Greenspan, J.S., Greenspan, D. and Winkler, J.R. (1992). Oral complications of HIV infection. In *The Medical Management of AIDS*, 3rd edn, eds Sande, M.A. and Volberding, Paul A., W.B. Saunders, Philadelphia, p. 161.
8. Greenspan, J.S. and Greenspan, D. (1994). Oral manifestations of HIV infection and AIDS. In *Textbook of AIDS Medicine*, eds Broder, S., Merigan, T.C. Jr. and Bolognesi, D., Williams & Wilkins, Baltimore, MD, p. 532.
9. Walzer, Peter D. (1993). Editorial review: *Pneumocystis carinii*: recent advances in basic biology and their clinical application. *AIDS* **7**(10), 1293–305.
10. Edman, J.C., Kovacs, J.A., Masur, H. *et al.* (1988). Ribosomal RNA sequence shows *Pneumocystis carinii* to be a member of the fungi. *Nature* **334**(5), 19.
11. Walzer, Peter D. (1991). *Pneumocystis carinii* – a new clinical spectrum? *New England Journal of Medicine* **324**, 263–5.
12. Opravil, M., Marincek, B., Fuchs, W.A. *et al.* (1994). Shortcomings of chest radiography in detecting *Pneumocystis carinii* pneumonia. *Journal of Acquired Immune Deficiency Syndromes* **7**(1), 39–45.
13. Ayliffe, G.A.J., Coates, D. and Hoffman, P.N. (1993). *Chemical Disinfection in Hospitals*, 2nd edn. Public Health Laboratory Service (PHLS), London.
14. Leigh, T.R., Parsons, P., Hume, C. *et al.* (1989). Sputum induction for diagnosis of *Pneumocystis carinii* pneumonia. *Lancet* 22 July, **ii**(8656), 205–6.
15. Nelson, M., Bower, M., Smith, D. and Gazzard, B.G. (1990). Life-threatening complication of sputum induction (correspondence). *Lancet,* 13 January, **335**, 112–13.
16. Wharton, J.M., Coleman, D.L., Wofsy, C.B. *et al.* (1985). Trimethoprim-sulfamethoxazole or pentamidine for *Pneumocystis carinii* pneumonia in the acquired immunodeficiency syndrome. *Annals of Internal Medicine* **105**, 37.
17. Smith, C.L. (1990). Nursing management of aerosolised pentamidine administration. *AIDS Patient Care*, February, **4**(1), 13–17.

18. Green, S.T., Nathwani, D., Christie, P.R. *et al.* (1990). Domiciliary nebulized pentamidine for secondary prophylaxis against *Pneumocystis carinii* pneumonia. *Journal of the Royal Society of Medicine* **83**(1), 18–19.
19. Montgomery, A.B., Luce, J.M., Turner, J. *et al.* (1987). Aerosolised pentamidine as sole therapy for *Pneumocystis carinii* pneumonia in patients with acquired immunodeficiency syndrome. *Lancet*, 29 August, **ii**(8557), 480–2.
20. Hopewell, P.C. (1990). Prevention of lung infections associated with HIV infection. In *Aids and the Lung*, eds Mitchell, D. and Woodcock, A., British Medical Journal, London, pp. 66–77.
21. Ungar, Beth L.P. (1994). *Cryptosporidium* and cryptosporidiosis. In *Textbook of AIDS Medicine*, eds Broder, S., Merigan, T.C. Jr. and Bolognesi, D., Williams & Wilkins, Baltimore, p. 335.
22. Centers for Disease Control (1986). Classification system for human T-lymphotropic virus type III/lymphadenopathy-associated virus infection. *Morbidity and Mortality Weekly Report (MMWR)*, 23 May, **35**(20), 334–9.
23. Ancelle Park, R.A. (1992). European AIDS definition. *Lancet*, 14 March, **339**, 671.
24. Anon. (1992). Changing case-definition for AIDS. *Lancet*, 14 November, **340**, 1199–201.
25. Centers for Disease Control (1992). Unexplained CD4+ T-lymphocyte depletion in persons without evident HIV infection – United States. *Morbidity and Mortality Weekly Report (MMWR)*, **41**, 541–5.
26. Smith, D.K., Neal, J.J. and Holmberg, S.D., Centers for Disease Control Idiopathic CD4+ T-Lymphocytopenia Task Force (1993). Unexplained opportunistic infections and CD4+ T-lymphocytopenia without HIV infection. An investigation of cases in the United States. *New England Journal of Medicine*, **328** 373–9.
27. Centers for Disease Control (1992). Update: CD4+ T-lymphocytopenia in persons without evident HIV infection – United States, *Morbidity and Mortality Weekly Report (MMWR)*, **41**, 578–9.
28. Ho, D.D., Cao, Y.Z., Zhu, T.F. *et al.* (1993). Idiopathic CD4+ T-lymphocytopenia – immunodeficiency without evidence of HIV infection. *New England Journal of Medicine* **328**(6), 380–5.
29. Heredia, A., Muller, J., Soriano, V. *et al.* (1994). Absence of evidence of retroviral infection in idiopathic CD4+ T-lymphocytopenia syndrome. *AIDS* **8**(2), 267–81.
30. World Health Organization (1992). Unexplained severe immunosuppression without evidence of HIV Infection. *Weekly Epidemiological Record* **67**, 309–11.

Further reading

Broder, S., Merigan, T.C. Jr., and Bolognesi, D. (1994). *Textbook of AIDS Medicine*. Williams & Wilkins, Baltimore, MD (ISBN 0–683–01072–7).

DeVita, V.T. Jr., Hellman, S. and Rosenberg, S.A. (1992). *AIDS: Etiology, Diagnosis, Treatment and Prevention*, 3rd edn. J.B. Lippincott, Philadelphia (ISBN 0–397–51229–5).

Muma, R.D., Lyons, B.A., Borucki, M.J. and Pollard, R.B. (1994). *HIV: Manual For Health Care Professionals*. Appleton & Lange, Norwalk, CT (ISBN 0–8385–0170–2).

Sande, M.A. and Volberding, P.A. (1992). *The Medical Management of AIDS*, 3rd edn. W.B. Saunders, Philadelphia (ISBN 0–7216–6752–X).

Wormser, G.P. (1992). *AIDS and Other Manifestations of HIV Infection*, 2nd edn. Raven Press, New York (ISBN 88167–881–3).

7

A Dangerous Liaison – Tuberculosis and HIV Disease

Tuberculosis is much more than a medical affliction caused by a specific bacterium. It is by turns a strange, a terrible and a fascinating entity, like the multi-layered mystery of the famous Russian doll. No sooner do we think we understand it, than a new form, as baffling and menacing as ever, appears to confound us.

Tuberculosis: The Greatest Story Never Told, Frank Ryan

Introduction

Tuberculosis has been a misery of mankind since the Stone Age[1] and accounts of the disease appeared in the earliest surviving literature. Various manifestations of tuberculosis have been recorded throughout the ages, including spinal tuberculosis, scrofula (enlarged, sometimes discharging, tuberculous lymph glands in the neck), and consumption, i.e. pulmonary tuberculosis. From the middle of the seventeenth to the end of the nineteenth century, pulmonary tuberculosis gained in epidemic force, becoming known as 'the white plague', sweeping through major cities in both Europe and North America (especially London and New York City), infecting half the world's population and killing 7 million people a year. During the twentieth century, a dramatic decline in cases was witnessed in North America and Europe, due to improved living conditions in the earlier part of the century and advances in medical treatment from the 1950s onwards.

Historical Background

The causative agent of tuberculosis, *Mycobacterium tuberculosis*, was identified by the German microbiologist, Robert Koch in 1882 and, in

1890, Koch unsuccessfully used an injection of killed tubercle bacilli ('old tuberculin') in an attempt to develop a therapeutic agent for tuberculosis. By 1907, however, the Austrian physician, Clemens von Pirquet, using old tuberculin, developed a skin test to diagnose infection by *M. tuberculosis*. Prior to Koch's discovery, the natural history of tuberculosis had been described in the early nineteenth century by the French physicians Gaspard Laurent Bayle and René Laënnec (both of whom died from the disease). A vaccine to prevent disease was developed and first used by the French bacteriologists Albert Léon Calmette and Camille Guérin (the BCG vaccine) in 1921 and, by 1944, streptomycin, the first drug which was truly effective in tuberculosis, was discovered by the Russian microbiologist Selman Abraham Waksman, working in America. This was quickly followed by the discovery of other drugs which, along with streptomycin, would prove to be almost miraculous in the treatment of tuberculosis, for example, PAS (para-aminosalicylic acid) and isoniazid. Since then, an impressive repertoire of drugs has been developed to treat tuberculosis, e.g. rifampicin, ethambutol and pyrazinamide.

Epidemiology

The World Health Organization estimates that one-third of the world's population, i.e. > 1.72 billion persons, are currently infected with *Mycobacterium tuberculosis* and, from this pool of infected persons, 8 million new cases of active tuberculosis (and 2.9 million deaths) are seen each year[2]. Although most (> 75 per cent) of these persons live in the developing world, tuberculosis, going hand in hand with poverty and HIV infection, is re-emerging in industrialized nations as a significant threat to public health. On a global scale, tuberculosis accounts for more preventable ill health and death than any other single pathogen in existence today. In addition, it is estimated that, worldwide, by early 1992, at least 4.6 million people were co-infected with HIV and *M. tuberculosis* (Fig. 7.1)[3].

The World Health Organization estimates that there will be more than 90 million new cases of TB in the 1990s and that 30 million people will die from TB, with a doubling of the mortality rates in Africa. The worst affected area is South and South-East Asia, where some 12 million deaths (Fig. 7.2) are expected, with a further 7 million deaths in East Asia and the Pacific. This increase is principally due to poor-quality control programmes, exacerbated by demographic factors (accounting for 75 per cent of the predicted increase),

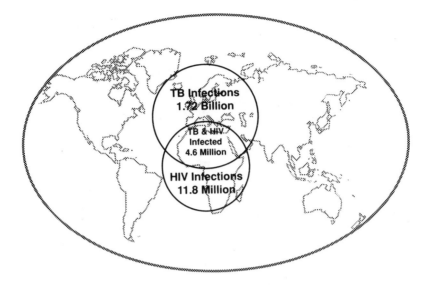

Fig. 7.1 Dual pandemics: tuberculosis and HIV infection (world population 5.6 billion)

but the escalation of HIV infection will account for 25 per cent of the projected increase[4].

In the USA, the incidence of individuals with tuberculosis continued to decline over the past several decades, from > 84 000 cases in 1953 to a nadir of approximately 22 000 cases in 1984[5]. Since that time, however, a resurgence has been seen in the USA, especially in the age range 25–40 years, principally due to the prevalence of HIV infection in this group, and homelessness[6]. Currently, it is suggested that approximately 10–15 million people in the USA are infected with *M. tuberculosis*[7].

In the UK, cases also continued to fall until the end of the late 1980s, when a slow, but steady increase in cases was observed. However, unlike the USA, there is no evidence as yet to suggest that HIV infection is responsible for this upsurge. The increase in notifications of tuberculosis in the UK is mainly due to tuberculosis in people who have recently immigrated, or whose families immigrated, into the UK from the Indian subcontinent (India, Pakistan, Bangladesh), where the prevalence and incidence of tuberculosis is high[8]. However, other groups in the UK who are at an increased risk for tuberculosis include the elderly, the homeless and any persons who are

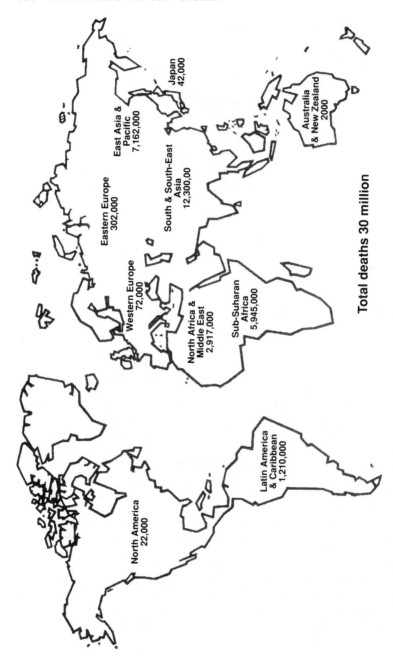

Fig. 7.2   Estimated cumulative tuberculosis deaths, 1990–99

immunocompromised, including those who are infected with HIV[9].

Aetiology

Tuberculosis is caused by some members of a group of bacteria known as 'mycobacteria'. These small (less than 0.5 μm in diameter) non-sporing, Gram-positive, aerophilic bacilli are slender, curved (often beaded) rods, enveloped by acid-fast surface lipids, and reproduce slowly by binary fission. As an aerobic intracellular microbe, it requires high oxygen tension environments to flourish, e.g. the lungs and kidneys. Tuberculosis refers only to disease caused by either *M. tuberculosis* (the most common), *M. bovis* or *M. africaneum*. Other environmental mycobacteria, e.g. *M. avium* and *M. intracellulare*, can cause human disease which often mimics tuberculosis, but these are not usually communicable and do not generally respond well to drugs which are effective against tuberculosis. In addition, another important mycobacterium (*M. leprae*) is the causative agent of leprosy (Hansen's disease) which causes disease worldwide in > 12 million people.

Transmission

M. tuberculosis is usually transmitted from one person to another by the respiratory route, i.e. by inhalation of tubercle bacilli released from an infected person as droplet nuclei during coughing, sneezing and talking. Once expelled, the bacilli can float in room air for several hours, remaining a potential threat to uninfected susceptible individuals who can become infected by breathing in these droplet nuclei. Fomites are not implicated in transmitting the tubercle bacilli. *M. bovis* is usually transmitted via contaminated milk from infected cows, causing lesions in the tonsils, lymph nodes, gastro-intestinal tract, bones and joints. As bovine tuberculosis has been brought under control, it is currently no longer a significant cause of mycobacterial disease in humans in most parts of the developed world. However, outbreaks of tuberculosis due to *M. bovis* in persons infected with HIV have been reported, including multi-drug resistant pulmonary tuberculosis and human-to-human transmission[10,11]. In some parts of the developing world, e.g. sub-Saharan Africa, where both infections are common, *M. bovis* may re-emerge as an important cause of tuberculosis in persons co-infected with HIV[12].

Definition

Not all those infected with *M. tuberculosis* develop clinically apparent disease. Thus a person may have active tuberculosis or may be healthy, yet carry the bacillus in his/her tissues. Consequently, it is useful to think of tuberculosis as having two components: **infection** and **disease**.

Infection During the initial phase of infection, a silent bacillemia (i.e. bacilli in the blood) commonly develops and other organs can be infected from the primary lesion in the lungs, i.e. extrapulmonary tuberculosis. In individuals with an intact, competent immune system, infection is usually well contained and is not contagious.

Disease In the Western world, active tuberculosis develops in approximately 10 per cent of infected persons following primary infection. Clinical disease, affecting the lungs and/or other sites (extrapulmonary tuberculosis) in adults is almost always the result of recrudescence, i.e. re-activation of earlier infection. Pulmonary tuberculosis is contagious.

Pathogenesis of tuberculosis

There are four 'possible' stages of the tuberculous process:

1. Primary or initial infection (not contagious)
2. Primary disease (not usually contagious)
3. Latent or dormant infection (not contagious)
4. Recrudescent or post-primary disease (may be contagious).

Primary tuberculosis infection

The inhalation of tubercle bacilli into the lungs of a non-infected, susceptible individual causes the development of an acute, local inflammatory lesion (known as the **Ghon focus**), usually in the lower or middle lung field. As bacilli begin to multiply at this site, some are ingested by macrophages and transported to the regional lymph nodes in the hilum or root of the lungs, causing these lymph nodes to enlarge. The Ghon focus and the enlarged hilar lymph nodes are together referred to as the **primary complex**. This inflammatory reaction attracts immunologically competent T lymphocytes (CD4+ helper cells) to the site of primary infection, where they secrete a variety of cytokines, e.g. interleukins and chemotactic factors. In response, monocytes are drawn into this area and are transformed by these cytokines, released from CD4+ helper cells, into activated macrophages and then into so-called **epithelioid cells**, which form a palisade, many cells thick, around the bacilli. This compact aggregate of epithelioid cells is termed the **granuloma** and is characteristic of many chronic infections. Granuloma formation is a generally successful attempt by the body to wall off and isolate a site of persistent infection. This promotes healing and the granulomas often become calcified (which may be seen in chest X-rays).

Unfortunately, not all tubercle bacilli within the granuloma are destroyed. Some, known as **persisters**, can survive for many years or decades, seeding recrudescence later in life[13]. However, in most people, cell-mediated immune responses are both efficient and effective in containing the infection at this stage and 90–95 per cent of primary infections go unrecognized, causing no symptoms or health problems and do not progress to active disease. The infection becomes dormant or latent, primary lesions heal and calcify and the tuberculin skin test becomes positive.

In primary infection, some bacilli may escape from the lungs via the lymphatic or bloodstream and, in a few individuals, this dissemination causes serious ill health (**primary extrapulmonary tuberculosis**) and significant mortality in infants and young children (and in immunocompromised adults), e.g. meningitis, renal tuberculosis and bone and joint involvement. The apices of the lungs may also be the site of disseminated infection, the tubercle bacilli leaving nodular scars (**Simon's foci**) which may serve as a breeding ground for later, active disease.

Active tuberculosis

Disease will develop in 5–10 per cent of individuals who, for a variety of reasons, do not successfully contain their infection in the primary stage. Although disease may develop within weeks or months following primary infection (primary tuberculosis), more commonly tubercle bacilli remain dormant for years and then begin multiplying, eventually causing **post-primary tuberculosis**. Approximately half of those individuals who develop disease will do so within 2 years of primary infection, the remaining half developing post-primary disease at any time from just over 2 years to many years later[14]. Precipitating factors leading to active disease following primary infection include the onset of diabetes mellitus, corticosteroid therapy, poor nutrition, intercurrent diseases, stress and HIV infection. Infected infants will often rapidly develop active tuberculosis, including disseminated disease, e.g. meningitis. Children over the age of 1 or 2 years who are infected will usually contain their infection, with the majority of those who are predestined to develop tuberculosis doing so in adolescence or young adulthood. Adults are at most risk of developing active disease within 3 years of primary infection[15]. HIV-infected individuals, who have not been infected with *M. tuberculosis* in the past, commonly develop primary tuberculosis within a few months of exposure to a source patient[16]. In Europe and North America, tuberculosis is more common in young adult females and, in later life, is seen more frequently in men; it is also seen in the elderly, in both sexes and in all races.

Immunopathology

Immunity in tuberculosis may be protective, leading to resolution of lesions, or tissue-damaging, leading, for example, to pulmonary cavitation and progression of disease. There is some evidence that protective immune reactions are mediated by Th1 CD4+ T lymphocytes and immunopathology by Th2 CD4+ T lymphocytes, or mixed Th1/Th2 T-cell activity[16,17].

In addition, in active disease, tumour necrosis factor (TNF) is released from activated macrophages and this cytokine is responsible for the extensive tissue necrosis in the upper lungs seen in post-primary pulmonary tuberculosis and the debilitating, wasting or cachexia ('consumption') seen in chronic, advanced disease. As TNF stimulates HIV replication, the large amounts produced in tuberculosis (and in other chronic mycobacterial infections, e.g. *M. avium-intracellulare*) may hasten the advent of AIDS by many years in otherwise asymptomatically HIV-infected persons[14]. As the immunopathology of tuberculosis, i.e. a dominance of Th2 activity, is similar to that seen in HIV disease (as discussed previously in Chapter 5), researchers are currently exploring therapeutic interventions that would facilitate a 'Th2 to Th1 shift'[17–19].

Pulmonary tuberculosis

In the early stages of pulmonary tuberculosis, although the individual may be feeling vaguely unwell and tired (fatigue), specific health problems may be ill-defined. Loss of appetite (anorexia) and progressive weight loss are eventually experienced, as are respiratory signs and symptoms. Chronic cough, a universal symptom in pulmonary tuberculosis, gradually becomes more productive of yellow or green mucus, especially in the morning upon awakening. Haemoptysis (blood in the sputum) is frequent, especially in advanced disease, and chest pain and dyspnoea can occur at any stage as a result of a pleural effusion or rupture of a lung (spontaneous pneumothorax). A tuberculous cavity may rupture into the pleural space, causing a tuberculous empyema and bronchopleural fistula. This event is extremely serious and requires urgent medical intervention, including pleural drainage. A low-grade fever is common, as are drenching night sweats, especially over the top part of the body.

As the disease progresses, wasting becomes more severe and the patient becomes seriously ill. Without effective treatment, up to one-third of non-HIV infected individuals with chronic illness will survive for many years, their lives alternating with periods of stability and relative well-being and exacerbations of active disease, involving more and more of the lung tissue. However, up to 60 per cent of untreated (or ineffectively treated) cases are fatal, the median survival period following onset of disease being approximately 2 and a half years[15].

HIV disease and tuberculosis

Co-infection with *M. tuberculosis* and HIV compounds the progressive loss of effective cell-mediated responses to both infections because of the dominance of Th2 cytokine activity and the progressive depletion of CD4+ T lymphocytes. Consequently, the clinical course of both infections is rapidly accelerated.

Individuals infected with HIV who are exposed to infection by tubercle bacilli are at significantly greater risk of progressing to active disease than are persons who are not infected with HIV. In addition, they are more likely to have a rapid, more severely progressive form of tuberculosis than non-HIV infected persons[5].

Tuberculosis is often the initial manifestation of HIV disease, often seen within the first 6 months following HIV infection, and may be the result of either earlier infection by the tubercle bacilli, i.e. post-primary disease, or recent exposure, i.e. primary disease[14]. In addition, extrapulmonary tuberculosis is much more common in individuals who are infected with HIV as the associated immunodeficiency facilitates bloodborne spread of tubercle bacilli (bacillemia) from the primary site of infection in the lungs[16].

A prominent aspect of pulmonary tuberculosis is that it is one of the few (and, by far, the most important) respiratory diseases seen in HIV-infected individuals which, unlike most opportunistic infections, can be transmitted to other susceptible individuals, including those who are not infected with HIV.

Extrapulmonary tuberculosis

The areas most commonly affected by this form of tuberculosis in persons co-infected with HIV are the lymphatic system, the gastro-intestinal and urogenital tracts and the bone marrow. Most patients with extrapulmonary lesions also have pulmonary disease[20].

Cytokine production in HIV-infected persons with tuberculosis

Tuberculosis, with its associated production of high levels of tumour necrosis factor (TNF), and other cytokines, will enhance transactivation and replication of HIV, further damaging immune function and significantly hastening the onset of end-stage HIV disease, i.e. AIDS[14,21,22].

Diagnosis of tuberculosis in persons infected with HIV

Tuberculosis is often seen before an individual is known to be infected with HIV and, consequently, appropriate counselling and serological testing for HIV infection should be considered for all patients with newly diagnosed TB[23] if their history suggests they may have been exposed to HIV. The early diagnosis of tuberculosis is essential in reducing the risk of transmission to others, including nosocomial transmission.

Investigations ordered by the physician to confirm a diagnosis of tuberculosis may include the following:

- Chest X-rays
- Tuberculin skin test
- Microscopy and culture of
    sputum
    urine
    blood
    cerebrospinal fluid
    faeces
    other body fluids
- Bronchoscopy
- Gastric washings.

Chest X-rays

Tuberculosis is often difficult to differentiate in chest X-rays from other pulmonary infections commonly seen in individuals with HIV disease. In tuberculosis, shadows in the upper zones of the lungs are common and lesions (infiltrates) above or behind the clavicle are frequently suggestive of a recrudescence in post-primary disease, especially in the older person. In younger adults, lesions may be identified anywhere in the lungs and pleural effusions (often unilateral) are commonly seen. As tuberculosis progresses, the centre of the lesions in the lungs become necrotic and resemble soft cheese (hence the term 'caseation'). If these lesions erode into a bronchus, the soft caseous material is discharged, resulting in a cavity which is usually clearly seen in a chest X-ray. Cavitation may be extensive and a source of haemoptysis and continuing disease. Serial chest films are usually needed to monitor both disease progression and response to treatment.

Individuals who are immunosuppressed as a result of HIV disease may have a fairly normal chest X-ray as their inflammatory reaction is reduced and there is, consequently, less cavitation of pulmonary lesions[24].

Tuberculin skin testing

Although not definitive, the tuberculin skin testing is helpful in identifying previous exposure to *M. tuberculosis*. The antigen used is known as **purified protein derivative** of tuberculin (**PPD**) and contains heat-treated products of the growth and lysis of tubercle bacillus.

PPD is measured in International Units, or IU, and comes in various strengths. Care must be taken to safeguard that the correct strength, as prescribed, is used. In addition, PPD must be stored in an appropriate refrigerator, between 2 and 10°C, ensuring that it is not frozen and that it is protected from light. It has a shelf-life of approximately 6 months if properly stored. Once an ampoule is opened, it must be used within 1 hour. As PPD can adsorb on to syringe surfaces, it should be drawn up in the syringe immediately prior to injecting, or used within 30 minutes after the syringe is filled.

Two types of PPD skin testing techniques are in common use: the **Mantoux test** (using diluted PPD) and a multiple puncture technique known as **Heaf test** (for which concentrated, i.e. undiluted PPD is used). Although the Heaf test is useful for mass screening, special infection control considerations apply to the disinfection of the puncture apparatus (known as the Heaf gun), which are discussed in other publications[25]. Newer Heaf guns use a disposable head apparatus which avoids both the need for disinfection and any risk of cross-infection.

Another multiple puncture technique in use, although not recommended for general use[25] in the UK, is the **tine test**. This is a 'use once and dispose' device with four metal tines (prongs) coated with dried tuberculin.

The Mantoux is the technique used in individual testing situations. For routine Mantoux testing, the PPD dilution strength used is 1 in 1000 (i.e. 100 IU/ml). In this strength, the unit dose in each 0.1 ml is 10 IU of PPD. The usual dose used in Mantoux testing in the UK is 10 units of PPD in 0.1 ml of solution. In the USA, 5 units of PPD in 0.1 ml of solution is more commonly used.

The Mantoux test is performed with a 1 ml syringe (tuberculin syringe) and a short bevel 25 or 26 gauge, 10 mm long intradermal needle. The solution is injected **intradermally** into the upper third of the flexor surface of the forearm . The nurse should document which arm is used for the injection so that there is no confusion 2–3 days later when the results are noted. This site may be cleaned, if necessary, with alcohol and allowed to dry prior to the injection. A correct intradermal injection will cause a small bleb (*peau d'orange*) or lump to be raised, typically of approximately 7 mm in diameter. If a bleb is not raised, the injection was not correctly given. The results (i.e. the diameter of the induration) will be read 48–72 hours later, but can be read up to 96 hours after the test[25].

A positive result, both in the UK and in the USA, consists of a transverse induration (i.e. a thickening of the skin, not the area of erythema) of ≥ 5 mm in diameter, as measured by a transparent ruler, in individuals known to be infected with HIV; anything less is considered a negative result[25]. In the USA, an induration of ≥ 10 mm indicates infection in non-HIV infected persons[24]. Some positive results may demonstrate an induration of up to 15 mm (or more) in diameter. The larger the size of the induration, the more positive is the result. A positive result will be found if the person tested has been exposed (i.e. infected) with *M. tuberculosis* and has relatively intact cell-mediated immunity. However, it is non-specific and may only indicate previous infection and not active tuberculosis. Infrequently, because of cross-reactivity between mycobacterial antigens, a positive reaction may be seen in individuals who have been exposed to other, non-tuberculosis mycobacteria in the environment. A strongly positive result in an adult, i.e. ≥ 15 mm, indicates that the person has active tuberculosis (or has received BCG vaccination in the past). Individuals who are infected with HIV may have lost significant cell-mediated immunity by the time they are tested and, although infected with *M. tuberculosis*, they often test negative, especially if their CD4+ T lymphocyte cell count is < 200 cells/μl. Control skin tests with at least two other antigens (e.g. candida, tetanus toxoid or mumps) may be used to establish whether or not the individual can mount a cell-mediated response to any antigen used for skin testing. Failure to react to any of the control skin test antigens indicates **anergy**, i.e. the immune system is too depressed to mount a reliable response to the skin test antigens. However, if the person reacts positively to the control antigens (indicating a functioning cell-mediated immune response) and is negative for the tuberculin skin test, it is unlikely that they are infected with *M. tuberculosis*.

Sputum microscopy and culture

The principal diagnostic procedure in pulmonary tuberculosis is smear and culture examinations of sputum (not saliva) specimens, collected daily on 3–5 (or more) consecutive days.

If the patient cannot produce a sputum specimen, following fasting (nothing by mouth), early morning aspiration of gastric contents can be collected, after the patient has coughed and swallowed for 10–15 minutes. Alternatively, fibre-optic bronchoscopy may be employed for broncho-alveolar lavage. If bronchoscopes are used, it is important that machines used for rinsing these instruments use sterile distilled water, not tap water which often contains environmental mycobacteria (e.g. *M. chelonei, M. avium, M. kansasii*) and which may contaminate the specimen.

Mycobacteria differ from other bacteria in that they are not decolorized by weak acids and/or alcohol after staining by certain dyes. Thus they are often termed **acid-fast bacilli (AFB)** or acid-alcohol-fast bacilli. To detect AFB, the most commonly used microscopic examination of sputum is the **Ziehl–Neelsen (ZN) technique**, which is based on the use of hot phenolic solution of fuchsin (carbol fuchsin). A positive sputum specimen means that the patient is 'smear positive' and is infectious to others. Not all persons with active tuberculosis will have positive smear results, especially if they are immunocompromised, and caution is needed in interpreting a negative smear.

Sputum is also cultured, i.e. the mycobacteria are grown and identified in culture. Unlike microscopy, where a result is immediate, a culture takes at least 2–3 weeks before the result is known. Radiometric culture techniques, e.g. BACTEC (Becton Dickinson) and biphasic culture systems, e.g. Septi-Chek (Roche) give sputum culture results much quicker and can also be used for rapid drug susceptibility testing. These techniques are also used to detect *M. avium-intracellulare* infection in blood.

Other body fluids

In patients who are infected with HIV, blood (and sometimes bone marrow) is frequently cultured for mycobacterial growth. Urine and faeces may also be collected for the detection of AFB. If urine specimens are requested, 50 ml of early morning urine (EMU) are collected on 3 consecutive days; 24-hour urine collections are no longer used for AFB detection[26]. Examination of faeces for AFB is often requested when HIV-infected patients are suspected of having disseminated disease due to non-tuberculosis mycobacteria, such as *M. avium*.

Other (non-tuberculosis) environmental mycobacteria

Other than the mycobacteria which cause tuberculosis in humans, and *M. leprae*, which causes leprosy, there are a variety of environmental, non-tuberculosis mycobacteria which can cause serious illness, especially in persons already immuncompromised as a result of HIV infection. They are sometimes referred to as 'atypical' mycobacteria. These bacteria are ubiquitous and widely distributed in nature, existing as saprophytes (i.e. living off dead or decaying plant or animal matter), principally in soil and water and also in the intestinal tract of animals and birds. They are not usually transmitted from person to person, although this may rarely occur in immunocompromised individuals. Generally, individuals become infected with these bacteria following source exposure to them in the environment (soil, dirt, swimming pools, drinking water, animals, aquaria, fish, etc.). The portal of entry following exposure is via the respiratory or, more commonly, the gastro-intestinal tract. Some mycobacteria which cause cutaneous diseases, such as *M. marinum*, *M. ulcerans* and (rarely) *M. kansasii*, are contracted through abraded skin, especially in swimming pools and exposure to aquaria.

These environmental mycobacteria are much less virulent than *M. tuberculosis* and exposure to them is common. Infection with non-tuberculosis mycobacteria does not usually cause any illness in individuals who have a competent, normally functioning immune system and who do not have any other serious predisposing illnesses, e.g.

Table 7.1 Important environmental (non-tuberculosis) mycobacteria in HIV disease

Mycobacteria		Notes
M. avium *M. intracellulare*	} 'MAC'	Accounts for about 90% of pulmonary disease, lymphadenopathy and disseminated disease
M. kansasii *M. xenopi* *M. malmoense* *M. fortuitum* *M. szulgai* *M. chelonae*		Causes similar localized or disseminated disease, but with much less frequency. Most clinical isolates are of doubtful clinical significance[32]

chronic lung disease, cancer, malnutrition, etc. However, in persons with HIV disease, infection with these bacteria can cause serious illness, including pulmonary conditions resembling tuberculosis and systemic, disseminated disease[27–29].

Important environmental mycobacteria commonly associated with patients with HIV disease are listed in Table 7.1. The most commonly involved environmental mycobacteria causing illness in patients with HIV disease are two closely related species, *M. avium* and *M. intracellulare*, often bundled together and referred to as either **MAI** (*M. avium-intracellulare*) complex, or, more commonly **MAC** (*M. avium* complex). For reasons that are not well-understood, most disease caused by environmental mycobacteria (about 90 per cent of cases), which may be localized or disseminated, in patients with coexisting HIV disease, is due to MAC. Occasionally, however, other environmental mycobacteria can cause disseminated disease in patients with HIV disease, as noted in Table 7.1.

Disseminated MAC disease is generally seen in patients with end-stage HIV disease who have a CD4+ T lymphocyte count < 100 cells/μl. Large natural history studies of MAC complicating HIV disease suggest that systemic MAC disease is virtually inevitable in patients with AIDS who live long enough[30].

Common health care problems seen in bacteraemic patients include severe fatigue and chronic malaise, weight loss (15–20 per cent of normal weight), fevers and drenching night sweats and, sometimes, diarrhoea[31].

Physicians use the same investigational tools to diagnose MAC, and other non-tuberculosis mycobacterial diseases, in patients infected with HIV as they use for tuberculosis. Blood cultures are especially important in patients with suspected disseminated disease due to MAC. Cultures of bone marrow, lymph nodes, spleen, exudates and abscesses will often show mycobacterial growth and tuberculosis must be excluded before treatment is prescribed.

Other non-tuberculosis environmental mycobacteria may cause human disease, especially of soft tissues, skin and surgical wounds, including *M. chelonei, M. ulcerans* and *M. marinum.* In addition, post-injection abscesses can be caused by *M. chelonei* and *M. fortuitum*, which may contaminate syringes, needles or injectable material. These are, however, no more commonly seen in patients with HIV disease than in any other members of the community.

Nursing implications related to drug treatment for mycobacterial diseases

There are several important principles associated with effective treatment regimens for mycobacterial disease.

- Once identified and cultured, the patient's isolate (specific infecting mycobacteria) is tested in the laboratory for susceptibility to a variety of antimycobacterial drugs. However, empirical treatment, based upon the physician's own previous experience, and standard guidelines, usually commences immediately mycobacterial disease is suspected.
- As mycobacteria quickly develop resistance to drugs used to treat tuberculosis and disease due to MAC, single drug therapy is never used. Multiple drugs are prescribed, using a three or four drug regimen, all given simultaneously for an extended period of time.
- Tuberculosis is treated in two phases: an 'initial phase', using three or four drugs for the first 2 months, and then a 'continuation phase', using two drugs for at least 4 months.
- In patients co-infected with HIV, both treatment phases may be prolonged and may continue for at least 9 months; at least for 6 months following sputum conversion from 'smear positive' to 'smear negative'[33]. Individuals infected with HIV respond just as well to antituberculosis treatment as those who are not infected with HIV[34]. Treatment or prophylaxis for disease due to MAC may continue for the rest of the patient's life[28].
- Patient understanding and compliance is absolutely essential to prevent the emergence of multiple drug-resistant organisms. In many instances, health care workers must directly supervise each

and every prescribed administration of medication, a practice now referred to as **directly observed therapy**, or **DOT**.

- Non-compliance with treatment may be related to the untoward side-effects of the drugs used and nurses play a critical role in helping patients adjust to these agents and in keeping the physician informed in relation to the occurrence of any side-effects. Ignorance and lack of personal interest by some physicians and other health care workers may also lead to non-compliance.

The nursing implications of current drugs used in the treatment and/or prophylaxis of both tuberculosis and disease due to MAC in patients infected with HIV are described in Table 7.2[35,36], including important drug interactions. An important nursing consideration in drug therapy is that patients with HIV disease have a higher rate of all types of adverse reactions to antimycobacterial drugs than patients who are not co-infected with HIV[34]. Consequently, an understanding by nurses of the likely side-effects of drugs used in the treatment of tuberculosis and disease caused by MAC is paramount.

Table 7.2 Drugs used in the treatment of tuberculosis and diseases due to MAC

Drug	Nursing implications
First line drugs used for tuberculosis	
Isoniazid (INH)	Usually given orally or, very rarely, intramuscularly. Peripheral neuropathy is the only common side-effect. More rarely, hepatitis and psychosis may be associated with INH administration. Insomnia, restlessness and muscle twitching can occur. Concomitant pyridoxine (vitamin B_6) administration is often prescribed to reduce the incidence of serious side-effects
	INH is always included in any antituberculosis regimen, unless specifically contraindicated
	INH may be used for tuberculosis prophylaxis in patients with HIV disease
	Prednisolone increases INH levels and INH administration will increase levels of phenytoin, carbamazepine, diazepam and warfarin
	INH may be given during pregnancy
	INH administration reduces serum levels of the antifungal drugs, ketoconazole and fluconazole

Table 7.2   *continued*

Drug	Nursing implications
Rifampicin	Usually given orally but may be given intravenously. Either given 30 minutes before breakfast or immediately prior to going to sleep in the evening. Like INH, always included in any antituberculosis regimen unless specifically contraindicated. Hepatitis may be associated with treatment during the first 2 months of therapy. On intermittent treatment, six toxicity syndromes have been described following rifampicin therapy: influenzal, abdominal, and respiratory symptoms, shock, renal failure and thrombocytopenic purpura (bleeding disorder)
	Rifampicin may be given during pregnancy
	Rifampicin therapy reduces the effectiveness of oral contraceptives. In addition, by its actions on the liver, rifampicin therapy accelerates the metabolism of several drugs, including: phenytoin, corticosteroids, oral coumarin anticoagulants, oral diabetic drugs, digoxin, methadone, morphine, phenobarbitone and dapsone
	Rifampicin therapy may decrease levels of zidovudine (AZT) and the antifungal drugs, ketoconazole and fluconazole
	Ketoconazole inhibits the absorption of rifampin
	Nurses must warn patients that this drug causes a red-orange discoloration of urine and other secretions, e.g. sweat, saliva and tears. This can cause staining of soft contact lenses and lens implants
Pyrazinamide	Usually only given during the first 2–3 months of treatment and is always given in tuberculosis meningitis. Is given orally and side-effects include hepatitis, gastro-intestinal disturbances, arthralgias and hyperuricemia (leading to gout)
	Pyrazinamide is not usually given during pregnancy as it may be teratogenic
Thiacetozone	Inexpensive drug commonly used in developing countries for treatment of tuberculosis, usually with INH and streptomycin. In patients with HIV disease, this drug can cause a severe cutaneous

Table 7.2 *continued*

Drug	Nursing implications
	hypersensitivity reaction known as Stevens–Johnson syndrome, which may be fatal[37]

Drugs used in drug-resistant tuberculosis

Drug	Nursing implications
Ethionamide	Similar to INH and is given orally. Side-effects include severe allergic cutaneous reactions and drug fever, liver damage and severe nausea, diarrhoea and abdominal pain. Nausea may be reduced if this drug is given in the evening, at bedtime. Anti-emetics may need to be prescribed
Fluorinated quinolones	Includes ciprofloxacin, perfloxacin, sparfloxacin, norfloxacin and ofloxacin. These agents are used principally in drug-resistant tuberculosis. Ofloxacin is the most commonly used drug of this class and is given orally (rarely, it can be given intravenously). Although ciprofloxacin is involved in various drug interactions, ofloxacin is not
Para-aminosalicylic acid (PAS)	Given orally with food as it may cause gastric disturbances, such as diarrhoea, abdominal pain and nausea. Other side-effects include goitre, crystalluria and allergic reactions, e.g. rashes, drug fever and haematological disorders
Ethambutol	Can cause visual disturbances, e.g. loss of acuity, colour blindness and restriction of visual fields, especially if the daily dosage is > 15 mg/kg. Nurses must advise patients to discontinue treatment with this drug immediately if they develop any signs of ocular toxicity and return to clinic for re-evaluation. If a nursing determination is made that an individual patient cannot understand this aspect of the treatment, alternative drugs can be discussed with the prescribing physician. This is especially important in children who may not be able to tell you that they are having visual problems. Ophthalmic examinations must be performed before, and at intervals during, treatment
	Ethambutol may be given during pregnancy
Streptomycin	Not commonly used any more in the UK. It is given intramuscularly and the standard dose is not more than 1 g/day in adults. The dose is reduced to 500–750 mg in patients weighing < 50 kg or those who are > 40 years of age. Children are given

Table 7.2 *continued*

Drug	Nursing implications
	doses in the range of 15–20 mg/kg daily. This drug causes ototoxicity and can cause deafness, vertigo and gait disturbances. Side-effects increase after a cumulative dose of 100 g and a nursing record of the cumulative dose given must be kept.
	Cutaneous hypersensitivity (skin rashes and fever) may occur, usually within 2–3 weeks of initiating treatment with this drug. If fever develops, the drug should be discontinued and the physician consulted
	Streptomycin treatment may rarely result in a chronic eczema involving the limbs, often seen after the eighth week of therapy
	Anaphylaxis (collapse and cardiac arrest) can occur following injection with streptomycin
	Streptomycin is not given to pregnant women because of the risk of foetal ototoxicity
	Nurses must wear gloves when preparing and administering streptomycin because of the risk of developing allergic skin reactions to this agent. Injection sites are alternated daily as it is a painful injection
	As streptomycin must be given by injection, ensuring an adequate supply of sterile needles may present problems
Kanamycin and amikacin	Related to streptomycin with a similar profile of side-effects. Both are given by injection
Capreomycin and viomycin	Multi-system side-effects are associated with these drugs, which are reserved for drug-resistant organisms, including kidney and liver damage, ototoxicity and hypersensitivity reactions. Both are given by injection. Monitoring of hearing and balance necessary
Cycloserine	Rarely used as toxicity is impressive, including vertigo, headache, convulsions, confusional states and psychosis (risk of suicide)

Drugs used for prophylaxis or treatment of disease due to MAC

Clarithromycin	Given orally to treat disseminated disease due to MAC. Side-effects include nausea, vomiting,

Table 7.2 *continued*

Drug	Nursing implications
	taste perversion, abdominal pain, diarrhoea, rash, headache and flatulence
	Drug interactions include decreased levels of zidovudine (AZT) during clarithromycin therapy/prophylaxis. Concomitant administration of erythromycin products increases potential interactions with a whole variety of other drugs, e.g. anticoagulants, triazolam and phenytoin
Rifabutin	Given orally. Side-effects and drug interactions are similar for rifampicin. Frequently used as prophylaxis and/or treatment for disease due to MAC
Clofazimine	Often used in treating patients with disease due to MAC (and (leprosy)
	Side-effects include severe gastro-intestinal disturbances and malabsorption and this drug is contraindicated in patients with a history of peptic ulcer disease
	Nurses must warn patients that clofazimine may cause a red discoloration of the skin, hair, urine and faeces. Patients should avoid exposure to sunlight while on clofazimine therapy. This drug is given orally

Of the many drug interactions encountered, of special note are those antimycobacterial drugs which reduce the activities of antiretroviral drugs, such as zidovudine (AZT) or antifungal drugs. In addition, some drugs commonly used in the management of opportunistic events in patients with HIV disease may decrease the effectiveness of antimycobacterial agents, e.g. ketoconazole inhibits the absorption of rifampicin and if these two drugs are taken together, a treatment failure is likely[6].

Antituberculosis drugs may be classified as 'first line' agents, which are used in drug-susceptible tuberculosis, and drugs principally reserved for suspected or known drug resistance. In addition, some antimycobacterial drugs are chiefly reserved for either prophylaxis or treatment of disease due to MAC.

Drugs and drug combinations more commonly used in the developing world are fully described in other texts[38–40].

In pregnancy, drugs commonly used to treat tuberculosis include isoniazid, rifampicin and ethambutol; streptomycin is contraindicated and pyrazinamide is generally avoided.

Corticosteroids

Corticosteroids, e.g. prednisolone, dexamethasone, etc., suppress the inflammatory response and are used with caution in the treatment of patients with tuberculosis. They are prescribed in some forms of tuberculosis to reduce inflammation and subsequent fibrosis which could compromise the function of vital structures, e.g. in tuberculous meningitis (to prevent arteritis and strangulation of cranial nerves by fibrosis of exudates) and in pericardial tuberculosis (to prevent constrictive pericarditis). They may also be used in other clinical situations, e.g. pleural and peritoneal effusions, tubercular lesions of the larynx, kidneys and the eye, and in patients who are so ill that they may die before antimycobacterial drugs can start to work. In addition, physicians may prescribe steroids as part of the management of severe allergic reactions to antimycobacterial drugs. Nurses must be familiar with the common side-effects associated with steroid administration, including fluid retention, moon-face, re-activation of peptic ulcer disease and occasionally, confusion and psychosis.

Multi-drug resistant tuberculosis

In the USA, Asia and Africa, the emergence of a significant increase in cases of multi-drug resistant tuberculosis is alarming. Mycobacteria become resistant to drugs normally used to treat tuberculosis chiefly either as a result of poor compliance, i.e. where patients stop taking one or more of their drugs, or as a consequence of incompetent or inappropriate prescribing by physicians. Factors leading to drug resistance are listed in Table 7.3. There are two types of drug resistance in tuberculosis: **initial (primary) drug resistance** and **secondary drug resistance**. Initial resistance is ʰhe result of being infected with drug-resistant tubercle bacilli following exposure to a person with drug-resistant tuberculosis. Secondary resistance is acquired by an individual as a result of either poor compliance or inadequate treatment. Poor compliance is often associated with those who are socially, economically and educationally deprived, including the homeless, drug users and alcoholics.

Multi-drug resistance is defined as tuberculosis resistant to both isoniazid and rifampicin, the two most effective drugs available for the treatment of tuberculosis, **as well as** resistance to other drugs[16]. Drug-resistant tubercle bacilli are transmitted in exactly the same way as drug-susceptible organisms. HIV infection does not, by itself, make an individual more likely to have multi-drug resistant tuberculosis. However, drug-resistant tuberculosis in an individual who is infected with HIV is associated with a high mortality rate[33]. Recently, outbreaks of multi-drug resistant tuberculosis have been reported in hospitals in which over 80 per cent of patients were also infected with HIV[41].

The nosocomial transmission of multi-drug resistant tuberculosis to health care workers and to and among HIV-infected patients, in both hospitals and out-patient clinics, is well documented and associated with extraordinarily high case-fatality rates, e.g. 72–89 per cent[42,43]. Outbreaks of multi-drug resistant tuberculosis have also occurred in prisons, involving both inmates and prison guards[5].

It is important to remember that multi-drug resistant tuberculosis is transmitted in exactly the same manner as drug-susceptible tuberculosis, i.e. by 'AFB smear positive' individuals who are coughing. It is no more nor more less infectious than drug-susceptible tuberculosis.

Several factors are related to the risk, both of transmission and the probability that an exposed person will become infected and develop tuberculosis following exposure. In addition to the infectiousness of the source patient, the risk of transmission is related to the closeness and intensity of exposure. Anyone sharing the same airspace for a prolonged period, e.g. family members, patients and health care workers, is at more risk of contracting infection than those individuals who are only briefly exposed to the source patient, e.g. one-time hospital visitors. However, exposure of any length in small, confined, poorly ventilated environments is dangerous. This may include facil-

Table 7.3 Factors associated with the development of drug resistance in the treatment of tuberculosis

Inappropriate medical treatment
Monotherapy (using just one drug)
Insufficient number of agents in the regimen
Suboptimal dosage
Prior inappropriate use of antituberculosis drugs, e.g. 'over-the-counter' availability and inclusion of antituberculosis drugs in cough medicines, etc. in developing countries

Inadequate administration of medication
Poor patient compliance, e.g. erratic drug ingestion
Poor drug absorption
Patient discontinuing one or more of the prescribed agents due to side-effects
Counterfeit drugs in developing countries

ities in hospitals and clinics used for cough-inducing procedures, e.g. physiotherapy, sputum induction, administration of aerosol therapy, bronchoscopy and endotracheal intubation. The likelihood that an exposed person will become infected with and develop tuberculosis is related to that person's susceptibility. The most important factor which will increase individual susceptibility to primary infection is immunodeficiency, including immunodeficiency secondary to HIV infection. Consequently, HIV-infected individuals, whether they are patients, staff or visitors, should not be exposed to individuals with tuberculosis, especially those patients with multi-drug resistant strains.

Prevention of multi-drug resistant tuberculosis

Of critical importance in prevention is ensuring that persons with drug-susceptible tuberculosis are identified and appropriately treated. Most probably this will include ongoing supervision to ensure both compliance and completion of therapy. The need for directly observed therapy (DOT) must be assessed in each instance and resources identified for this strategy when it is required.

Multiple-drug preventive therapy is recommended for individuals who are infected with HIV (or otherwise immunocompromised) and who have been exposed to multi-drug resistant tuberculosis (single drug preventive treatment, e.g. INH, is generally felt sufficient following exposure to drug-sensitive tuberculosis). Active tuberculosis **must be excluded** prior to initiating any preventive chemotherapy. The duration of this preventive therapy in HIV-infected persons is 12 months and chest X-ray evaluations are carried out every 3 months[5].

Treatment issues associated with multi-drug resistant tuberculosis

Sputum specimens are cultured for drug susceptibility and the physician will prescribe appropriate drugs. These drugs are usually more expensive and more likely to cause side-effects than first-line antimycobacterial agents. Treatment regimens may include ethionamide, PAS, ciprofloxacin, ofloxacin, clofazimine, cycloserine, capreomycin, kanamycin and amikacin. The nursing implications of these drugs, and side-effects associated with them are described in Table 7.2. Treatment usually continues for 2 years, although injectable drugs are usually discontinued after the first 4 months[41]. Surgical intervention, e.g. pneumonectomy, may be appropriate in some cases[44].

Infection control measures must be developed and consistently implemented to prevent nosocomial transmission, and these are discussed later. Education, training and information dissemination to both patients and health care workers is of equal importance in preventing multi-drug resistant tuberculosis. Caring for patients with mycobacterial diseases, especially in the context of HIV co-infection, must be addressed in both pre- and post-registration nursing (and medical school) curricula and more in-depth training given to health care personnel who are directly caring for patients with both HIV and mycobacterial infections.

Bacillus Calmette–Guérin (BCG) vaccination

The BCG vaccine was developed in France in 1921. This is a live vaccine which is produced from a weakened (attenuated) strain of *M. bovis*. It is inexpensive and is available in a freeze-dried preparation in a rubber-capped vial with the diluent in a separate ampoule. It is simple to administer, transport and store and, in general, gives relatively good protection against tuberculosis in some circumstances. The vaccine is stored, protected from light, in a refrigerator (between 2 and 8°C and never frozen) and has a shelf-life of approximately 12–18 months.

The vaccination is administered intradermally using a separate tuberculin syringe and 25 g or 26 g 3/8th inch needle for each patient. The recommended site for the injection is at the insertion of the deltoid muscle near the middle of the left upper arm. In girls, for cosmetic reasons, the upper and lateral surface of the thigh may be preferred. A correctly given intradermal injection results in a tense, blanched raised bleb, typically of 7 mm in diameter following a standard injecting dose of 0.1 ml (0.05 ml for infants < 3 months).

Jet injectors must not be used for BCG immunization. In neonates, infants and very young children only, the percutaneous route (using a modified Heaf gun) may be used as an alternative to the intradermal method. Several (18–20) needles and a BCG vaccine which has been specifically prepared for percutaneous use is needed. Percutaneous BCG immunization is not recommended for older children, teenagers and adults.

BCG vaccination has been available for general use in the UK since 1953 when a national immunization programme was initiated, targeted at children aged 13 years. However, the protection afforded by BCG vaccination is variable and is the subject of much controversy. In the UK, conclusive evidence is available which indicates that the BCG vaccination offers good protection against tuberculosis whilst in other countries BCG may confer less effective protection[45]. Even so, it is probable that BCG vaccination in the newborn protects against the more serious forms of tuberculosis, e.g. meningeal and disseminated disease.

BCG vaccination is only given to individuals who have a negative tuberculin skin test, except for babies, who may be given BCG vaccination during the first 3 months of life without first having a tuberculin skin test. In the UK, government guidelines[25] recommend BCG vaccination for school children between the ages of 10 and 13 years, all students, including trainee teachers and student nurses, and all health service staff who may have contact with infectious patients or their specimens. In addition, contacts of 'AFB smear positive' cases of active tuberculosis are vaccinated, unless the contacts are known to be infected with HIV. BCG vaccination may also be offered to new immigrants to the UK from areas of high prevalence of tuberculosis, e.g. the Indian subcontinent) or to those travelling to these areas and planning to remaining there for an extended period.

Contraindications to BCG vaccination are as in Table 7.4:

Table 7.4   Contra-indications to BCG Vaccination

BCG vaccination should not be given to persons:
- who have a positive tuberculin skin test;
- who are receiving corticosteroid or other immunosuppressive treatments, including general radiation;
- suffering from a malignant condition such as lymphoma, leukaemia, Hodgkin's disease or other tumours of the reticuloendothelial system;
- in whom the normal immunological mechanism may be impaired, as in hypogammaglobulinaemia;
- who are known to be infected with HIV;
- who are pregnant;
- with pyrexia;
- with generalized septic skin conditions (but if eczema exists, an immunisation site should be chosen that is free from skin lesions.

It is not safe to give BCG vaccination to persons who are infected with HIV. Individuals who are immunosuppressed may not be able to limit the BCG infection to the site of vaccination. Consequently, the bacilli may then spread throughout the body, causing disease, i.e. **disseminated BCG infection**. In addition, immunosuppression may negatively affect the effectiveness of any vaccine, including BCG. Finally, BCG is a powerful activator of T lymphocytes and it may, by stimulating them, increase HIV replication and subsequent disease progression[46].

In the UK, BCG vaccination is not given to individuals known or suspected to be infected with HIV, including infants born to HIV-infected mothers. HIV-infected contacts of 'AFB smear positive' cases of tuberculosis are referred to specialist physicians for consideration of antimycobacterial chemoprophylaxis, rather than being given BCG vaccination[46]. Recommendations in relation to administering BCG vaccinations vary in different parts of the world. The World Health Organization recommends that in countries where tuberculosis in children remains a significant problem, BCG should continue to be given to all well children, including those whose mothers are known to be infected with HIV[38].

The protective efficacy of BCG vaccination varies in different countries and this is probably related to exposure to local environmental mycobacteria which sensitize local populations and modifies the protective response to BCG. In addition, it is important to remember that any protection afforded by BCG vaccination in childhood diminishes with time and adults may be susceptible to primary infection.

A more effective vaccine against tuberculosis is needed to prevent the unfolding global tragedy being contemplated as a result of escalating numbers of persons co-infected with tuberculosis and HIV, and the spectre of multiple-drug resistant tuberculosis. Researchers are currently exploring a new vaccine, based on a killed suspension of a strain of *M. vaccae*, which may also be immunotherapeutic[17,47,48].

Preventing nosocomial transmission of tuberculosis in health care settings

A variety of guidelines have now been produced in relation to preventing the transmission of tuberculosis, especially in health care settings[46,49,50]. CDC recommendations are reprinted in full in Appendix 4. The salient points of all these guidelines, which must be considered in preventing nosocomial transmission of *M. tuberculosis* in health care facilities caring for patients with HIV disease, are discussed below.

Policies and procedures

All health care facilities must have developed local operational policies and procedures in relation to preventing nosocomial transmission of tuberculosis. These policies must be based on accepted guidelines and periodically reviewed. Approaches to policy development should be multi-faceted and focus on the issues in Table 7.5:

Table 7.5　Policies for Preventing Nosocomial Transmission of Tuberculosis

---

Issues
- Protocols for early diagnosis and treatment of patients with active tuberculosis
- Infection control ('Respiratory Precautions') policies and procedures
- Engineering approaches to ensure the provision of appropriate and safe environments in which to care for patients with active tuberculosis
- Medical surveillance of transmission of tuberculosis to health care workers
- In-service education and quality assurance monitoring

Both nursing services and occupational health departments must be closely involved with the development, implementation and monitoring of policies and procedures.

Identification of persons with active tuberculosis

One of the most important aspects of all prevention strategies is the rapid detection, isolation and treatment of persons with active tuberculosis. Preventing the generation of infectious droplet nuclei is accomplished by identifying those who have open tuberculosis and initiating appropriate antituberculosis chemotherapy.

Infectiousness is greatest among patients with pulmonary or laryngeal tuberculosis, who have a productive cough, pulmonary cavitation on chest X-ray and who are AFB smear positive.

Appropriate antituberculosis chemotherapy is just as effective in HIV-infected persons as in individuals who are not infected with HIV, and patients generally become non-infectious after 2–3 weeks of treatment[49]. The greatest risk of exposure to infection is from those patients with unsuspected tuberculosis or those patients who are not receiving (or compliant with) adequate chemotherapy. Physicians will have a high index of suspicion of tuberculosis in any patient with HIV disease who has a persistent, productive cough or other symptoms suggestive of tuberculosis, as discussed previously. Diagnostic protocols may include those investigations discussed previously. It is important to remember that active tuberculosis can occur simultaneously with other pulmonary conditions, such as pneumocystosis or bacterial pneumonia.

AFB respiratory precautions

Source-control methods

M. tuberculosis is dispersed into the air as small particles, known as 'droplet nuclei', when an individual with active pulmonary tuberculosis coughs, sneezes or talks. Droplet nuclei are so small (1–5 μm) that they are kept airborne by normal currents of air and can easily spread throughout a room or building. Patients with active pulmonary tuberculosis are infectious until sputum specimens have been reported as 'smear negative' on three consecutive days. Patients with extra-pulmonary tuberculosis are not usually infectious, unless they have non-pulmonary disease located in the respiratory tract or oral cavity or extrapulmonary disease that includes an open abscess or lesion, especially if drainage is extensive. MAC infection is of very little risk to non-immunocompromised patients and the actual risk of MAC transmission among HIV-infected persons is not known. Patients with HIV disease who have active pulmonary tuberculosis are no more or no less infectious than are patients who are not infected with HIV. Infection control measures which are designed to reduce the spread of droplet nuclei into the general air circulation are referred to as **source control methods** because they are designed to entrap these infectious particles as they are emitted by the patient, or 'source'.

Respiratory isolation rooms

All patients with active pulmonary tuberculosis, or suspected of having the disease, must be cared for in **respiratory isolation rooms** which are adequately ventilated and kept at negative pressure relative to the surrounding areas, until they are non-infectious. This prevents the release of infectious droplet nuclei into the hallways and other areas of the wards (although it does not protect health care staff who enter the room!). Negative pressure means that air flows into the room, not out of the room. CDC recommendations[49] are that room air is exhausted directly from the room to the outside of the building. If it is recirculated (e.g. in accident and emergency rooms), it should first pass through an air cleaner, e.g. high efficiency particulate air (HEPA) filters, which will remove most suspended droplet nuclei. The maintenance of negative pressure in the room is essential and manometers incorporating both visible displays and audible alarms that activate when the negative pressure fails are recommended[51].

Respiratory isolation booths
Booths are useful as a source control method of infection control and are used for sputum induction or administration of aerosolized medications, e.g. pentamidine. Booths must be equipped with exhaust fans that remove nearly 100 per cent of airborne particles during the time interval between patients. Booths must maintain a negative pressure inside the booth and the air from the booth is exhausted directly to the outside of the building.

Patient use of a mask or PR
Only in some limited circumstances is it practical for patients to wear a properly fitted surgical mask or disposable, valveless particulate respirator (PR) to reduce the spread of infectious droplet nuclei, e.g. when being transported within or between medical facilities.

Patient education
A simple, but effective source control technique is to teach the patient to cover all coughs and sneezes with a tissue. This will capture and contain most liquid drops and droplets before evaporation can occur. These tissues must be properly disposed of and patients taught to wash their hands frequently and effectively. A small plastic sputum jar, with cover, should be carried by patients so that any sputum produced is expectorated into the jar rather than somewhere else. These jars must be properly disposed of, preferably by incineration. Restriction of immunocompromised visitors while the patient is infectious, e.g. HIV-infected friends and relatives, must be discussed with the patient.

Other infection control measures

A variety of other respiratory precautions are used to reduce microbial contamination of air shared by infectious patients and health care staff and other patients.

Disposable masks and particulate respirators (PRs)
The use of disposable effective high filtration surgical masks may provide additional protection against transmission of tubercle bacilli and are worn to protect the face from sputum contamination. The use of disposable particulate respirators (PRs), usually similar to cup-shaped surgical masks, provide a better facial fit and filtration capability and are preferred to surgical masks[52]. Disposable PRs offer

good protection against inhalation of particles as small as 1μm in diameter. They must be worn by all staff when appropriate ventilation is not available.

In addition, PRs must be worn by staff when caring for patients undergoing procedures which may produce bursts of aerosolized infectious particles or result in copious coughing or sputum production. PRs should also be worn by health care staff when caring for infectious patients with productive coughs who are unable or unwilling to cover their mouths when coughing[49]. PRs must fit the face snugly, with no gaps, otherwise they will function more like a funnel than a filter as air will preferentially flow through the gaps. PRs which do not fit the face properly offer no protection and may be counter-productive as they induce a false sense of confidence[53].

Other barrier precautions
Other barrier precautions, such as gowns, eye protection and disposable gloves, are appropriate in some circumstances when caring for patients with tuberculosis. Wearing gowns may assist in maintaining general cleanliness as they can be more easily changed than a uniform when visibly soiled. Contaminated hands of health care staff are often responsible for transmission of nosocomial infections, especially involving immunocompromised patients, and wearing gloves when assisting with various procedures, e.g. bronchoscopy, endotrachael suctioning, etc., seems sensible, as does the use of eye protection, to protect against splashing. HIV-infected patients with active tuberculosis may also have other concurrent infections and effective handwashing technique is just as important in this arena as it is in general nursing. All of the elements of **Universal Infection Control Precautions**, as described in Chapter 12, apply in caring for all patients, including those with active tuberculosis.

Decontamination
Decontamination includes cleaning, disinfecting and sterilizing equipment. Critical items, such as needles, surgical instruments, cardiac catheters, etc. that are introduced directly into the bloodstream or other normally sterile areas of the body must be sterilized before use. Semi-critical items, e.g. non-invasive flexible and rigid fibre-optic endoscopes or bronchoscopes, endotracheal tubes, or anaesthesia breathing circuits should preferably be sterilized or subjected to high-level disinfection processes (see Chapter 12). High-level disinfection will destroy tubercle bacilli if painstaking physical cleaning before either sterilization or high-level disinfection is carried out. *M. tuberculosis* and environmental mycobacteria, e.g. *M. chelonei* and *M. avium-intracellulare* have been transmitted by

contaminated bronchoscopes and invariably this has been attributed to inadequate cleansing or inappropriate disinfection of the broncho-scope[54]. Appropriate disinfection procedures for endoscopes used for patients with active (or suspected) tuberculosis, co-infected with HIV, as adapted from current guidelines and expert advice[55] are as follows:

- All endoscopes must be thoroughly cleaned with a neutral deter-gent, either by hand or by 'automated washer disinfectors', prior to disinfection.
- Certain items of equipment, e.g. those with hollow lumina or complex spiral structures, e.g. biopsy forceps and cytology brushes, can only be reliably cleaned by using an ultrasonic cleaner. They are sonicated in detergent or a proprietary ultra-sonic fluid (not disinfectant) for 10 minutes prior to being cleaned in the usual way.
- After cleaning, endoscopes should be immersed in 2 per cent alkaline glutaraldehyde for 1 hour; formaldehyde and butan-1,4-dial/2,5-dimethoxytetrahydrofuran (Gigasept®) is an acceptable alternative to alkaline glutaraldehyde.
- Idophors, cetrimide and chlorhexidine have little mycobac-tericidal activity and should not be used.
- Endoscopes should be disinfected prior to use on immunocompromised patients and rinsed in either sterile water (not tap water) or 70 per cent ethanol.

Engineering considerations

Maintaining negative pressure respiratory isolation rooms and ensuring that they are exhausted appropriately, i.e. away from air-intake vents, people, animals, and in accordance with any environmental health regulations, requires ongoing support from specialist engineers. Additional engineering approaches include the following[49]:

Reducing microbial contamination of air   Droplet nuclei are elimin-ated or reduced in number by appropriate general ventilation and engineering advice is needed to ensure ventilation standards for indoor air quality are consistently met. This includes ensuring that ventilation is effective in diluting and removing airborne contami-nants and that air mix, air flow and air pressures requirements are adhered to.

Air filtration   High-efficiency particulate air (HEPA) filters are able to remove almost 100 per cent of droplet nuclei and they are often used in units caring for patients with active tuberculosis. They must be used if air in respiratory isolation rooms is to be recirculated (which is **not** recommended). They must be properly installed and maintained if they are to be effective. Filters are replaced and carefully disposed of by engineering staff at regular intervals.

Germicidal ultraviolet radiation Germicidal ultraviolet (UV) lamps are recommended by CDC as a supplement to ventilation in facilities caring for patients with tuberculosis, or where the risk of tuberculosis transmission is high[49]. Although their use remains controversial, many experienced tuberculosis clinicians and mycobacteriologists continue to support their use[56,57]. Shielded germicidal UV lamps are used either attached to the walls or suspended from ceilings. Unshielded germicidal UV lamps are often incorporated into the inside of ventilation system ducts, disinfecting air entering or leaving an area.

More detailed engineering information can be found in the CDC guidelines in Appendix 4.

Medical surveillance of transmission of tuberculosis to health care workers

A tuberculosis screening and prevention programme for all staff employed in health care facilities should be established. Policies and protocols must be developed in relation to chemoprophylaxis for staff who become infected with *M. tuberculosis* but who do not have active disease. All staff should have a tuberculin skin test when they are employed, including those with a history of BCG vaccination. Staff who have a negative skin test should receive BCG vaccination if they are working in areas in which patients with either HIV disease or tuberculosis are cared for, unless BCG vaccination is contraindicated. More detailed advice can be found in the CDC guidelines in Appendix 4.

In-service education and quality assurance

Studies have shown that delays in implementing respiratory pre-cautions due to employee unawareness of policies and procedures can result in increased risk of nosocomial transmission[58]. In-service education initiatives must ensure that staff are familiar with these policies and that routine quality assurance mechanisms are used to monitor the consistent application of recommended procedures. Any institution or health care facility which is caring for patients with HIV disease must develop and implement continuing in-service education and training programmes for staff in relation to both caring for patients with tuberculosis within the context of HIV disease, and associated infection control measures.

Conclusion

Stephen Joseph[59] remarked that 'Waxing and waning in recent Western consciousness, tuberculosis, like the poor whom it seeks out, is always with us.' Second only to HIV disease itself, tuberculosis is set to re-emerge as a continuing, significant threat to the public health, truly the terrible synergistic twin of the AIDS pandemic. Once again, all nurses are required to increase their competence in developing prevention and care strategies in relation to tuberculosis, an often forgotten plague.

References

1. Evans, C.C. (1994). Historical background. In *Clinical Tuberculosis*, ed. Davies, Peter. Chapman & Hall, London, pp. 1–17.
2. Kochi, A. (1991). The global tuberculosis situation and the new control strategy of the World Health Organization. *Tubercule* **72**, 1–6.
3. Mann, J., Tarantola, D.J.M. and Netter, Thomas W. (eds) (1992). *AIDS in the World: A Global Report*. Harvard University Press, London, pp. 148–63.
4. WHO (1994). Press Releases. WHO/6 (21 January 1994), WHO/9 (26 January 1994). World Health Organization, Geneva.
5. Centers for Disease Control (1992). National Action Plan to Combat Multidrug-Resistant Tuberculosis; Meeting the Challenge of Multidrug-Resistant Tuberculosis. Summary of a Conference, Management of Persons Exposed to Multidrug-Resistant Tuberculosis. *Morbidity and Mortality Weekly Report (MMWR)*, 19 June, **41**(RR-11), 6.
6. Barnes, Peter F., Block, Alan B., Davidson, Paul T. *et al.* (1991). Review article – current concepts: Tuberculosis in patients with human immunodeficiency virus infection. *New England Journal of Medicine*, 6 June, **324**(23), 1644–50.
7. Centers for Disease Control (1990). The use of preventive therapy for tuberculous infection in the United States: Recommendation of the Advisory Committee for Elimination of Tuberculosis. Morbidity and Mortality Weekly Report (*MMWR*) **39**, 9–12.
8. Watson, John M. (1993). Editorial: Tuberculosis in Britain today. *British Medical Journal*, 23 January, **306**(6872), 221–2.
9. PHLS Communicable Diseases Surveillance Centre (1993). Tuberculosis in England and Wales. *Communicable Disease Report* **3**, 85.
10. Bouvet, E., Casalino, E., Mendoza-Sassi, G. *et al.* (1993). A nosocomial outbreak of multidrug-resistant *Mycobacterium bovis*

among HIV-infected patients: A case-control study. *AIDS*, **7**, 1453–60.

11. Dankner, W.M., Waecker, N.J., Essey, M.A. *et al.* (1993). *Mycobacterium bovis* infections in San Diego: a clinicoepidemiological study of 73 patients and a historical review of a forgotten pathogen. *Medicine* **72**, 11–37.

12. Daborn, C.J. and Grange, J.M. (1993). HIV/AIDS and its implication for the control of animal tuberculosis. *British Veterinary Journal* **149**, 405–17.

13. Grange, John M. (1992). The mystery of the mycobacterial persister. *Tubercle and Lung Disease* **73**, 249–51.

14. Festenstein, F. and Grange, John M. (1991). Tuberculosis and the acquired immune deficiency syndrome: A review. *Journal of Applied Bacteriology* **71**, 19–30.

15. Daniel, Thomas M. (1991). Tuberculosis. In *Harrison's Principles of Internal Medicine*, 12th (International) edn, eds Wilson, J.D., Braunwald, E., Isselbacher, K.J. *et al.*, Vol. 1. McGraw-Hill, New York, pp. 637–48.

16. Barnes, Peter F. and Barrows, Susan, A. (1993). Tuberculosis in the 1990s. *Annals of Internal Medicine*, 1 September, **119**(5), 400–10.

17. Stanford, J.L., Onyebujoh, P.C., Rook, G.A.W., *et al.* (1993). Old plague, new plague, and a treatment for both? *AIDS* **7**(9), 1275–7.

18. Rook, G.A.W. (1991). Mobilising the appropriate T-cell subset: the immune response as taxonomist? *Tubercle* **72**, 253–4.

19. Clerici, Mario and Shearer, Gene M. (1993). Viewpoint: A Th1 to Th2 switch is a critical step in the etiology of HIV infection. *Immunology Today* **14**(3), 107–11.

20. Chaisson, Richard E. and Slutkin, Gary (1989). Tuberculosis and human immunodeficiency virus infection. *Journal of Infectious Diseases*, 1 January, **159**(1), 96–100.

21. Wallis, Robert S., Vjecha, Michael, Amir-Tahmasseb, Manijeh *et al.* (1993). Influence of tuberculosis on human immunodeficiency virus (HIV-1): Enhanced cytokine expression and elevated b2-microglobulin in HIV-1-associated tuberculosis. *Journal of Infectious Disease*, 1 January, **167**(1), 43–8.

22. Daley, C.L., Small, P.M., Schecter, G.F. *et al.* (1992). An outbreak of tuberculosis with accelerated progression among persons infected with the human immunodeficiency virus. An analysis using restriction-fragment-length polymorphisms. *New England Journal of Medicine* **326**, 231–5.

23. Subcommittee of the Joint Tuberculosis Committee of the British Thoracic Society (1992). Education and Debate: Guidelines on the management of tuberculosis and HIV infection in the United Kingdom. *British Medical Journal*, 9 May, **304**(6836), 1231–3.

24. Berkow, R. and Fletcher, A.J. (eds) (1992). *The Merck Manual of Diagnosis and Therapy*, 16th edn. Merck Research Laboratories, New Jersey.

25. Department of Health, Welsh Office, Scottish Office Home and Health

Department, DHSS (Northern Ireland) (1992). *Immunisation against Infectious Disease*. HMSO, London, pp. 81–7.

26. Jenkins, P.A. (1994). The microbiology of tuberculosis. In *Clinical Tuberculosis*, ed. Davies, Peter. Chapman & Hall, London, p. 35.

27. Masur, H. and the USA Public Health Service Task Force on Prophylaxis and Therapy for *Mycobacterium avium* Complex (1993). Recommendations on prophylaxis and therapy for disseminated *Mycobacterium avium* complex disease in patients infected with the human immunodeficiency virus. *New England Journal of Medicine* **329**(12), 898–904.

28. Centers for Disease Control (1993). Recommendations on Prophylaxis and Therapy for Disseminated *Mycobacterium avium* Complex for Adults and Adolescents Infected with Human Immunodeficiency Virus. *Morbidity and Mortality Weekly Report (MMWR)*, 25 June, **42**(RR-9), 17–20.

29. Carlin, Elizabeth (1993). Editorial comment on papers of outstanding interest. *Current AIDS Literature*, December, **6**(12), 432–3.

30. Nightingale, S.D., Byrd, L.T., Southern, P.M. *et al.* (1992). Incidence of *Mycobacterium avium-intracellulare* complex bacteremia in human immunodeficiency virus-positive patients. *Journal of Infectious Diseases* **165**, 1982–5.

31. Young, Lowell S. (1994). Atypical mycobacteria. In *Textbook of AIDS Medicine*, eds Broder, S., Merigan, T.C. Jr. and Bolognesi, D., Williams & Wilkins, Baltimore, pp. 283–94.

32. Yates, M.D., Pozniak, A. and Grange, J.M. (1993). Isolation of mycobacteria from patients seropositive for the human immunodeficiency virus (HIV) in south east England: 1984–92, *Thorax* **48**, 990–5.

33. Centers for Disease Control (1993). Initial Therapy for Tuberculosis in the Era of Multidrug Resistance: Recommendations of the Advisory Council for the Elimination of Tuberculosis. *Morbidity and Mortality Weekly (MMWR)*, 21 May, **42**(RR-7), 1–8.

34. Small, Peter M., Schecter, Gisela, F., Goodman, Philip, C. *et al.* (1991). Treatment of Tuberculosis in Patients with Advanced Human Immunodeficiency Virus Infection. *New England Journal of Medicine*, 31 January, **324**(5), 289–94.

35. Winstanley, P.A. (1994). The clinical pharmacology of anti-tuberculosis drugs. In *Clinical Tuberculosis*, ed. Davies, Peter. Chapman & Hall, London, pp. 129–40.

36. British Medical Association and Royal Pharmaceutical Society of Great Britain (1994). *British National Formulary*, No. 27 (March 1994).

37. Nunn, Paul, Kibuga, Daniel, Gathua, Sam *et al.* (1991). Cutaneous hypersensitivity reactions to thiacetazone in HIV-1 seropositive patients treated for tuberculosis. *Lancet*, 16 March, **337**(8742), 627–30.

38. Harries, A.D. (1994). The association between HIV and tuberculosis in the developing world. In *Clinical Tuberculosis*, ed. Davies, Peter. Chapman & Hall, London, pp. 241–64.

39. Crofton, Sir John, Horne, Norman and Miller, Fred (1992). *Clinical*

Tuberculosis, Macmillan, London.
40. WHO (1993). *Treatment of Tuberculosis: Guidelines for National Programmes*, World Health Organization, Geneva.
41. Dooley, S.W. Jr. and Simone, Patricia M. (1994). The extent and management of drug-resistant tuberculosis: The American experience. In *Clinical Tuberculosis*, ed. Davies, Peter. Chapman & Hall, London, pp. 171–89.
42. Centers for Disease Control (1990). Nosocomial transmission of multidrug-resistant tuberculosis to health-care workers and HIV-infected patients in an urban hospital – Florida. *Morbidity and Mortality Weekly (MMWR)* 39(40), 718–22.
43. Centers for Disease Control (1991). Nosocomial transmission of multidrug-resistant tuberculosis among HIV-infected persons – Florida, 1988–1991. *Morbidity and Mortality Weekly (MMWR)* 40(34), 585–91.
44. Donnelly, R.J. and Davies, P.D.O. (1994). Surgical management of pulmonary tuberculosis. In *Clinical Tuberculosis*, ed. Davies, Peter. Chapman & Hall, London, pp. 171–89.
45. Citron, K.M. (1993). BCG vaccination against tuberculosis: editorial. *British Medical Journal*, 23 January, 306(6872), 222–3.
46. Ormerod, L.P., Skinner, C., Darbyshire, J.H. *et al.*(1992). Guidelines on the management of tuberculosis and HIV infection in the United Kingdom: Education and Debate – A report by the Subcommittee of the Joint Tuberculosis Committee of the British Thoracic Society. *British Medical Journal*, 9 May, 304(6836), 1231–3.
47. Standford, J.L., Grange, J.M. and Pozniak, A. (1991). Is Africa Lost? *The Lancet*, 31 August, 338(8766), 557–8.
48. Standford, J.L. and Grange, J.M. (1994). The promise of immunotherapy for tuberculosis. *Respiratory Medicine* 88, 3–7.
49. Centers for Disease Control (1990). Guidelines for Preventing the Transmission of Tuberculosis in Health-Care Settings, with Special Focus on HIV-Related Issues, *Morbidity and Mortality Weekly (MMWR)*, 7 December, 39(RR-17).
50. PHLS Communicable Diseases Surveillance Centre (1992). Nosocomial transmission of tuberculosis in AIDS care centres. *Communicable Disease Report*, 22 May, 2(6), R71–2.
51. Nicas, M., Sprinson, J.F., Royce, S.E. *et al.* (1993). Isolation rooms for tuberculosis control. *Infection Control and Hospital Epidemiology*, November, 14(11), 619–22.
52. Hutton, Mary D. and Polder, Jacquelyn A. (1992). Guidelines for preventing tuberculosis transmission in health care settings: What's new? *American Journal of Infection Control*, February, 20(1), 24–6.
53. Pippin, D.J., Verderame, R.A. and Weber, K.K. (1987). Efficacy of face masks in preventing inhalation of airborne contaminants. *Journal of Oral Maxillofacial Surgery* 45, 319–23.
54. Nelson, K.E., Larson, P.A., Schranfragel, D.E. *et al.* (1983). Transmission of tuberculosis by flexible fibrebronchoscopes. *American Review of Respiratory Diseases* 127, 391–2, as cited in Hanson, Peter J. and Collins, John V. (1990). AIDS and infection control in

respiratory units. In (1990) *AIDS and the Lung* (articles reprinted from *Thorax*), eds Mitchell, David and Woodcock, Ashley. *British Medical Journal*, London, pp. 1–12.

55. Hanson, Peter J. and Collins, John V. (1990). AIDS and infection control in respiratory units, in *AIDS and the Lung* (articles reprinted from *Thorax*), eds Mitchell, David and Woodcock, Ashley. *British Medical Journal*, London, pp. 1–12.

56. Macher, Janet M. (1993). The use of germicidal lamps to control tuberculosis in healthcare facilities. *Infection Control and Hospital Epidemiology*, December, **14**(12), 723–8.

57. Iseman, Michael D. (1992). Perspective: A lead of faith: What can we do to curtail intra-institutional transmission of tuberculosis? *Annals of Internal Medicine*, 1 August, **117**(3), 251–3.

58. Lin-Greenberg, Alan and Anez, Thelma (1992). Delay in respiratory isolation of patients with pulmonary tuberculosis and human immunodeficiency virus infection. *American Journal of Infection Control*, February, **20**(1), 16–18.

59. Joseph, Stephen (1993). Public Health Policy Forum: Editorial: Tuberculosis, again. *American Journal of Public Health*, May, **83**(5), 647–8.

Further reading

Centers for Disease Control (1990). Guidelines for Preventing the Transmission of Tuberculosis in Health-Care Settings, with Special Focus on HIV-Related Issues. *Morbidity and Mortality Weekly Report (MMWR)*, 7 December, **39**(RR-17).

Crofton, Sir John, Horne, Norman and Miller, Fred (1992). *Clinical Tuberculosis*. Macmillan, London (ISBN 0-333-56690-4).

Davies, Peter D.O. (ed.) (1994). *Clinical Tuberculosis*. Chapman & Hall, London (ISBN 0-412-48630-X).

Festenstein, F. and Grange, John M. (1991). Tuberculosis and the acquired immune deficiency syndrome: A review. *Journal of Applied Bacteriology* **71**, 19–30.

Mitchell, David and Woodcock, Ashley (eds) (1990). *AIDS and the Lung* (articles reprinted from *Thorax*). *British Medical Journal*, London.

Ryan, Frank (1992). *Tuberculosis: The Greatest Story Never Told*. Swift Publishers, Bromsgrove (ISBN 1-874082-00-6).

WHO (1993). *Treatment of Tuberculosis: Guidelines for National Programmes*. World Health Organization, Geneva (ISBN 92-4-154451-1).

8

HIV Disease and the Nervous System

It is now well established that HIV acquisition is frequently associated with a variety of neuropsychiatric syndromes[1]. Neuropsychiatric syndromes refer to both central nervous system (CNS) diseases and organic mental disorders and may be due to opportunistic infections, neoplastic processes or the primary effect that HIV has on the CNS. In assessing and planning care, it is essential that the nurse has a sound knowledge of the potential neurological consequences of HIV infecion. Neuropsychiatric manifestations of HIV infection include those listed in Table 8.1.

Neurological dysfunction may be the first manifestation of HIV infection. Early neurological syndromes include atypical aseptic meningitis, acute encephalitis and acute peripheral neuropathy. These syndromes may appear soon after HIV infection at the time of seroconversion.

Atypical aseptic meningitis

Aseptic meningitis is a febrile meningeal inflammation due to early CNS infection with HIV. Patients frequently seek medical advice

Table 8.1 Neuropsychiatric manifestations of HIV infection

Atypical aseptic meningitis	
Acute encephalitis	
Peripheral neuropathy	
Autonomic neuropathy	Due to neurotrophic effects of HIV
Vacuolar myelopathy	
Landry–Guillain–Barré syndrome	
Subclinical cognitive dysfunction	
Organic mental disorders	
CNS opportunistic infections	
CNS neoplastic disease	
Cerebrovascular disorders	

because of various meningeal signs, such as:

- Fever
- Drowsiness
- Stiff neck
- Headache
- Vomiting.

The aseptic meningitis associated with HIV infection is complicated by additional features not generally seen in patients with aseptic meningitis (i.e. it is **atypical**). These atypical features include cranial nerve dysfunction, especially involvement of cranial nerves V, Vll and VIII[2]. Involvement of the trigeminal (V) and facial (Vll) nerves may evoke facial numbness, palsy and paralysis and trigeminal neuralgia. Involvement of the auditory (VIII) nerve may produce tinnitus, deafness and vertigo. Other atypical features include the tendency for this type of meningitis to recur and to become chronic.

Investigations include lumbar puncture and head CT (computerized tomography) scanning. A CT scan is desirable in patients in which HIV infection is being considered to exclude intracerebral abscess caused by *Toxoplasma gondii*, which may present in a similar fashion. Lumbar puncture then might be contraindicated due to the risk of a change in the CSF pressure, caused by the sudden withdrawal of fluid from the spinal canal, precipitating herniation of the medulla and cerebellar tonsils into the foramen magnum (i.e. **coning**) with fatal results.

CSF obtained from lumbar puncture usually shows a normal glucose level (50–100 mg/100 ml), a normal or only slightly elevated protein content (20–45 mg/100 ml), an increase in mononuclear or polymorphonuclear white cells, lymphocytic pleocytosis (i.e. an excessive number of lymphocytes in the CSF) and the absence of bacterial growth on culture. HIV has been detected in the CSF in patients with atypical aseptic meningitis[3].

Atypical aseptic meningitis may be either acute or chronic and, in general, complete recovery can be expected. Medical treatment is entirely symptomatic (e.g. analgesics and antipyretics), although zidovudine (Retrovir – AZT) may be used. Fluid balance is maintained but care is taken not to overhydrate the patient.

Acute encephalitis

Acute encephalitis is an acute inflammatory disease of the brain due to direct HIV invasion and/or hypersensitivity initiated by HIV infection of the brain. Like acute atypical meningitis, acute encephalitis occurs most frequently soon after HIV infection, at the time of seroconversion[4]. Acute encephalitis differs from atypical aseptic meningitis in that there is evidence of cerebral dysfunction which is independent of signs of meningeal inflammation. Signs of cerebral dysfunction commonly observed include:

- Alterations in level of consciousness
- Personality change
- Seizures
- Paresis
- Focal neurological signs.

Investigations include a CT scan and lumbar puncture to exclude cryptococcal meningitis and intracerebral abscess caused by *Toxoplasma gondii*. Acute encephalitis is a more serious condition than atypical aseptic meningitis and, although recovery can be expected, high-dependency nursing care is required to maintain a safe environment for the patient to recover. The patient's need for nutrition, adequate hydration and to maintain a normal body temperature, must be carefully assessed and facilitated. Antipyretics and anticonvulsant medications may be prescribed and zidovudine (Retrovir – AZT) may be used. Both atypical aseptic meningitis

Table 8.2 HIV encephalopathy: indicators of cortical dysfunction

Disorders of intellect
Memory loss
Short attention span and impairment in ability to concentrate
Deterioration in learning abilities and ability to abstract
Slow and difficult thinking
Blunting of perception and errors of judgement

Disorders of behaviour
Social withdrawal
Disinhibited or embarrassing and anti-social behaviour
Deterioration in self-care (e.g. lack of attention to personal cleanliness, dress and nutrition)

Disorders of mood
Labile emotions (easily frustrated, irritable, quickly changing mood)
Anxiety
Depression

Disorders of personality
Former personality traits accentuated
Interpersonal relationships altered
Demanding behaviour and egocentricity

and acute encephalitis are medical emergencies and patients must be admitted to hospital for immediate treatment and to assist them to meet their safety needs.

Peripheral neuropathy

HIV infection of peripheral nerves (e.g. cranial and spinal nerve) may cause symptoms either prior to or after the development of ARC or fully expressed AIDS (often seen in patients with subacute encephalitis). Peripheral neuropathy may be either acute, subacute or chronic.

There is symmetrical involvement of both sensory and motor nerves (i.e. **symmetrical sensorimotor neuropathy**) and patients frequently complain of the occurrence of spontaneous pains (**dysaesthesia**) and pain which is provoked by gentle, light touch or temperature stimulation (**hyperaesthesia**).

There may be weakness and wasting in the arms and legs (i.e. **distal atrophy**). Involvement of the spinal nerve roots may produce pain referred to the back of the thigh and leg below the knee, weakness, flaccidity and eventually atrophy of the legs (**radicular syndrome**).

Involvement of a peripheral nerve on one side of the body (**asymmetric**) is characterized by a sensation of numbness, prickling or tingling (i.e. **paraesthesia**), pain and weakness. This condition is known as **mononeuritis multiplex** and may present prior to the development of AIDS.

Acute peripheral neuropathy may present as a facial paralysis and involve only one side of the face (**Bell's palsy**).

Zidovudine (Retrovir – AZT) may be used to treat this condition.

Vacuolar myelopathy

HIV frequently has a direct effect on both motor and sensory nerves in the spinal cord in patients with AIDS and produces a paraesthesia, weakness and spasticity of the legs. There may be a failure or irregularity of muscular coordination, especially manifested when voluntary muscular movements are attempted (ataxia). Urinary incontinence may develop. This condition is known as **vacuolar myelopathy** and may be seen in patients with subacute encephalitis. Zidovudine (Retrovir – AZT) may be used to treat this condition.

Autonomic neuropathy

Damage to the autonomic nervous system can result in erectile failure, some cases of unexplained diarrhoea or cardiovascular instability. The latter may lead to postural hypotension, fainting and cardiovascular arrest. Erectile failure may be treated with alpha-adrenoceptor blocking agents such as yohimbine. Diarrhoea due to autonomic neuropathy may respond to treatment with adrenergic neurone blocking drugs such as guanethidine (Ismelin®). Hypotension associated with autonomic neuropathy may be effectively treated with fludrocortisone (Florinef®).

Other neurological syndromes

Landry–Guillain–Barré syndrome

This is an acute, rapidly progressive form of polyneuropathy characterized by muscular weakness and various disorders of movement, due to involvement of the spinal roots and peripheral nerves, which may also be seen in patients with AIDS[5].

Subclinical cognitive dysfunction

Most patients with AIDS, without known neurological complications, will develop impairment of reasoning, perception, intuition, memory, language and ability to learn. This is probably due to diffuse cerebral dysfunction of the dominant hemisphere[5].

Organic mental disorders

Organic mental disorders (OMD) are extremely common in patients with AIDS, being seen in upwards of 70 per cent of all patients. They are classified as being either acute or chronic[6].

Acute organic mental disorders

Delirium is the major acute OMD seen in patients with AIDS and is characterized by an altered and/or fluctuating level of consciousness. Delirium has an acute onset and is secondary to underlying conditions seen in patients with AIDS, such as:

- CNS opportunistic infections
- Meningitis (e.g. atypical aseptic meningitis)

- HIV encephalopathy
- CNS neoplasms
- Seizure disorders and post-seizure states
- Septicaemia
- Cerebral hypoxia
- Electrolyte imbalance (e.g. hyponatraemia, hypokalaemia, hyper- or hypoglycaemia)
- Cerebral oedema
- Cerebrovascular infarction or haemorrhage
- Pyrexia
- Brain abscess
- Environmental factors (e.g. isolation, distress, sleep deprivation) Drugs (side-effects) and alcohol.

Typically, it resolves completely within a week without any ill effects.

Treatment is aimed at correcting the underlying cause and maintaining a safe environment for the patient during this period. Sedatives and analgesics should not be given during this episode as they further depress the cerebral cortex.

Chronic organic mental disorders

Chronic organic mental disorders are more frequently encountered in individuals infected with HIV than acute OMD. **Dementia** is the predominant chronic OMD seen in patients with AIDS and, like acute OMD, has a multifactorial aetiology, the causes including:

- HIV encephalopathy
- Progressive encephalitis due to other viruses (e.g. CMV, herpes simplex, varicella zoster and JC virus)
- Space-occupying lesions caused by B-cell lymphoma or (rarely) Kaposi's sarcoma
- Space-occupying lesions caused by infectious agents (e.g. *Candida albicans, Toxoplasma gondii, Cryptococcus neoformans*)
- Cerebrovascular accidents.

The most common cause of dementia is the direct effect of HIV infection on either cerebral cortical or subcortical structures of the brain. This is referred to as **HIV encephalopathy** (AIDS dementia complex, or ADC).

Dementia due to HIV encephalopathy has an insidious onset. There is a progressive loss of cognitive function, beginning with problems coping with complicated tasks and ending with a bedbound, incontinent individual. A careful nursing assessment will reveal various indicators of cortical dysfunction (Table 8.2). The clinical staging of HIV encephalopathy is described in Table 8.3.

The objective of medical management is to treat the underlying cause. Zidovudine (Retrovir – AZT) may produce significant improvement in patients with HIV encephalopathy.

Opportunistic infections of the CNS

Opportunistic CNS infections account for many of the neurological syndromes seen in individuals with AIDS. The most frequent causes of opportunistic CNS infections in patients with AIDS are:

- *Toxoplasma gondii*
- *Cryptococcus neoformans*
- Herpes simplex
- Cytomegalovirus
- *Candida albicans*
- *Mycobacterium tuberculosis*
- *Mycobacterium avium-intracellulare*
- Papovavirus

Table 8.3 Clinical staging of HIV encephalopathy

Stage	Characteristics
Stage 0 (normal)	Normal mental and motor function
Stage 0.5 (equivocal/ subclinical)	Either minimal or equivocal evidence of motor impairment; can work and perform activities of daily living
Stage 1.0 (mild)	Unequivocal evidence of functional impairment; able to do all but demanding tasks
Stage 2.0 (moderate)	Cannot work but can perform basic activities of self-care
Stage 3.0 (severe)	Major intellectual incapacity or motor disability
Stage 4.0 (end stage)	Nearly vegetative

Toxoplasma gondii

Intracerebral abscess caused by the protozoon *Toxoplasma gondii* is one of the most common opportunistic CNS infections seen in patients with AIDS. It is manifested by an insidious onset of confusion and lethargy prior to the development of focal neurological deficits (e.g. seizures) or a diminished level of consciousness. The clinical diagnosis is confirmed by head computerized tomography (CT) scans, magnetic resonance imaging (MRI) scans and lumbar puncture. CT scans frequently demonstrate cerebral ring-enhancing lesions and MRI scans may be positive. CNS fluid from lumbar punctures may show an increased concentration of protein (i.e. more than 20–45 mg/100 ml) and it may be possible to isolate the organism from the CSF. However, lumbar puncture may be contraindicated due to the risk of 'coning'.

A toxoplasma serology (indirect immunofluorescence assay or Sabin–Feldmann dye inclusion test) may be positive and a brain biopsy may be required to confirm the diagnosis. Treatment of CNS toxoplasma infection incorporates the use of pyrimethamine and sulfadiazine. Clindamycin, spiramycin and sulfadoxine may also be used[7]. Dexamethasone or mannitol and/or diuretics are given if there is cerebral oedema. Maintenance treatment is required for the rest of the patient's life as relapse after cessation of treatment is common. Maloprim, a combination of dapsone (a bacteriostatic sulphone) and pyrimethamine, is commonly used for maintenance therapy. Toxoplasma infection of the CNS is associated with a high mortality in patients with AIDS. Toxoplasma may also cause visual dysfunction (chorioretinitis).

Cryptococcus neoformans

A granulomatous meningitis, with granulomas or cysts developing in the cerebral hemispheres, typically results from cryptococcal fungal infection of the CNS. Patients present with a history of headache, high fever, nausea and vomiting and photophobia. Some may also experience seizures. CNS fluid from lumbar puncture may be normal or show an increased number of cells (pleocytosis), increased protein and a lowered glucose content (i.e. less than 50–100 mg/100 ml). CT scans are usually normal, although they may show hydrocephalus and/or cerebral atrophy. The diagnosis is confirmed by indian ink staining of CSF fluid, cultures of CSF or the detection of cryptococcal antigens in CSF fluid or serum.

Medical treatment consists of amphotericin B and 5-flucytosine by intravenous infusion through a central line. Amphotericin B has significant side-effects, which include rigors, fever and renal damage (e.g. hypokalaemia). Antihistamine cover with chlorpheniramine maleate (Piriton®) is common while patients are being treated with amphotericin B. Relapse is common and can be predicted by a rise in serum cryptococcal antigen titre. Therefore, monthly maintenance treatment (with the same drugs via a peripheral line) for the rest of the patient's life is usual. Fluconazole (Diflucan®) is now replacing amphotericin B and 5-flucytosine as the treatment of choice for cryptococcal meningitis as it can be given either orally or intravenously and has few side-effects. Therapy with fluconazole is initiated with a single dose of 400 mg (either orally or intravenously) on the first day, followed by 200 mg once daily for 10–12 weeks after the CSF has become culture negative. Like CNS toxoplasma infection, cryptococcal CNS infection is associated with a high mortality rate in patients with AIDS.

Herpes simplex virus

Disseminated infection with herpes simplex virus frequently causes an encephalitis. Typical signs may include lethargy, alterations in level of consciousness, muscle weakness and/or paresis, seizures, disturbances of balance and personality changes. The clinical diagnosis may be confirmed by atraumatic lumbar puncture, which may show the presence of erythrocytes in the CSF and, if necessary, by recovery of the virus (or immunological techniques to demonstrate the virus) from cerebral tissue obtained by brain biopsy (the virus rarely being present in the CSF). The antiviral drug acyclovir will treat this condition effectively in most patients.

Cytomegalovirus (CMV)

Chorioretinitis, leading to impaired visual acuity in patients with AIDS, is most frequently caused by cytomegalovirus. CMV may also cause encephalitis. CT scans may demonstrate ring-enhancing lesions. The specific medical treatment for CMV conditions is the antiviral drug ganciclovir. Foscarnet (Fascavir®) may also be used.

Mycobacteria and *Candida albicans*

Both of these opportunists may cause mass CNS lesions (CT scans showing ring-enhancing lesions). *Mycobacterium tuberculosis* causes tuberculous meningitis or tuberculomas. *Mycobocterium avium-intracellulare* may also cause CNS infection. Treatment is with maximum antituberculosis chemotherapy (e.g. ansamycin, clofazimine, cycloserine, ethionamide and ethambutol) and, possibly, corticosteroids. Systemic candidiasis, caused by *Candida albicans* may also manifest as meningitis. Fluconazole, amphotericin B (and, sometimes, 5-flucytosine) are used to treat this condition.

Papovavirus (JC virus)

Infection with papovavirus may cause **progressive multifocal leucoencephalopathy (PML)** in patients with AIDS. PML has a gradual or insidious onset, the patient frequently presenting with hemiparesis progressive intellectual impairment, aphasia, dysarthria and hemianopia. CT scans and EEG may be useful in confirming this diagnosis but the definitive diagnostic investigation is identifying the JC virus in brain tissue (obtained by brain biopsy), using immunofluorescence antibody (IFA) staining or electron microscopic agglutination. The course of this disease is relentlessly progressive, the duration from onset of symptoms to death being usually 1–4 months. Cytosine or adenine arabinoside have been helpful in treatment in a few cases. However, there is currently no effective therapy for most individuals who develop PML.

CNS neoplastic diseases

Approximately 5 per cent of patients with AIDS develop CNS neoplasms. The most common is **B-cell lymphomas**, usually primary but may be secondary to systemic lymphomas. CNS neoplasms, due to **Kaposi's sarcoma**, may also occur and cause CNS bleeding.

Space-occupying lesions often present with a history of weakness, lethargy or confusion and focal neurological deficits or seizures.

Diagnostic tests include CT and MRI scans and examination of CSF fluid. Additionally, brain biopsy may be undertaken. *Toxoplasma gondii* infection may also cause mass lesions in the CNS and this diagnosis should be excluded as it is a potentially treatable CNS infection. Often patients are treated empirically for *T. gondii* infection for a month to see if there is an improvement which may save the patient from requiring a brain biopsy.

Standard anti-cancer drugs (e.g. vincristine, vinblastine and etoposide – VP-16) do not readily cross the blood–brain barrier and treatment consists of total head deep X-ray treatment (DXT) by external beam radiotherapy. Dexamethasone or mannitol and/or diuretics are given to counteract the initial cerebral oedema caused by DXT.

Cerebrovascular disorders

CNS bleeding related to emboli from non-bacterial endocarditis, immune thrombocytopenic purpura (ITP) or cerebral arteritis, is sometimes seen in patients with AIDS.

Onset of symptoms is usually abrupt with headache followed by steadily increasing neurological deficits. Hemiparesis is seen in major bleeds located in the hemispheres. Symptoms of cerebellar or brainstem dysfunction (e.g. conjugate eye deviation or ophthalmoplegia, stertorous breathing, pinpoint pupils and coma) occur when the bleed is located in the posterior fossa. Nausea and vomiting, focal or generalized seizures and loss of consciousness are all common.

The diagnosis is made by CT scans. Lumbar puncture is usually contraindicated as the change in CSF pressure during lumbar puncture may precipitate transtentorial herniation.

Treatment is symptomatic.

Caring for patients with neuropsychiatric syndromes

The problems associated with neuropsychiatric syndromes can be summarized as shown in Table 8.4.

Objectives of care

The primary objectives of care are to:

- maintain a safe environment in which the patient can recover;
- prevent complications from neurological assault;
- maintain vital functions; patent airway;
- provide support to the patient, family and friends;
- assist the patient to regain maximum independence; and
- assist the patient to meet self-care requisites.

Nursing intervention

Assessment

A functionally orientated nursing neurological evaluation, as

Table 8.4 Problems associated with neuropsychiatric syndromes

Problem	Origin of problem
Actual problems	
Alterations in maintaining self-care requisites	Nervous system dysfunction
Potential problems	
Fever, headache, nausea and vomiting, drowsiness, stiff neck	CNS opportunistic infections and meningeal inflammation
Alterations in level of consciousness, focal neurological signs, seizures, paresis, personality changes	Cerebrovascular accidents and cerebral dysfunction
Pain, weakness and wasting in arms and legs, flaccidity and atrophy of legs, paraesthesia, facial paralysis	Peripheral neuropathy
Paraesthesia, weakness and spasticity of legs, ataxia, urinary incontinence	Vacuolar myelopathy
Erectile failure, diarrhoea, hypotension	Autonomic neuropathy
Muscular weakness, disorders of movement	Polyneuropathy
Impairment of reason, perception, intuition, memory, language and ability to learn	Subclinical cognitive dysfunction
Delirium, dementia, impaired cognitive function, incontinence	Organic mental disorders
Pressure sores	Incontinence, immobility
Emotional lability	Cerebral dysfunction
Disturbances in gait and sense of balance	Neuropathy, cerebellar dysfunction
Airway obstruction	Unconsciousness

described by Mitchell and Irvin[8], is useful in patient assessment (Table 8.5).

Table 8.5 Organization of a functionally oriented nursing neurological evaluation

General category	Functional category	Examples of specific function which may be tested
Consciousness	Arousing (reticular activating system)	Arousability, response to verbal and tactile stimuli
Mentation	Thinking (general cortical function plus specific regional functions)	Educational level Content of conversation Orientation Fund of information Insight, judgement, planning
	Feeling (affective)	Mood and affect Perception and reaction to ability, disability
	Language	Content and quantity of speech Ability to name objects Ability to repeat phrases Ability to read, write, copy
	Remembering	Attention span Recent and remote memory
Motor function	Seeing (cranial nerves II, III, IV, VI)	Acuity Visual fields Extra-ocular movement Pupil size, shape, reactivity Presence or absence of diplopia, nystagmus
	Eating (cranial nerves V, IX, X, XII)	Chewing Swallowing Gag (if swallowing impaired)
	Expressing facially (cranial nerve VII)	Symmetry of smile, frown
	Speaking (cranial nerves VII, IX, X, XII)	Clarity Presence or absence of nasality
	Moving (motor and cerebellar systems)	Muscle tone, mass, strength Presence or absence of involuntary movements

Table 8.5 *continued*

General category	Functional category	Examples of specific function which may be tested
		Coordination: heel-to-toe walk, observing during dressing Posture, gait, position
Sensory function	Smelling (cranial nerve I)	Ability to detect odours
	Blinking (cranial nerve V)	Corneal reflex
	Hearing (cranial nerve VIII)	Acuity, presence or absence of unusual sounds
	Feeling (sensory pathways)	Pain – pinprick Touch, stereognosis Temperature – warm, cold

Altered level of consciousness

Information for the nursing assessment will need to be obtained from a variety of sources, including family, friends and neighbours, as the patient will not be able to provide a reliable history. The assessment must take into consideration any medications or non-prescription drugs the patient may be using. A Glasgow Coma Scale[9,10] is initiated (Fig. 8.1) to compare changes in the patient's level of consciousness over a given period of time. This scale assesses three aspects of behavioural response – eye-opening, verbal response and motor response – which indicate the general functioning or dysfunction of the brain.

Eye-opening
Spontaneously – patient opens eyes when nurse approaches bed.
Opening to speech – patient opens eyes in response to his/her name, either at normal speaking voice or increased volume.
Opening to pain – patient opens eyes in response to painful stimuli.
No eye-opening – eyes do not open to speech or painful stimuli.

				Date								
				Time								
GLASGOW COMA SCALE	Eye opening		4. Spontaneously								Eyes closed due to swelling = C	
			3. To speech									
			2. To pain									
			1. None									
	Best verbal		5. Oriented								Endotracheal tube or tracheostomy = T	
			4. Confused									
			3. Inappropriate									
			2. Incomprehensible									
			1. None									
	Best motor		6. Obeys commands								Usually record best arm response	
			5. Localizes to pain									
			4. Flexion/withdrawal to pain									
			3. Abnormal flexion									
			2. Abnormal extension									
			1. None									
	Pupils	Right eye	Size								+ = Reacts − = No reaction C = Eyes closed	
			Reaction									
		Left eye	Size									
			Reaction									
LIMB MOVEMENT	Arms		Normal power								Record right (R) and left (L) separately if there is a difference between the two sides	
			Mild weakness									
			Severe weakness									
			Spastic flexion									
			Extension									
			No response									
	Legs		Normal power									
			Mild weakness									
			Severe weakness									
			Extension									
			No response									

Pupil scale mm

1 •
2 •
3 ●
4 ●
5 ●
6 ●
7 ●
8 ●

Blood pressure

Systolic = V
Diastolic = Λ
Blue   = Lying
Red   = Sitting
           Standing

Pulse = •
   (Red)

	BP/Pulse						Temp °C
	210						42
	200						41
	190						40
	180						39
	170						38
	160						37
	150						36
	140						35
	130						34
	120						33
	110						32
	100						31
	90						30
	80						
	70						
	60						
	50						Temperature = •
	40						(Blue)

Respirations = •
   (Blue)

	Resp						Temp
	30						30
	25						25
	20						20
	15						15
	10						10

Comments

Fig. 8.1 The Glasgow Coma Scale for the assessment of level of consciousness

Best verbal response
Response is recorded to simple, direct questions (light touch or painful stimuli may be used).

Best motor response
Response to commands to raise his/her arm or two fingers is noted. Asking the patient to grasp the nurse's fingers is unreliable as the grasp reflex may still be present.
Ability to localize pain is noted when the patient moves a limb in response to painful stimuli.
Flexion withdrawal to pain occurs when the arm bends at the elbow in response to painful stimuli (e.g. pressure on the patient's fingernail bed).
Abnormal flexion is noted and refers to the arm flexing at the elbow and the turning of the hand so that the palm faces downwards or backwards, making a fist (i.e. pronation).
Abnormal extension to pain occurs when the patient straightens the elbow and moves the arm away from the body (i.e. abduction), often with internal rotation, in response to painful stimuli to the fingernail bed.

Other responses assessed on the Glasgow Coma Scale are:

Pupils   Pupil size is measured by comparing it to the pupil scale on the chart and pupil reaction is measured in response to light (i.e. a direct beam from an ophthalmoscope or pen light). In health, pupils are of equal size and constrict briskly when stimulated by a direct beam of light.

Limb movement   Limb movement is assessed by noting the movement of both arms and legs to verbal commands or painful stimuli.
Weakness, either mild or severe, is noted by comparing one limb against the other.
Spastic flexion of the arms is noted if there is a slow, stiff movement of the arm, bending at the elbow and the hand held against the body.
Extension occurs when, in response to painful stimuli, the knee or elbow are straightened.
No response is recorded when there is no movement in response to painful and varied stimuli.

Vital signs   Vital signs are recorded frequently or continuously monitored. Potential problems associated with unconsciousness have been comprehensively described by Kim et al.[11] and are shown in Table 8.6.

Table 8.6 Potential problems relevant to the patient with an altered level of consciousness

Problem	Causative factors	Signs and symptoms
Altered sensation: Visual, auditory, kinaesthetic, gustatory, tactile and olfactory	Abnormal metabolic processes Supratentorial lesions Infratentorial lesions Psychogenic	Disoriented in time or place Disoriented with persons Altered abstraction Altered conceptualization Altered problem-solving abilities Altered behaviour or communication patterns Anxiety Irritability Reports auditory or visual hallucinations
Alterations in thought processes	Abnormal metabolic processes Supratentorial lesions Infratentorial lesions Psychogenic	Disorientation to time, place, person, circumstances and events Altered perception Lack of concentration Memory deficit Hyper/hypovigilance Impaired ability to make decisions Impaired ability to reason
Airway clearance ineffective	Loss of gag reflex Immobility Impaired perception and awareness	Cough ineffective Rapid respirations Râles and rhonchi present on auscultation of lungs Cyanosis Dyspnoea Secretions in oral pharynx
Impaired physical mobility	Neuromuscular impairment Immobilization Impaired perception or awareness	Altered muscle tone Decreased range of joint movement Impaired coordination Decreased muscle strength

Table 8.6   *continued*

Problem	Causative factors	Signs and symptoms
Potential for injury	Lack of awareness of environmental hazards Potential for complications from invasive therapeutic measures	Bruises and skin abrasions Altered mobility Impaired coordination Disorientation to circumstances and events
Potential impairment of skin integrity	Immobility Altered muscle tone/ spasticity Altered sensation Weight loss Inadequate nutrition Use of restraints, splints, and other devices Urinary incontinence	Redness, oedema, or breaks in skin Immobility Use of restraints, splints or other devices Spasticity Urinary incontinence Decreased sensation
Alterations in nutrition: less than body requirements	Immobility Loss of gag reflex Loss of control of voluntary movement Impaired awareness	Weight loss Decreased daily food/fluid intake Decreased skin thickness Aspiration of food/fluids
Alterations in patterns of urinary elimination: incontinence	Immobility Impaired awareness Sensory motor impairment Neuromuscular impairment	Involuntary voiding
Alteration in bowel elimination: incontinence	Immobility Neuromuscular impairment Impaired awareness Alteration in nutrition	Involuntary passage of stools
Self-care deficit: feeding, bathing/ hygiene, dressing/ grooming, toileting	Impaired perception and awareness Neuromuscular impairment Decreased strength and endurance	Inability to feed, bathe, dress, groom or toilet self Lack of coordination Inability to follow instructions

Assisting with self-care requisites

Patients with altered levels of consciousness and other manifestations of neurological dysfunction will need assistance with self-care requisites as described in Chapter 14. The need for a safe environment is paramount. Cot sides (bed-rails) are always kept in the upright position for patients with altered levels of consciousness and for patients who are confused. Special attention to the care of the eyes and mouth is vital, as is positioning. Unconscious patients are placed in the lateral or semiprone position and the body properly aligned. Patients must be turned every 2 hours and pressure area care given. They will require assistance with their need for adequate hydration and nutrition and for faecal and urinary elimination. Frequent reality orientation is essential.

Assistance with all self-care requisites is continuously evaluated and care continued or replanned according to the patient's response and the dynamics of the underlying neuropsychiatric processes.

Caring for patients with neuropsychiatric conditions in psychiatric hospitals

Patients may be safely and competently cared for in psychiatric hospitals, when appropriate. This requires aggressive in-service nursing education and the creation of policies and procedures for patients with HIV-related illness which are as thorough as those for district general hospitals.

From time to time it may be necessary to detain patients with neuropsychiatric syndromes in either district general hospitals or psychiatric hospitals, either to protect them from harm, or, more rarely, to protect the community. Patients may be detained in hospital either under the Mental Health Act of 1983 or the Public Health (Control of Diseases) Act of 1984 (inclusive of the statutory regulations made by the Secretary of State on 22 March 1986).

Mental Health Act 1983 (Part II)

The following sections of the Mental Health Act 1983 (Part II) can be used, if required, to detain a patient in hospital.

Section 2 A patient may be admitted to hospital for assessment, for a period not exceeding 28 days, either for his or her own health or safety, or with a view to the protection of other persons.

Section 4   A patient may be admitted to hospital for emergency assessment for a period of 72 hours.

Section 5   Under 5(2), a patient, who is already an in-patient in hospital, may be further detained in hospital for a period of 72 hours. This will allow the consultant in charge to have the patient detained on the ward and will give medical staff an opportunity to decide on further action and, if appropriate, application for detention under other sections of the Mental Health Act.

Further sections of the Act can be used to detain patients for varying periods of time.

Public Health (Control of Diseases) Act 1984

Statutory regulations made by the Secretary of State (22 March 1986) provide for AIDS being a notifiable disease for the purposes of Sections 35, 38, 43 and 44 of the Act. This Act allows for the provisions for compulsory medical examination and for compulsory removal of a patient to hospital, where the interest of the sufferer, his or her family and the public appear to justify that such action should be taken. Section 38 of the Act allows for the compulsory detention in hospital of a patient already in hospital.

Obviously, the detention of any citizen in hospital against his or her will is a serious event which, fortunately, is rarely required. However, there are circumstances when, either for the good of the patient or the good of the community, compulsory admission may be appropriate. It may be necessary initially to have the patient evaluated in a district general hospital to rule out treatable neurological syndromes (e.g. opportunistic CNS infections). If the patient is suffering from intercurrent psychosis (e.g. depressive or hypomanic phase of an existing manic depressive illness) or if a patient with a chronic psychosis develops AIDS and requires in-patient care, this care is best delivered in a psychiatric hospital.

Clearly, nurses have a profound duty to ensure that the legalities of compulsory admission have been properly enacted and to support the patient, family and friends during this frightening period.

Long-stay patients in psychiatric hospitals who are infected with HIV are, of course, able to sexually transmit this infection to other individuals. Sexual activity in psychiatric in-patients in long-stay units is probably quite common, perhaps compounded by the effect, of chronic psychosis which may diminish judgement and self-control[12]. Considerable vigilance is required from nursing staff to circumvent this risk. The potential risk of violence is always real in individuals who are frightened, confused and have an altered mental state.

References

1. Price, Richard W. and Worley, John M. (1994). Neurological complications of HIV-1 infection and AIDS. In *Textbook of AIDS Medicine*, eds Broder, S., Merigan, T.C. Jr. and Bolognesi, D., Williams & Wilkins, Baltimore, MD, pp. 489–505.
2. Carne, C.A. (1987). ABC of AIDS: Neurological manifestations. *British Medical Journal*, 30 May, **294** 1399–401.
3. Ho, D., Rota, T.R., Schooley, R.T. *et al.* (1985). Isolation of HTLV-III from cerebrospinal fluid and neural tissue of patients with neurologic syndromes related to the acquired immunodeficiency syndrome. *New England Journal of Medicine* **313** 1493–7.
4. Rosenblum, M.L., Levy, R.M. and Bredesen, D.E. (1988). *AIDS and the Nervous System*. Raven Press, New York.
5. Wolcott, D., Fawzy, F. and Pasnau, R. (1985). Acquired immune deficiency syndrome (AIDS) and consultation–liaison psychiatry. *General Hospital Psychiatry* **7**, 280–92.
6. Egan, V. (1992). Neuropsychological aspects of HIV infection: Editorial review. *AIDS Care* **4**(1), 3–10.
7. Israelski, D.M. and Remington, J.S. (1992). AIDS-associated toxoplasmosis. In *The Medical Management of AIDS*, 2nd edn, eds Sande, M.A. and Volberding, P.A., W.B. Saunders, London, pp. 319–45.
8. Mitchell, P.H. and Irvin, N. (1977). Neurological examination: nursing assessment for nursing purposes. *Journal of Neurosurgical Nursing* **9**(1), 23–8.
9. Teasdale, G. (1975). Acute impairment of brain function – Part 1, Assessing conscious level. *Nursing Times* **71**(24), 914–17.
10. Teasdale, G., Galbraith, S. and Clarke, K. (1975). Acute impairment of brain function – Part 2, Observation record chart. *Nursing Times* **71**(25), 972–3.
11. Kim, M.J., McFarland, G.K. and McLane, A.M. (eds) (1984). *Pocket Guide to Nursing Diagnosis*. C.V. Mosby, St Louis.
12. Fenton, T.W. (1986). AIDS and psychiatry: practical, social and ethical issues – practical problems in the management of AIDS-related psychiatric disorder. *Journal of the Royal Society of Medicine*, May, **80**(5), 271–4.

Further reading

Dilley, J.W. (1992). Management of neuropsychiatric disorders in HIV-spectrum patients. In *The Medical Management of AIDS*, 3rd edn, eds Sande, M.A. and Volberding, P.A., W.B. Saunders, London (ISBN 0-7216-6752-X).

Holland, J.C., Jacobsen, P., Breitbart, W. (1992). Psychiatric and psychosocial aspects of HIV infection. In *AIDS: Etiology, Diagnosis, Treatment and Prevention*, 3rd edn, eds DeVita, V.T. Jr., Hellman, S. and Rosenberg, S.A., J.B. Lippincott, Philadelphia, (ISBN 0-397-51229-5).

Koppel, B.S. (1992). Neurological complications of AIDS and HIV infection: An overview. In *AIDS and Other Manifestations of HIV Infection*, ed. Wormser, Gary P., Raven Press, New York (ISBN 0-88167-881-3).

Lechtenberg, R. and Hollenberg Sher, J. (1988). *AIDS in the Nervous System*. Churchill Livingstone, London (ISBN 0-443-08616-8).

Price, Richard W. and Worley, John M. (1994). Neurological complications of HIV–1 infection and AIDS. In *Textbook of AIDS Medicine*, eds Broder, S., Merigan, T.C. Jr. and Bolognesi, D., Williams & Wilkins, Baltimore, MD, (ISBN 0-683-01072-7).

Rosenblum, M.L., Levy, R.M. and Bredesen, D.E. (1988). *AIDS and the Nervous System*. Raven Press, New York (ISBN 0-88167-259-9).

Worley, J.M. and Price, R.W. (1992). Management of the Neurologic Complications of HIV–1 Infection and AIDS. In *The Medical Management of AIDS*, 3rd edn, eds Sande, M.A. and Volberding, P.A., W.B. Saunders, London (ISBN 0-7216-6752-X).

9

Acute Viral Hepatitis and HIV Disease

Acute viral hepatitis, the characteristic inflammation of the liver, can be caused by many infectious and non-infectious agents, but the most common causes are viruses. Currently (1994), there are seven viruses recognized as causing acute hepatitis. Two are **herpes – viruses** cytomegalovirus (CMV) and Epstein–Barr virus (EBV) – and the remaining five are **hepatotropic viruses**:

- Hepatitis A virus (HAV)
- Hepatitis B virus (HBV)
- Hepatitis C virus (HCV)
- Hepatitis D virus (HDV) (Delta)
- Hepatitis E virus (HEV)
- ? Other non-A, non-B hepatitis viruses.

Hepatitis A virus (HAV)

Hepatitis A virus has an RNA genome and is transmitted enterically (faecal–oral route of transmission). HAV is only found in faeces and this virus is not present in the blood or other body fluids. Infection with HAV is most common where sanitation and hygiene are poor, and as these improve, as has happened in the developed world, the incidence of infection and the prevalence of natural antibody to this virus, fall. In the UK, a high proportion of people (around 70 per cent in some regions) reach the age of 50 years without acquired natural antibodies to hepatitis A and so remain susceptible to infection. HAV can also be transmitted sexually, e.g. oral–anal sexual activity.

HAV disease has a short incubation period, symptoms starting to present within 10–15 days following exposure. Complete recovery usually occurs within 24 weeks and progression to chronic hepatitis is rarely, if ever, seen. The severity of the illness ranges from asymptomatic infection, through clinical hepatitis (with or without jaundice) to fulminant hepatic failure. In areas of high prevalence, most children have antibodies to HAV by the age of 3, and these infections are generally asymptomatic or very mild. In later life, infections tend to be more serious: 70–80 per cent of adults develop jaundice, preceded typically by malaise, anorexia, nausea and fever. Patients over 49 years of age, and those with existing liver disease have a higher risk of both morbidity and mortality.

Following primary infection, IgM antibodies to HAV appear and are present for some months, before disappearing, being replaced by IgG HAV antibodies. The presence of IgM antibodies is indicative of primary infection, whereas the presence of IgG antibodies indicates previous exposure and immunity from further attacks.

HAV infection is not associated with a carrier state. Faecal excretion of the virus declines rapidly once clinical symptoms appear and usually ceases within 2 weeks of the onset of clinical hepatitis. HAV infection is prevalent throughout the world and is maintained in the human population through oral–faecal contamination routes. Passive immunization is available from the use of **human normal immunoglobulin (HNIG)** and, since April 1992, active immunization is available by the use of a new **inactivated virus vaccine** (Havrix® – SmithKline Beecham). Individuals should be tested for anti-HAV IgG prior to either form of immunization if time allows and if they are over 50 years of age (especially if they have lived overseas) or have a history of jaundice.

Hepatitis E virus (HEV)

This virus also has an RNA genome and is similarly transmitted enterically. It is clinically and epidemiologically similar to HAV infection. The incubation period is probably the same as in HAV infection. However, this virus has only been identified within the last 3–4 years and much is still unknown. It is probably the major cause of community-acquired, enterically transmitted non-A, non-B hepatitis in the developing world.

Epidemics caused by HEV have been described recently in which the infection was mild and self-limiting in all those infected, except pregnant women, in whom high mortality rates (up to 40 per cent) may be seen[1]. This virus is endemic in tropical and subtropical developing countries, where infection is highly associated with contaminated water. HEV infection is probably not associated with a carrier state or progression to chronic liver disease.

Hepatitis B virus (HBV)

Hepatitis B virus infection is uniquely dangerous in that primary infection is associated with an impressive titre of virus in the blood, e.g. 500 μg/ml of viral antigen and 10 trillion extra viral particles (surface antigen, also known as **Australia antigen**) in each millilitre of blood[2]. HBV has a DNA genome with at least four distinct, intimately related Ag–Ab (antigen–antibody) systems (Fig. 9.1).

HBV surface antigen (HBsAg)   This is associated with the viral surface coat; its presence in serum usually provides the first evidence of acute HBV infection. Excess viral coat protein (HBsAg, or 'Australia antigen') is produced and these extra pieces of HBsAg outnumber the intact hepatitis B virion (the **Dane particle**). HBsAg characteristically appears during the incubation period, usually 1–6 weeks before

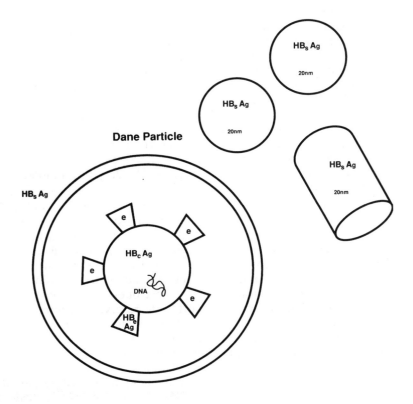

Fig. 9.1   Structure of the hepatitis B virus

clinical or biochemical illness develops, and disappears during convalescence. The corresponding Ab (anti-HBs) appears only weeks or months later, after clinical recovery, and usually persists for life. In up to 10 per cent of patients, HBsAg persists after acute infection and anti-HBs does not develop. These patients usually develop chronic hepatitis or become asymptomatic carriers of the virus.

HBcAg (core Ag)   This is associated with the viral inner core. Antibody to the core appears at the onset of clinical illness, with gradually diminishing titres thereafter, usually for years or life.

HBeAg (the 'e' Ag)   This appears to be a peptide derived from the viral core. It is found only in HBsAg+ serum and its presence reflects more active viral replication and is generally associated with greater infectivity of blood (and other body fluids, e.g. semen) and a greater likelihood of progression to chronic liver disease. In contrast, presence of the corresponding Ab (anti-HBe) points to relatively lower infectivity and usually portends a benign outcome.

HDV (hepatitis delta virus)   This is a unique, defective RNA virus that can replicate only in the presence of HBV, **never alone!** It occurs as either a co-infection with acute HBV infection or a superinfection in established chronic hepatitis B. Injecting drug users are at a relatively high risk of acquiring HDV infection in Europe and North America. In other parts of the world, HDV is more commonly acquired following sexual exposure. Clinically, HDV infection is typically manifested by unusually severe (e.g. fulminant) acute hepatitis B; acute exacerbation in chronic HBV carriers (superinfection); or a relatively aggressive course of chronic hepatitis B. Hepatitis D infection is diagnosed by detecting antibodies to the virus (**anti-HDV**) in the blood.

HBV is found in almost every body fluid, e.g. blood, saliva, tears, seminal fluid, cerebrospinal fluid, breast milk and urine. HBV is transmitted parenterally, typically by contaminated blood or blood products. Non-parenteral spread occurs, including sexual transmission between both heterosexual and homosexual partners. Sexual exposure is the most frequent method of transmission in the UK. The role of transmission by insect bites remains unclear. Chronic HBV carriers provide a worldwide reservoir of infection. Vertical transmission, i.e. infected mother to child, either *in utero*, intrapartum or post-partum (breast milk), also occurs and, in some parts of the developing world and the Far East, is the most important mode of HBV perpetuation in the population.

HBV infection is diagnosed by identifying HBsAg in blood and its presence indicates **acute primary HBV infection**. The corresponding antibody, **anti-HBs,** appears after recovery and persists for life.

Consequently, its presence indicates previous exposure and immunity from further attacks.

The incubation period ranges from 50 to 160 days following exposure to the virus. Progression to chronic liver disease will occur in 5–10 per cent of patients. HBV disease is one of the most serious, persistent viral infections on earth, infecting 200 million people worldwide, and is second only to HIV infection in causing morbidity and mortality.

Active immunization with a genetically derived HBsAg (Engerix B® – Smith, Kline & French) and passive immunization with hepatitis B immunoglobulin are both available.

Hepatitis C virus (HCV)

Hepatitis C virus has an RNA genome and, like HBV, is transmitted parenterally. Sexual transmission of HCV does occur, albeit rarely[3]. However, coexisting HIV infection may increase the efficiency of sexually transmitting hepatitis C virus[4].

Hepatitis C virus is a major cause of post-transfusion, non-A, non-B hepatitis in the world and has an incubation period of approximately 8 weeks. (Note: This is shorter than HBV disease.) HCV infection is diagnosed by identifying antibodies to the virus (**anti-HCV**) in the blood. Although the disease is clinically similar to HBV hepatitis, the acute phase is usually less severe. Up to 50 per cent of HCV-infected patients will progress to chronic liver disease, often benign and subclinical. However, 20 per cent of these patients will eventually develop cirrhosis[5].

Nursing assessment

The nursing history and ongoing nursing observations will elicit the typical signs and symptoms of acute viral hepatitis (Table 9.1).

Nursing intervention

The treatment of acute viral hepatitis is symptomatic and nursing interventions are focused on predictable patient problems, including activity intolerance, altered nutrition and potential fluid volume deficit. Ongoing evaluation of care and continuing nursing observations will detect signs of complications, especially **fulminant hepatitis with encephalopathy** (Table 9.2). This is a rare condition, often

Table 9.1   Acute viral hepatitis: clinical presentation[2,5-7]

Pre-icteric phase
'Prodromal' or incubation phase occurs 3–10 days before the onset of jaundice

Sudden onset: Progressive worsening of anorexia, malaise, nausea and vomiting, fever, distaste for cigarette smoking (if a smoker)
Sometimes urticarial, pruritic hives, maculopapular lesions and/or fleeting, irregular patches of erythema; arthralgias occasionally occur, especially in HBV infection
Myalgias, chills and right, upper quandrant abdominal pain may occur

Icteric phase
Lasts 1–3 weeks

Jaundice: Dark urine and jaundice: eyes show scleral icterus, and faeces may be clay-coloured
Temperature usually normal, as are vital signs, however there may be a bradycardia if the patient has severe hyperbilirubinaemia
Serum bilirubin may increase to 20 times normal; hepatic transaminases levels (AST, ALT) may increase to 100 times normal and an increase in alkaline phosphatase (1–3 times normal) may also be seen
Systemic symptoms begin to regress and the patient feels better, despite worsening jaundice

Recovery phase
Jaundice gradually recedes during a 2–4 week recovery phase

---

associated with HBV or HCV infection. Although survival from this complication is rare, it does occur, usually because of highly skilled nursing care. Patient education initiatives might centre on reducing risk to other bloodborne viruses, i.e. safer sexual behaviour and harm-reduction techniques used for injecting drugs. Hepatitis B immunization may be indicated.

Medical treatment of acute viral hepatitis

There is no specific treatment for acute viral hepatitis. If HBV or HCV infection become chronic, alpha-interferon may be prescribed. It is only given subcutaneously, daily for up to 6 months[7]. During acute illness, supportive treatment focuses on intravenous fluid replacement, anti-emetics, mild analgesia if required, and antipyretics. Drugs which are potentially hepatotoxic, e.g. paracetamol (USA

Table 9.2   Fulminant hepatitis with encephalopathy[5,6]

Onset:	Sudden rapid clinical deterioration with the onset of hepatic encephalopathy. Patient becomes lethargic and somnolent, with personality and behavioural changes. Coma may develop within hours. An early sign is **asterixis**, the irregular flapping of forcibly dorsiflexed, outstretched hands. Bleeding is common, resulting from liver failure and DIC (disseminated intravascular coagulation). An increasing prothrombin time is a grave prognostic indicator
Prognosis:	Meticulous nursing care and competent medical management of each specific complaint is required. Survival in adults is rare, although when it does occur, survivors recover completely without permanent liver damage

– acetaminophen) should be avoided, as should alcohol. There is no substantial evidence to suggest that either dietary or activity restrictions have any benefit for patients with acute hepatitis. The patient's appetite usually returns to normal during the icteric phase.

Infection control

Universal Precautions or Body Substance Isolation are sufficient to prevent nosocomial transmission in health care settings. Needlestick and other sharp instrument injuries are extremely serious, as the risk of acquiring hepatitis B infection from a patient with active disease is far greater than the risk of HIV acquisition. This is evidenced by a case where a needlestick injury involved a patient infected with both HIV and HBV. Hepatitis B virus was transmitted to the health care worker, but HIV was not[9].

Relationship of hepatotropic viruses to HIV infection

Active HBV infection is present in approximately 10 per cent of HIV-infected patients (some, co-infected with HDV)[10]. Patients with HIV disease who are negative for serological markers of previous HBV infection should be considered for active immunization, although their response to vaccination may be variable, depending on the degree of immunosuppression that exists at the time of immunization.

Co-infection with HCV is very common (> 50 per cent) among HIV-infected injecting drug users and haemophiliacs[11,12].

Re-activation of hepatitis B virus infection during the course of HIV disease has been well documented[8] and the severity of the disease is impressive. Liver failure and death may quickly result from this event. The usual serological markers for HBV infection, i.e. HBsAg, may be absent in re-activating hepatitis in patients who are co-infected with HIV, and physicians may need to test for HBV DNA.

References

1. Anon. (1990). Editorials: The A to F of viral hepatitis. *Lancet*, 10 November, **336**(8724), 1158–60.
2. Dienstag, J.L., Wands, J.R. and Illselbacher, K.J. (1991). Acute hepatitis. In *Harrison's Principles of Internal Medicine*, 12th edn, International Edition, eds Wilson, J.D., Braunwald, E., Isselbacher, K.J. *et al.*, McGraw-Hill, London, pp. 1322–37.
3. Skidmore, S.J., Collingham, K.E. and Drake, S.M. (1994). Brief report: Sexual transmission of hepatitis C. *Journal of Medical Virology* **42**, 247–8.
4. Eyster, M.E., Alter, J.J., Aledort, L.M. *et al.* (1991). Heterosexual co-transmission of hepatitis C virus and human immunodeficiency virus. *Annals of Internal Medicine* **115**, 764–8.
5. Berkow, R. and Fletcher, A.J. (1992). *The Merck Manual of Diagnosis and Therapy*, 16th edn. Merck Research Laboratories, Rahway, NJ, pp. 897–904.
6. Grimes, D. (1991). *Infectious Diseases*. Mosby-Year Book, St Louis, pp. 105–15.
7. Paar, D.P. (1994). Hepatitis. In *HIV: Manual For Health Care Professionals*, eds Muma, R.D., Lyons, B.A., Borucki, M.J. and Pollard, R.D., Appleton & Lange, Norwalk, CT, pp. 77–86.
8. McNair, A., Main, J., Goldin, R. *et al.* (1994). Liver disease and AIDS. In *Textbook of AIDS Medicine*, eds Broder, S., Merigan, T.C. and Bolognesi, D., Williams & Wilkins, Baltimore, MD, pp. 581–95.
9. Gerberding, J.L., Hopewell, P.C., Kamingky, L.S. *et al.* (1985). Transmission of hepatitis B without transmission of AIDS by accidental needlestick. *New England Journal of Medicine* **312**, 56.
10. Wormser, G.P. and Horowitz, H. (1992). Care of the adult patient with HIV infection. In *AIDS and Other Manifestations of HIV Infection*, 2nd edn, ed. Wormser, G.P., Raven Press, New York, p. 177.
11. Wormser, G.P., Forseter, G., Joline, C. *et al.* (1991). Hepatitis C in HIV-infected intravenous drug users and homosexual men in suburban New York City. *Journal of the American Medical Association* **265** 2958.
12. Esteban, J., Esteban, R., Viladomio, L. *et al.* (1989). Hepatitis C virus antibodies among risk groups in Spain. *Lancet* **2**, 294–7.

10

The Impact of HIV Infection on Women

A decade ago, women and children seemed to be on the periphery
of the AIDS epidemic. Today, . . . women and children are at the
centre of our concern. AIDS has not spared them. On the contrary,
the epidemic wave has affected millions of women and their
children, and millions more are threatened.

Dr Michael Merson, Executive Director, WHO Global
Programmes on AIDS 1993

Introduction

All over the world, AIDS is becoming a leading cause of death among
women. In many societies, in many cultures, being a woman is a
significant risk factor for HIV acquisition. As more and more women
become infected with HIV, an ever increasing number of children will
be born, similarly infected with this virus, eventually being robbed of
their mothers, their childhood and ultimately, their lives. Uninfected
children will be destined to the world of the 'AIDS orphans'. Women
are central to the concept of family; to nurturing, protecting and
caring. They have complex relationships and structures in their daily
lives and sophisticated and subtle responsibilities and commitments.
Their demise, consequent to HIV disease, will increasingly rock the
stability of communities in every country where AIDS exists.

Epidemiology

By mid-1994, the World Health Organization (WHO) estimated that
there were over 3 million adolescent and adult persons with AIDS
in the world and over 16 million adolescents and adults infected with
either HIV-1 or HIV-2[1], including at least 5 million women[2]. By
the year 2000, there will be almost 40 million persons in the world infected with HIV, including 2.3 million children[2,3]. Approximately
one-third of current AIDS cases, i.e. 1 million, are women, and, by

the year 2000, it is estimated that the number of men and women infected will be equal globally, i.e. 20 million women infected[4]. More than 1 million women became infected in 1993 alone and at least 4 million women will have died as a result of HIV infection within the next five years[5].

Risk factors and female vulnerabilities

As a group, women are more vulnerable to becoming infected with HIV than are men for a variety of reasons, including socio-economic status, biological influences, sexual practices and epidemiological factors.

Socio-economic status

Women may be both socially and culturally vulnerable to HIV infection as they are often economically dependent on men. Throughout the world, their status is lower than that of men and they have fewer opportunities for education and to acquire financial independence and personal freedom. This often means that they have little power or control over decisions relating to the sexual behaviour of their partner, e.g. condoms and safer sex, and accessing primary prevention information. Women are vulnerable to coerced sex, including marital and non-marital rape, sexual abuse in and outside of the family, and/or being forced into the sex industry. In most cultures, women are expected to be passive and submissive in their sexual relationships, which are invariably controlled by men. They lack the skills and confidence to discuss sexual behaviour with their partners and have little bargaining power within their sexual relationships. This sexual subordination of women makes it impossible for them to protect themselves from sexually transmitted HIV infection. In many industrialized countries, such as in Western Europe and North America, injecting drug use is a major contributor to HIV infection in women. However, heterosexual exposure to the virus in these countries will soon come to dominate the mode of transmission.

Biological influences

Men are more efficient at transmitting HIV to women than are women to men, and women are biologically more vulnerable to HIV infection than are men. As the receptive partner, women have a larger mucosal surface exposed during sexual intercourse.

In addition, semen contains a higher volume and concentration of virus than that present in vaginal or cervical secretions. The presence of covert, pelvic inflammatory disease or genital infection increases the risk of HIV acquisition, as does any factor which disrupts the vaginal or cervical epithelium, e.g. sexual trauma, chemical damage, hormonal influences, etc. Other factors which have been implicated in increasing the susceptibility of women to HIV infection include cervical ectopy, use of oral contraceptives, defloration, dyspareunia (painful coitus), perimenopausal status, and the use of intrauterine devices (IUD) for contraception[6,7].

Young women are particularly susceptible to infection as their genital tract is not mature at the time they begin to menstruate. The mucous membrane changes from being a thin, single layer of cells to a thick, multi-layer wall. This transition may not be completed until their late teens or early twenties. The intact but immature genital tract surface in young women is less efficient as a barrier to HIV than the mature genital tract of older women. Finally, in postmenopausal women, the mucous membrane becomes thinner and so it is also a less efficient barrier to the virus[8].

Sexual practices and epidemiological factors

Women tend to have sex with, and often marry, men who are older then they are. Men usually have had more partners (and more opportunities to become infected) than the women with whom they have sex. Consequently, women are becoming infected at an earlier age than are men and are being diagnosed as having AIDS when they are, on average, 10 years younger than men[8]. Sex during menses and anal sex increases the risk of HIV infection if the male partner is infected. The disease stage and immunological status of the infected male partner influences the risk; the danger to the female is greatest either during early male primary infection or when the male partner has symptomatic (late) HIV disease.

Women are also vulnerable to HIV infection via contaminated blood transfusions. Throughout the world, women are the major recipients of blood transfusions, which are used primarily to treat anaemia caused by repeated pregnancies and diseases, such as malaria, and to respond to the complications of childbirth, e.g. postpartum haemorrhage. Screening blood for HIV infection is beyond the reach of most developing countries, and this places the entire female community at considerable risk.

Drug use (both injectable and non-injectable drugs) increases the likelihood of entering into more high-risk sexual encounters in order to support their dependency, including prostitution. The feminization of poverty limits the economic options open to women, especially single mothers and young girls, and forces many into the sex industry. Here, it seems only a matter of time before they become infected. A comparatively new phenomenon of international sex tourism has, along with drug use, firmly seeded HIV infection in the South Pacific basin, an area where most of the world's population reside.

Rape, a common form of violence, perpetuated against women by men all over the world, adds to the risk of infection. The more violent the assault, the greater the peril of HIV transmission if the attacker is infected.

Health care problems in women with HIV disease

There often seems to be many barriers to early diagnosis and treatment for women, including poor access to health care facilities. In the industrialized countries of the world, women often do not perceive themselves as being at risk of HIV infection. This low index of suspicion is frequently mirrored in providers of health care for women, leading to a delay in establishing a correct diagnosis. Even in developing countries, a lack of targeted health education may leave many women unaware of early symptoms of HIV disease.

Women are prone to the same opportunistic infections and neoplasms seen in men (Chapter 6). *Candida* oesophagitis and *Pneumocystis carinii* pneumonia are the most frequent AIDS-defining events in women who are infected with HIV[9]. In addition, there are several gynaecological conditions which are now associated with HIV disease in women, including:

- **vulvovaginal candidiasis** – persistent, frequent or poorly responsive to treatment;
- **cervical dysplasia** – from moderate to invasive;
- **pelvic inflammatory disease** – especially those with tubo-ovarian abscess; and
- **herpes simplex lesion** – lasting more than 1 month.

Invasive cervical cancer

In 1993, the Centers for Disease Control and Prevention in the USA added **invasive cervical cancer** to the list of AIDS indicator diseases in the expanded surveillance case definition for AIDS[10]. Several studies had identified an increased prevalence of cervical dysplasia, a precursor lesion for cervical cancer, among HIV-infected women[11,12]. In addition, several studies have found that a higher prevalence of cervical dysplasia among HIV-infected women is associated with a greater degree of immunosuppression[12,13]. Finally, HIV infection may adversely affect the clinical course and treatment of cervical dysplasia and cancer[14,15].

Cervical dysplasia is caused by some strains of **human papillomavirus (HPV)** and is a precursor lesion for cervical cancer. HPV infection is a common sexually transmitted infection, and also causes anogenital warts (condyloma acuminata). Cervical dysplasia is usually asymptomatic but can be detected by gynaecological screening, including **Papanicolaou (Pap) smears**. HIV-infected women should have Pap smears every 6–12 months. Those with abnormal smears should be monitored more closely and treated more aggressively than women who are not infected with HIV[16]. Colposcopic biopsy may be more reliable than Pap smears in detecting intra-epithelial neoplasia in HIV-infected women and colposcopy should be performed following either inadequate or abnormal Pap smears[17,18].

Women with invasive cervical cancer may complain of abdominal pain, vaginal bleeding and discharge, and lymphadenopathy. A variety of treatment options are available for the various stages of cervical cancer, including local cone excision, cryotherapy and laser therapy. The treatment of choice for locally invasive disease is surgery[9,17].

Candidiasis

Recurrent **vulvovaginal candidiasis** is a common health care problem in women infected with HIV. There may be five or six recurrences a year, which may be treated by standard antifungal agents, such as clotrimazole, ketoconazole or fluconazole. If ketoconazole is prescribed, liver function should be monitored.

Pelvic inflammatory disease

Pelvic inflammatory disease (PID) refers to infection of the fallopian tubes (**salpingitis**), although the term is often used to include infections of the cervix (**cervicitis**), uterus (**endometritis**) and ovaries (**oophoritis**). PID is caused by a variety of pathogenic micro-organisms, including *Chlamydia trachomatis* and *Neisseria gonorrhoeae*. Numerous aerobic and anaerobic micro-organisms may also cause PID.

Women with PID present with progressively more severe, usually bilateral, lower abdominal pain. Fever, vaginal discharge and irregular vaginal bleeding are also associated with PID. Abscesses may develop in the fallopian tubes, involving the ovary (tubo-ovarian abscess) and the tubes (one or both) may fill with pus (pyosalpinx). Immediate treatment is with antibiotics, e.g. cefoxitin, ceftriaxone and/or doxycycline.

Sexual contacts of women with PID should be traced and examined, and treated if infected. Symptoms which persist, despite adequate treatment, may be a result of a progressively worsening immune status.

Herpes simplex lesion

In HIV-infected women, genital herpes infection caused by the herpes simplex virus may persist, disseminate and be more painful than lesions in women who are not infected with HIV[19]. Any lesion in an HIV-infected person puts their sexual partner(s) at an increased risk of HIV infection. Treatment is with acyclovir (Zovirax) and severe disease may require intravenous administration. Acyclovir-resistant strains of herpes simplex virus are not uncommon in women who are infected with HIV and other drugs may be prescribed, such as ganciclovir (Cymevene®) and foscarnet (Foscavir). If foscarnet is prescribed, nurses must ensure adequate hydration throughout therapy to minimize the risk of nephrotoxicity. Although acyclovir is remarkably free of side-effects, ganciclovir may cause neutropenia and the patient's white cell count must be closely monitored. Antibiotics may be prescribed if lesions are infected with other micro-organisms.

Pregnancy

Women who become infected with HIV tend to do so early in their reproductive years. On average, worldwide, about one-third of babies born to HIV-infected mothers are themselves infected[5]. There is no conclusive evidence to date that pregnancy accelerates disease progression in HIV-infected mothers and most clinicians agree that the risk is low[20]. However, the risk of pregnancy accelerating HIV disease is increased in those women with low CD4+ T-cell counts or with symptomatic disease.

Many women learn of their HIV status from prenatal screening. If infected with HIV, an assessment protocol can be used to monitor and screen for potential health care problems, such as that developed by the University of Texas Medical Branch at Galveston, Texas[18] (Table 10.1).

Aerosolized pentamidine may be used for PCP prophylaxis in pregnant women throughout their pregnancy. Sulphamethoxazole

Table 10.1   Evaluation of pregnant HIV-infected women[18]

Prenatal
Initial visit: Antibodies to toxoplasma and cytomegalovirus
                 Tuberculosis skin testing (Mantoux)
                 Cervical cultures for *Neisseria gonorrhoeae* and *Chlamydia trachomatis*
                 Hepatitis B surface antigen
                 VDRL
                 Cryptococcal antigen
                 Beta-2 microglobulin
                 SMA 12
Thereafter: CD4+ T-lymphocyte counts every 3 months (monthly if < 300 mm³)
                 Administer Pneumovax® vaccine

Delivery
Urine or cervical culture for cytomegalovirus
Repeat toxoplasma titres for seronegative patients

Prenatal and postpartum therapy
If CD4+ T-lymphocyte count < 500 mm³, discuss zidovudine (AZT) therapy
If CD4+ T-lymphocyte count < 200 mm³, encourage PCP prophylaxis and zidovudine therapy

may cause bilirubin toxicity and kernicterus in the infant and is generally reserved for PCP prophylaxis in the first and second trimesters only (aerosolized pentamidine being given in the third trimester)[9]. Zidovudine (AZT) treatment, especially if the woman's CD4+ T-lymphocyte count is <500 mm³, should be discussed fully so that she can make an informed decision as to potential benefits and risks.

Contraception

Women must have access to information in relation to contraception and surgical sterilization should neither be encouraged nor discouraged[18]. Various contraceptive methods are available[21].

Barriers

Male condom

HIV cannot pass through the intact latex membrane of the male condom[22]. However, some condoms allow leakage[23] and some fail physical tests to assess reliability[24]. In addition, oil-based lubricants, such as petroleum jelly, baby oil or lotion and oil-based vaginal preparations can damage condoms. Most condom failure is likely to be due to incorrect use rather than poor condom quality. Condoms can be ripped or split during use, be torn with fingernails or slip off before withdrawal. Some men find standard condoms too small or too difficult to put on. Larger size condoms are available and men can practise putting condoms on by themselves, outside of the stress and urgency of sexual intercourse.

Properly used, the condom is the only feasible way of reducing HIV transmission during oral or anal intercourse. Its main disadvantage is that the use of the male condom ultimately relies on men, and women may be unable to ensure that it is used.

Female condom

In recent years, a female condom, known as Femidom®, has been developed in the UK and marketed throughout the world. It is made from polyurethane, which is impermeable to HIV[25]. Femidom cannot be used without men knowing it is being used. Consequently, women may not even be in control of this protection as it will frequently require male permission. Because of its expense and general unavailability in the developing world, Femidom is unlikely to play a major role in HIV prevention, but for some women it increases the options.

Diaphragm and cervical cap

It is not certain what efficacy these methods have in preventing HIV transmission. However, case-control studies on cervical gonorrhoea and trichomoniasis suggest that their use might reduce transmission rates by 50 per cent[26]. Although these methods prevent semen from reaching the cervix, they offer no protection to the vagina.

Intra-uterine contraceptive device (IUD)

IUDs should be discouraged in women who are at risk of infection or who are already infected with HIV. Various studies have shown that the risk of male-to-female transmission of HIV was 3 times higher in couples using an IUD and the risk of women becoming infected was again trebled if they used an IUD[27,28].

Oral contraceptives

It is not clear whether oral contraception affects the risk of HIV infection or transmission. Studies in prostitutes using oral contraceptives show that the risk of HIV infection is doubled or trebled[29,30]. Other studies, in women who are not prostitutes, suggest that women are protected[31,32]. Both progestogen and progestogen plus oestrogen are weakly immunosuppressive. However, it is not clear if this is significant in relation to HIV infection[21].

Injectable contraceptives

It is not known if injectable progestogens, such as medroxy-progesterone acetate (Depo-Provera®) increase the risk of HIV infection or transmission[21].

Spermicides

The most commonly used spermicide in the UK is nonoxynol-9[33]. This spermicide can easily inactivate HIV and other viruses and bacteria *in vitro*[34,35]. However, research has not established the safety of spermicides containing nonoxynol-9, specifically with regard to local toxicity to the genital and rectal epithelia[36]. Studies in female prostitutes indicate that nonoxynol-9 may paradoxically increase the risk of HIV infection by causing vaginal irritation and microscopic mucosal breaks[37,38]. It is difficult to offer advice on this particular spermicide except that the above studies were conducted on women who used large amounts of nonoxynol-9 (in sponges). It is probable that ordinary use of products containing nonoxynol-9 as a sexual lubricant, e.g. C-Film®, Delfen®, Duragel®, etc., and male condoms which are pre-lubricated with nonoxynol-9, offer additional protection against HIV infection[35] to women who are not sex industry workers.

Primary prevention

Primary prevention targeted at both men and women could focus on HIV awareness and education, access to effective health care, the prevention and control of sexually transmitted diseases, safer sex and safer injecting techniques. National AIDS programmes must continue to strive for a comprehensive screening service for blood transfusions. The development of an inexpensive, widely available, safe and effective vaginal virucide or microbicide, active against HIV and other pathogenic micro-organisms is a high priority for WHO-sponsored biomedical research. This would be a potent preventative weapon, the use of which would be under female control. Finally, women will continue to be at risk of HIV infection unless men everywhere help put an end to cultural traditions and socio-economic conditions which lead to women's subordination.

References

1. World Health Organization (1994). AIDS data at 31 October 1993 and the current global situation of the HIV/AIDS pandemic. *Weekly Epidemiological Record* **69**, 5–8.
2. Mann, J., Tarantola, D.J. and Netter, T.W. (1992). *AIDS in the World: A Global Report*. Harvard University Press, London.
3. Global programme on AIDS (1993). *The HIV/AIDS Pandemic: 1993 Overview*. World Health Organization, Geneva.
4. MacDonald, M.G., Magann, E.F., and Morrison, J.C. (1993). Overview of medical management of HIV-seropositive pregnant women. *Pediatric AIDS and HIV Infection: Fetus to Adolescent* **4**(1), 3–7.
5. WHO (1993). *Press Release*. WHO/69, 7 September, World Health Organization, Geneva.
6. European Study Group on Heterosexual Transmission of HIV (1992). Comparison of female-to-male and male-to-female transmission of HIV in 563 stable couples. *British Medical Journal* **304**, 809–13.
7. Haverkos, H.W. and Battjes, R. (1992). Female-to-male transmission of HIV. *Journal of the American Medical Association* **268**, 1855.
8. The United Nations' Development Programme (1994). Editorial: Young women: Silence, susceptibility, and the HIV epidemic. *AIDS and HIV Infection: Fetus to Adolescent* **5**(1), 1–9.
9. Newman, T. and Martens, M.G. (1994). Women and HIV. In *HIV: Manual For Health Care Professionals*, eds Muma, R.D., Lyons, B.A., Borucki, M.J. and Pollard, R.B., Appleton & Lange, Norwalk, CT, pp. 138–47.
10. Centers for Disease Control and Prevention (1992). 1993 Revised Classification System for HIV Infection and Expanded Surveillance Case Definition for AIDS Among Adolescents and Adults. *Morbidity and Mortality Weekly Report (MMWR)*, 18 December, **41**(RR-17), 1–19.
11. Laga, M., Icenogle, J.P., Marsella, R. *et al.* (1992). Genital papillomavirus infection and cervical dysplasia – opportunistic complications of HIV infection. *International Journal of Cancer* **50**, 45–8.
12. Schafer, A., Friedmann, W., Mielke, M. *et al.* (1991). The increased frequency of cervical dysplasia – neoplasia in women infected with the human immunodeficiency virus is related to the degree of immunosuppression. *American Journal of Obstetrics and Gynecology* **164**(2), 593–9.

13. Feingold, A.R., Vermund, S.H., Burk, R.D. *et al.* (1990). Cervical cytologic abnormalities and papillomavirus in women infected with human immunodeficiency virus. *Journal of Acquired Immune Deficiency Syndromes* **3**, 896–903.
14. Maiman, M., Fruchter, R.G., Serur, E. *et al.* (1990). Human immunodeficiency virus infection and cervical neoplasia. *Gynecological Oncology* **38**, 377–82.
15. Klein, R.S., Adachi, A., Fleming, I. *et al.* (1992). A prospective study of genital neoplasia and human papillomavirus (HPV) in HIV-infected women (abstract). Vol. 1. Presented at the VIII International Conference on AIDS/111 STD World Congress, Amsterdam, The Netherlands, 19–24 July, 1992.
16. Gifford, A.L. (1993). The new AIDS definition: TB, pneumonia, cervical cancer. *Focus* **8**(6), 1–4.
17. Spinillo, A., Tenti, P., Zappatore, R. *et al.* (1992). Prevalence, diagnosis and treatment of lower genital neoplasia in women with human immunodeficiency virus infection. *European Journal of Obstetrics, Gynecology, and Reproductive Biology* **43**(3), 235–41.
18. Minkoff, H.L. and DeHovitz, J.A. (1991). Care of women infected with the human immunodeficiency virus. *Journal of the American Medical Association* **266**, 2253–8.
19. Allen, M.H. (1990). Primary care of women infected with the human immunodeficiency virus. *Obstetric and Gynecologic Clinics of North America* **17**, 557–69.
20. Cotton, D.J. (1994). AIDS in women. In *Textbook of AIDS Medicine*, eds Broder, S., Merigan, T.C., and Bolognesi, D., Williams & Wilkins, Baltimore, pp. 161–8.
21. Anon. (1993). Women, contraception and HIV. *Drug and Therapeutics Bulletin*, 6 December, **31**(25), 97–8.
22. Liskin, L., Wharton, C. and Blackburn, R. (1990). Condoms – now more than ever. *Population Report (Series H)* **8**, 1–36.
23. Carey, R.F., Herman, W.A., Retta, S.M. *et al.* (1992). Effectiveness of latex condoms as a barrier to human immunodeficiency virus-sized particles under conditions of simulated sex. *Sexually Transmitted Diseases* **19**, 230–4.
24. Anon. (1993). Condoms on test. *Which? way to Health*, August, 119–23.
25. Anon. (1993). Femidom® – a condom for women. *Drugs and Therapeutics Bulletin* **31**, 15–16.
26. Cates, W. Jr. and Stone, K.M. (1992). Family planning, sexually transmitted diseases and contraceptive choice: a literature update – part 1. *Family Planning Perspective* **24**, 75–84.
27. Lazzarin, A., Saracco, A., Musicco, M. *et al.* (1991). Man-to-woman sexual transmission of the human immunodeficiency virus. Risk factors related to sexual behaviour , man's infectiousness and woman's susceptibility. *Archives of Internal Medicine* **151**, 2411–16.
28. Kapiga, S., Hunter, D.J., Shao, J.F. *et al.* (1992). Contraceptive practice and HIV-1 infection among family planning in Dar-es-Salaam,

Eighth International Conference on AIDS. *Conference Abstracts*, PG C302 (PC 4343), 19–24 July, Amsterdam.
29. Plummer, F.A., Simonsen, J.N., Cameron, D.W. *et al.* (1991). Cofactors in male-female sexual transmission of human immunodeficiency virus type 1. *Journal of Infectious Diseases* **163**, 233–9.
30. Simonsen, J.N., Plummer, F.A., Ngugi, E.N. *et al.* (1990). HIV infection among lower socio-economic strata prostitutes in Nairobi. *AIDS* **4**, 139–44.
31. Musicco, M., Saracco, A., Nicolosi, A. *et al.* (1991). Assessment of incidence and risk factors for male-to-female HIV transmission. *Conference Abstracts*, Seventh International Conference on AIDS, PG 20(abstract MC4), 16–21 June, Florence, Italy.
32. Allen, S., Lindan, C., Serufilira, A. *et al.* (1991). Human immunodeficiency virus infection in urban Rwanda: Demographic and behavioural correlates in a representative sample of childbearing women. *Journal of the American Medical Association* **266**, 1657–63.
33. Chantler, E. (1992). Vaginal spermicides: some current concerns. *British Journal of Family Planning* **17**, 118–19.
34. Hicks, D.R., Martin, L.S., Getchell, J.P. *et al.* (1985). Inactivation of HTLV-III/LAV-infected cultures of normal human lymphocytes by Nonoxynol-9 in vitro. *Lancet*, 21–28 December, ii(8469–70), 422–3.
35. Polsky, B., Baron, P.A., Gold, J.W.M. *et al.* (1988). In vitro inactivation of HIV-1 by contraceptive sponge containing nonoxynol-9. *Lancet*, 25 June, i(8600), 1456.
36. Bird, K.D, (1991). The use of spermicide containing nonoxynol-9 in the prevention of HIV infection. *AIDS* **6**, 599–601.
37. Rekart, M.L. (1992). The toxicity and local effects of the spermicide nonoxynol-9. *Journal of Acquired Immune Deficiency Syndromes* **5**, 425–7.
38. Kreiss, J., Ngugi, E., Holmes, K. *et al.* (1992). Efficacy of nonoxynol-9 contraceptive sponge use in preventing heterosexual acquisition of HIV in Nairobi prostitutes. *Journal of the American Medical Association* **268**(4), 477–82.

Further reading

Berer, M. and Ray, S. (1993). *Women and HIV/AIDS: An International Resource Book*. Pandora Press, London (ISBN 0-04-440876-5).
Bury, J., Morrison, V. and McLachlan, S. (1992). *Working with Women & AIDS: Medical, Social & Counselling Issues*. Tavistock/Routledge, London (ISBN 0-414-07659-5).
Johnson, M.A. and Johnstone, F.D. (1993). *HIV Infection in Women*. Churchill Livingstone, London (ISBN 0-443-04885-1).
Mercey, Danielle, Bewley, Susan and Brocklehurst, Peter (1993). *A Guide to HIV infection & Childbearing*. The AIDS Education & Research Trust (AVERT), West Sussex, UK (Available from: AVERT, 11

Denne Parade, Horsham, West Sussex, RH12 1JD, UK, FAX UK 0403 211001).

Sherr, Lorraine (1991). *HIV and AIDS in Mothers and Babies: A Guide to Counselling*. Blackwell Scientific, Oxford (ISBN 0-632-02834-3).

11

Children and HIV Disease

Early in the pandemic, infants and children accounted for only a small number of patients with AIDS. However, as HIV spread into the female population, the number of children with AIDS has increased in countries all over the world. Heterosexual HIV transmission continues to escalate, and, worldwide, five out of every eleven newly infected adults are now women[1]. Mother-to-child transmission is also growing in importance. By the beginning of 1992, 1.1 million children had been infected with HIV and nearly 575 000 children had progressed to end-stage disease, i.e. AIDS. Between 1992 and 1995, 900 000 children will die of AIDS and millions more are destined to become infected[2].

HIV transmission to infants and children

The vast majority of infants and children who are infected with HIV have become so as a result of vertical transmission, i.e. from their HIV-infected mothers. Most infants become infected perinatally, either *in utero* or during delivery (intrapartum). The frequency for successful HIV transmission from an infected mother to her child varies in different parts of the world, but on average the vertical transmission rate is 30–40 per cent[3]. The fetus can become infected *in utero* /as early as the 13th week of pregnancy[4].

A smaller (and decreasing) number of children have become infected via contaminated blood products or blood transfusions, and newborn children may become infected in the early postpartum period from infected breast milk[5]. Injecting drug use in very young children has been reported which may expose them to HIV infection. HIV transmission to small children as a result of sexual abuse has also been documented[6].

The misuse of injectable drugs is the primary risk factor for HIV infection among women in the developed world. More than half of infected women contracted HIV infection either directly by using blood-contaminated injecting equipment, or indirectly through heterosexual contact with infected injecting drug users[4]. The explosion of cocaine (and its derivative, 'crack') use is also associated with increased high-risk sexual behaviour and may be responsible for exposing even more women to HIV infection.

Definition of pediatric AIDS/HIV infection

By definition, paediatric AIDS or HIV infection refers to children under the age of 13 years. Serological diagnosis of paediatric HIV infection is fraught with difficulties. All children born to HIV positive mothers will also be antibody positive for HIV because of the normal maternal transfer of antibodies *in utero*. Therefore, a standard HIV antibody test for IgG antibodies (e.g. ELISA, HIV immunoassays, etc.) is not a reliable indicator of infection in infants until after the age of 18 months. However, during this early period, HIV infection in the infant may be serologically diagnosed by a combination of tests, including virus cultures, antigen detection (usually p24), complete Western blot analysis and polymerase chain reaction tests (PCR). These tests are described in more detail in Chapter 19. Virus cultures, especially those performed 2–3 weeks after birth, are capable of identifying up to 80 per cent of children with HIV infection[7]. It is essential to remember that parents must give true, informed consent prior to their child having a serological test for HIV infection.

In addition to serological tests, the appearance of clinical symptoms are also important indicators of possible HIV infection in the infant. The main signs and symptoms seen in paediatric AIDS are listed in Table 11.1 and further described in the CDC case definition for AIDS (Table 11.2) and the CDC classification system for HIV infection in children under 13 years of age with which all paediatric nurses and midwives should be familiar[8].

Table 11.1   Principal signs and symptoms in paediatric AIDS

Recurrent and serious bacterial infections
Diarrhoea (persistent or recurrent)*
Oral candidiasis (recurrent, chronic)
Failure to thrive
Lymphoid interstitial pneumonitis (LIP)
Serious opportunistic infection, e.g. PCP
Fever*
Parotitis*
Hepatomegaly*
Splenomegaly*

Skin diseases (candidiasis and seborrhoea)
Chronic otitis media
Chronic sinusitis
Neurological disease, e.g. acquired microcephaly and/or brain atrophy, progressive symmetrical motor deficits

---

*Persisting for more than 2 months.

Table 11.2   CDC case definition for AIDS in children under 13 years of age

---

For the limited purposes of epidemiologic surveillance, CDC defines a case of paediatric AIDS as a child under 13 years of age who has had:
1. a reliably diagnosed disease at least moderately indicative of underlying cellular immunodeficiency, *and*
2. no known cause of underlying cellular immunodeficiency or any other reduced resistance reported to be associated with that disease.

The diseases accepted as sufficiently indicative of underlying cellular immunodeficiency are:
  Candidiasis of the oesophagus, trachea, bronchi, or lungs
  Cryptococcosis, extrapulmonary
  Cryptosporidiosis with diarrhoea persisting for more than 1 month
  Cytomegalovirus disease of an organ other than liver, spleen or lymph nodes in a child more than 1 month of age
  Herpes simplex virus infection causing a mucocutaneous ulcer that persists longer than 1 month; or bronchitis, pneumonitis, or oesophagitis for any duration in a child more than 1 month of age
  Lymphoid interstitial pneumonia and/or pulmonary lymphoid hyperplasia (LIP/PLH complex) affecting a child less than 13 years of age
  Mycobacterium avium complex or *M. kansasii* disease, disseminated (at a site other than or in addition to lungs, skin, or cervical or hilar lymph nodes)
  Pneumocystis carinii pneumonia
  Progressive multifocal leucoencephalopathy
  Toxoplasmosis of the brain affecting a child more than 1 month of age
  Bacterial infections, multiple or recurrent (any combination of at least two within a 2-year period), of the following types affecting a child less than 13 years of age:* septicaemia, pneumonia, meningitis, bone or joint infection, or abscess of an internal organ or body cavity (excluding otitis media or superficial skin or mucosal abscesses), caused by *Haemophilus, Streptococcus* (including *Pneumococcus*), or other pyogenic bacteria
  Coccidioidomycosis, disseminated (at a site other than or in addition to lungs, or cervical or hilar lymph nodes)*
  HIV encephalopathy*
  Histoplasmosis, disseminated (at a site other than or in addition to lungs or cervical or hilar lymph nodes)*
  Isosporiasis with diarrhoea persisting for more than 1 month*
  Kaposi's sarcoma at any age
  Lymphoma of the brain (primary) at any age*

Other non-Hodgkin's lymphoma of B cell or unknown immunologic phenotype*

*Indicates a diagnosis of AIDS only if there is also laboratory evidence of HIV infection

Specific conditions that must be excluded in a child are:
1. Primary immunodeficiency diseases – severe, combined immunodeficiency (SCID), DiGeorge syndrome, Wiskott–Aldrich syndrome, ataxia telangiectasia, graft-versus-host disease, neutropenia, neutrophil function abnormality, agammaglobulinaemia, or hypogammaglobulinaemia with raised IgM
2. Secondary immunodeficiency associated with immunosuppressive therapy, lymphoreticular malignancy or starvation

HIV infection in adolescents

AIDS and HIV infection also occurs in adolescents (age 13–18 years). Young adults presenting with AIDS in their twenties have most likely become infected (either sexually or through injecting substance misuse) as teenagers. Currently, there is an increase in all forms of sexually transmitted diseases in adolescents and in many countries they are a prime target for drug misuse (especially 'crack'). In both the United States and Europe, the majority of adolescents practise high-risk sexual behaviour at one time or another[9,10]. Consequently, a substantial rise in HIV infection in now being seen in teenagers[11]. Adolescents are diagnosed and classified as adults (*see* Chapter 7), however they present more unique legal and ethical problems. Although adolescents can give consent in the United States and in the United Kingdom in all issues involving sexually transmitted diseases, it is far from clear if they can consent to treatment with potentially toxic and, in many cases, experimental drugs. It is also not clear if an adolescent can refuse consent to disclose a diagnosis of HIV infection or AIDS to his or her parents.

Proposed 1994 paediatric HIV classification system

By the end of the summer, 1994, CDC will publish a new paediatric HIV classification system[12]. In the proposed system, children are categorized using three parameters: infection status, clinical status and immunological status. The categories are mutually exclusive. Once classified in a more severe category, a child is **not** reclassified in a less severe category even if the clinical or immunologic status improves. The proposed classification grid is shown in Table 11.3.

Table 11.3 Proposed 1994 paediatric HIV classification

Immune categories	Clinical categories			
	(N) No signs/ symptoms	(A) Mild signs/ symptoms	(B) Moderate signs/ symptoms	(C) Severe signs/ symptoms
(1) No evidence of suppression	N1	A1	B1	C1
(2) Evidence of moderate suppression	N2	A2	B2	C2
(3) Severe suppression	N3	A3	B3	C3

Children whose HIV infection status is not confirmed are classified using the above grid with a letter E (vertically Exposed) placed in front of the classification, e.g. 'E/N2'.

Immune category classification

The immune category classification is based on the CD4 count or CD4 percentage. If the use of both the CD4 count and the CD4 percentage result in classification into different categories, the child should be classified into the more severe category. CD4 values resulting in a change in classification should be confirmed by a second determination. Values thought to be in error should not be used. A child should not be reclassified to a less severe category regardless of subsequent CD4 determinations.

The purpose of the three categories in the immune axis is to categorize children by the severity of immunosuppression attributable to HIV. Age adjustment of the CD4 absolute count category is necessary because it varies with age. The proposed CD4 count and CD4 percentage categories for the immune categories by age group are shown in Table 11.4.

Determination of infection status

For the purposes of the classification system, the proposed definitions for infection status are as shown in Table 11.5.

Table 11.4 Proposed CD4 count and CD4 percentage categories by age group

Immune categories	Age groups		
	0–11 months	1–5 years	6–12 years
(1) No evidence of suppression	≥ 1500 > 25%	≥ 1000 > 25%	≥ 500 > 25%
(2) Evidence of moderate suppression	750–1499 15–25%	500–999 15–25%	200–499 15–25%
(3) Severe suppression	< 750 < 15%	< 500 < 15%	< 200 < 15%

Table 11.5 Proposed definitions for infection status

HIV infected
1. A child < 18 months of age, who is known to be HIV seropositive or born to an HIV-infected mother who:
   has positive results on two separate determinations (excluding cord blood) using one or more of the following HIV detection tests:
      HIV virus culture
      HIV polymerase chain reaction (PCR)
      HIV antigen (p24) *or*
   meets diagnosis of AIDS based on the 1987 AIDS case definition
2. A child ≥ 18 months of age born to an HIV-infected mother or a child infected by blood or blood products who:
   is HIV antibody positive by repeatedly reactive enzyme immunoassay (EIA) and confirmatory test (e.g. Western blot, immunofluorescence assay) *or*
   meets any of the criteria in 1 above

Vertically exposed (Prefix E)
A child who does not meet the criteria above who:
   is HIV seropositive by EIA and confirmatory test (e.g. Western blot, or IFA) and < 18 months old at the time of test *or*
   was born to an HIV-infected mother, but has unknown antibody status

Seroreverter (Prefix SR)
A child born to an HIV-infected mother who:
   has been documented to be HIV antibody negative (two or more negative EIA tests after 6 months of age) *and*
   has no other laboratory evidence of infection (has not had two positive viral detections tests if performed) *and*
   has not had an AIDS defining condition *and*
   does not have any evidence of significant immune suppression (N2 or N3) unexplained by other causes of immune deficiency

Clinical category classification

Children determined to be HIV-infected or vertically exposed to HIV may be classified into one of four mutually exclusive clinical categories based on signs, symptoms, or diagnoses related to HIV infection. Signs and symptoms related to other underlying causes (infectious, inflammatory, drug-related) should not be used to classify children. For example, a child with hepatitis B virus infection should not be classified as Category B based on hepatitis. However, a child with recurrent salmonella diarrhoea should be classified as Category B when the salmonella infection is thought to be related to HIV infection.

The criteria for diagnosis of some conditions and the determination of whether a child's sign, symptom, or diagnosis is related to HIV infection may not be clear in all cases. In some cases, classification may require judgement of the clinicians and researchers using the classification system. The proposed clinical categories are given in Table 11.6.

Table 11.6 Proposed clinical categories

Category N: Not symptomatic
Children with no signs or symptoms felt to be the result of HIV infection and/or are indicative of immunologic deficits attributable to HIV infection, or have only one of the conditions listed in category A

Category A: Mildly symptomatic
Children who have two or more of the conditions listed below. Conditions listed in categories B and C must not have occurred.
- Lymphadenopathy ($\geq$ 0.5 cm at $\geq$ 2 sites; bilateral = 1 site)
- Hepatomegaly
- Splenomegaly
- Dermatitis
- Parotitis
- Recurrent/persistent URI or sinusitis
- Recurrent/persistent otitis media

Category B: Moderately symptomatic
Children who have symptomatic conditions other than those listed for Category A or C which are attributed to HIV infection and/or are indicative of immunologic deficits attributable to HIV infection. Examples of conditions in clinical category B include, *but are not limited to*:
- Anaemia (< 8 g/ml), neutropenia (< 1000), and thrombocytopenia (< 100 000)
- Bacterial meningitis, pneumonia, or sepsis (single episode)
- Candidiasis, oropharyngeal (thrush), persistent (> 2 months) in child > 6 months of age

- Cardiomyopathy
- Cytomegalovirus infection, with onset *before* 1 month of age
- Diarrhoea, recurrent or chronic
- Hepatitis
- Herpes stomatitis, recurrent ($\geq$ 2 episodes within one year)
- HSV bronchitis, pneumonitis, or esophagitis with onset *before* 1 month of age
- Herpes zoster (shingles) involving at least two distinct episodes or more than one dermatome
- Lymphoid interstitial pneumonia or pulmonary lymphoid hyperplasia complex (LIP/PLH)
- Nephropathy
- Nocardiosis
- Persistent varicella zoster
- Persistent fever > 1 month
- Rhabdomyosarcoma
- Toxoplasmosis, onset *before* 1 month of age
- Varicella, disseminated (complicated chickenpox)

Category C: Severely symptomatic
Children who have any condition listed in the 1987 surveillance case definition for AIDS, with the exception of LIP

Treatment of children with AIDS

Aggressive, supportive treatment can decrease both morbidity and mortality in children with AIDS. The treatment programme developed at the Children's Hospital of New Jersey, as described by Connor *et al.*[13], serves as a model to provide maximum supportive care and is described in Tables 11.7 and 11.8.

As always, paediatric nursing care requires not only the care of the child but the care of the entire family who will require support throughout the illness of their child. In most cases, the mother is herself infected with HIV.

The management of children with HIV infection has previously concentrated on supportive care, i.e. the medical treatment of developing opportunistic infections and the relevant nursing care. The nursing care of children with HIV-related conditions is exactly the same as for any other seriously ill child. Care is assessed, planned, delivered and continuously evaluated as per the identified health care deficits of the infant or child. As for any other child, the parents are involved in all stages of the process of care, including the setting of short-term, medium-term and long-term goals.

The advent of specific antiretroviral therapy for HIV infection and increasing sophistication in the prophylaxis of common paediatric AIDS-related opportunistic infections, has increased both the length

Table 11.7   The goals of the multidisciplinary AIDS programme

1. Treat the disease/symptoms of immune deficiency resulting from HIV infection:
   - Aggressive treatment of infections
   - Nutritional support (total parenteral nutrition, ongoing nutritional assessment)
   - Periodic assessment of growth and development
   - Regular neurologic examination and testing for evidence of progressive encephalopathy
   - Supportive treatment of chronic lung disease

2. Prevent the disease process and treatment regimen from interfering with the development of the child:
   - Provide parents with specific information about the condition and treatment
   - Assist the parents to understand and manage the illness and its symptoms
   - Assist parents to identify and utilize resources within the health care system and the community
   - Assist the child in coping with and understanding the illness at an appropriate age level

3. Prevent the illness and its treatment regimens from disrupting the family unit:
   - Assist parents to develop an awareness of their rights within the system
   - Act as an advocate for the family with schools and other social agencies
   - Educate the professional and lay public

Table 11.8   Therapeutic protocol for paediatric HIV infection

Vigorous nutritional support
Hospitalize for parenteral feeding, hyperalimentation or nasogastric tube feeding

Antimicrobial therapy for intercurrent infection
Hospitalize for parenteral therapy as needed

Short course steroid for interstitial pneumonia
If patient is hypoxic ($PO_2 < 65$ mmHg on room air)

IV gamma-globulin
Full replacement dose every 3–4 weeks

and quality of life of many infants and children with HIV-related conditions. It is recognized that paediatric AIDS progresses more rapidly than adult AIDS; the median survival time from diagnosis to death is 14 months[4].

Consequently, the earlier an infant is serologically identified as being infected with HIV, the earlier an improved quality of medical monitoring, treatment and prophylaxis can be initiated.

In US, French and Italian studies[14-16] zidovudine (Retrovir – AZT) was reported to significantly improve the condition of many children with symptomatic HIV infection. Improvements were seen in growth, weight and height, neuropsychological function and immunological status. Children with early symptomatic disease tolerated zidovudine well, neutropenia being the main side-effect. Although the paediatric dose for zidovudine has not yet been established, a daily dose of 5 mg/kg[14] and twice daily administration may be sufficient[16].

The above studies are currently being extended to establish if zidovudine treatment during pregnancy can prevent *in-utero* (or intrapartum) HIV transmission to the foetus. In addition, they are exploring the efficacy of zidovudine treatment within 24 hours of birth to neonates born to HIV-infected mothers in interrupting HIV transmission.

Other antiretroviral agents are now in various phases of clinical studies[17] and hopefully during the late 1990s, increasingly effective and specific treatment for this disease will evolve. Zidovudine and other antiretroviral drugs are discussed more fully in Chapter 19.

Immunization and children infected with HIV

Children infected with HIV are at an increased risk from infectious diseases and should be vaccinated as a matter of priority. They should follow the approved schedule for routine immunizations as given in Table 11.9. Vaccine efficacy may be reduced in children who are infected with HIV and they may additionally need passive immune protection from the use of human normal immunoglobulin (HNIG) or specific immunoglobulins. If an HIV-infected child is receiving full-replacement therapy with intravenous gamma-globulin (i.e. HNIG), an immune response to live virus vaccines (e.g. MMR, polio) may be reduced. Children who are infected with HIV may safely have all of the vaccines listed in Table 11.9 (as can adults), providing that there are no clinical contraindications to immunizations. Immunization should not proceed in children who:

- have had a severe or general reaction to a preceding dose (all vaccines);
- are hypersensitive to eggs (influenza vaccine);
- have had previous anaphylactic reaction to eggs (MMR, influenza, yellow fever);
- are suffering from an acute illness and are febrile (all vaccines); or
- are suffering from vomiting and diarrhoea (polio).

In the UK, children who are asymptomatically infected with HIV may receive live polio vaccine (OPV) but excretion of the vaccine virus in the faeces may continue for longer than in normal individuals. Household contacts should be warned of this and the need for strict personal hygiene, including hand-washing after nappy changes for an HIV-positive infant. Inactivated polio vaccine (IPV) is generally used for children with symptomatic HIV infection, although OPV may be used.

Table 11.9   Routine immunization schedule UK (1990)

Vaccine	Age
Diphtheria, tetanus, pertussis (DTP) and polio (OPV or IPV)	2 months (1st dose) 3 months (2nd dose) 4 months (3rd dose)
Measles, mumps, rubella (MMR)	12–18 months
Booster diphtheria and polio	4–5 years
Rubella	10–14 years (girls only)
Booster tetanus and polio	15–18 years

In developing countries where the incidence of poliomyelitis remains high, the lack of evidence of side-effects to OPV support the WHO policy for its continued administration to all children.

In the United States, IPV is recommended for children with both symptomatic and known HIV asymptomatic infection, i.e. OPV is not used.

Other vaccines which HIV-infected children may receive, if necessary, are:

- Typhoid
- Cholera
- Meningococcal
- H. influenzae type b conjugate (HbC)
- Hepatitis B
- Influenza
- Pneumococcal.

In the United Kingdom (and the United States), the bacillus Calmette–Guérin (BCG) vaccine used for primary prevention of tuberculosis is never given to children (or adults) known to be infected with HIV as serious vaccine dissemination has been reported. However, in developing countries where the risk of tuberculosis is high, BCG vaccination at birth is still recommended by the WHO.

Yellow fever vaccine is also not given to children (or adults) known to be infected with HIV.

It is axiomatic that parents must give true, informed consent prior to their child being immunized. Mothers who know that they themselves are infected with HIV or who have children being investigated for HIV infection, are extremely anxious in relation to immunizations for their children. Nurses who care for these children should have a clear understanding of current recommendations[18–20].

References

1. Merson, M.H. (1993). *The HIV/AIDS Pandemic: Global Spread and Global Response*. Opening address: IXth International Conference on AIDS, 7–11 June, Berlin.
2. Mann, J., Tarantola, D.J.M. and Netter, T.W. (1992). *AIDS in the World: A Global Report*. Harvard University Press, Cambridge, MA. References
3. Bradbeer, C. (1990). Human immunodeficiency virus and its relationship to women, editorial review. *International Journal of STD and AIDS*, July, **14**, 233–8.
4. PHS – National Institute of Child Health and Human Development (1990). *The New Face of AIDS: A Maternal and Pediatric Epidemic*, June, US Department of Health and Human Services.
5. WHO (1987). Global Programme on AIDS on Special Programme of Research, Development and Research Training in Human Reproduction: Joint Statement – *Contraceptive Methods and HIV Infection*, SPA/INF/87.9. World Health Organization, Geneva.
6. Rubinstein, A. and Bernstein, L. (1986). The epidemiology of pediatric acquired immunodeficiency syndrome. *Clinical Immunology and Immunopathology* **40**, 115–21.
7. Rouzioux, C. (1989). Methods of early diagnosis. In *Aspects of Paediatric HIV Management* (International Seminar Series), ed. McFadzean,

W., Colwood House Medical Publications, UK, pp. 14–18.
8. Centers for Disease Control (1987). Classification System for Human Immunodeficiency Virus (HIV) Infection in Children Under 13 Years of Age. *Morbidity and Mortality Weekly Report (MMWR)*, 24 April, **36**(15), 225–32.
9. DiClemente, R., Durbin, M., Siegel, D. *et al.* (1990). An inverse relation between number of sex partners and condom use frequency among middle adolescents: Cause for concern. *Vl International Conference on AIDS – Abstracts*. Th.D.897, San Francisco.
10. Nieuwinckel, St., Knops, N., Poppe, E. *et al.* (1990). Belgian adolescents and AIDS – A survey of risk behaviour and prevention. *VI International Conference on AIDS – Abstracts*. Th.D.776, San Francisco.
11. Kilbourne, B.W., Chus, S.Y., Oxtoby, M.J. *et al.* (1990). Mortality due to HIV infection in adolescents and young adults. *Vl International Conference on AIDS – Abstracts*. Th.C.743, San Francisco.
12. Centers for Disease Control and Prevention (CDC) (1994). Proposed CDC Revised Pediatric Classification System – 1994 (Blake Caldwell, *personal communication*).
13. Connor, E.M., Minnefor, A.B. and Oleske, I.M. (1987). Human immunodeficiency virus infection in infants and children. In *Current Topics in AIDS*, Vol. 1, eds Gottlieb, M.S., Jeffries, D.J., Mildvan, D. *et al.*, John Wiley & Sons, UK, p. 193.
14. Griscelli, C. (1990). The French zidovudine open study. In *Aspects of Paediatric HIV Management* (International Seminar Series), ed. McFadzean, W., Colwood House Medical Publications, UK, pp. 33–6.
15. Wilfert, C. (1990). Review of US clinical trials. In *Aspects of Paediatric HIV Management* (International Seminar Series), ed. McFadzean, W., Colwood House Medical Publications, UK, pp. 37–41.
16. Giaquinto, C. (1990). Italian experience and future trials. In *Aspects of Paediatric HIV Management* (International Seminar Series), ed. McFadzean, W., Colwood House Medical Publications, UK, pp.42–5.
17. Johnson, R.P. and Schooley, R.T. (1989). Update on antiretroviral agents other than zidovudine. In *AIDS*, **Vol. 3**(suppl. 1). Current Science, UK, pp. 5145–51.
18. UK Departments of Health (1992). *Immunisation against Infectious Disease*, 1992 edn. HMSO, London.
19. Centers for Disease Control (1993). Recommendations of the Advisory Committee on Immunization Practices (ACIP): Use of Vaccines and Immune Globulins for Persons with Altered Immunocompetence. *Morbidity and Mortality Weekly Report (MMWR)*, 9 April, **42**(RR-4), 1–18.
20. Centers for Disease Control (1994). General Recommendations on Immunization: Recommendations of the Advisory Committee on Immunization Practices (ACIP). *Morbidity and Mortality Weekly Report (MMWR)*, 28 January, **43**(RR-1), 1–27.

Further reading

Claxton, R. and Harrison, T. (1991). *Caring for Children with HIV and AIDS.* Edward Arnold, London (ISBN 0-340-55256-5).

Pizzo, P.A., and Wilfert, C.M. (1994). *Pediatric AIDS: The Challenge of HIV Infection in Infants, Children and Adolescents.* Williams & Wilkins, Baltimore MD, Second edition. (ISBN 0-683-06894-6).

Scott, G.B. (1994). Special considerations in children. In *Textbook of AIDS Medicine*, eds Broder, S., Merigan, T.C. Jr. and Bolognesi, D., Williams & Wilkins, Baltimore MD, (ISBN 0-683-01072-7).

12

A Strategy for Infection Control in Nursing Practice

It is axiomatic that in assessing and planning nursing care for patients with an infectious disease, an extensive understanding of appropriate infection control (IC) procedures is required. Comprehensive guidelines for infection control have been published in both the United Kingdom and the United States and all nurses should be fully conversant with these documents[1-3]. The CDC Recommendations for the prevention of transmission of HIV (and other bloodborne pathogens) in health care settings are reprinted in full in Appendix 3. The information in this chapter is compatible with this guidance and is in a large part based on current guidelines issued by the UK Departments of Health[3].

Models of infection control

There are four systems of infection control precautions which complement each other. These are:

- Category-specific precautions
- Body substance isolation
- Universal precautions
- Disease-specific precautions.

In caring for patients with HIV disease, category-specific and disease-specific precautions may be appropriate in certain illnesses, e.g. respiratory isolation precautions for patients with active pulmonary tuberculosis, and the 'strict isolation' for patients with varicella (chickenpox). In general, however, the two major infection control systems are **universal precautions** and **body substance isolation**.

With the escalating numbers of individuals presenting for care who are asymptomatically infected with HIV (or other bloodborne viruses, e.g. hepatitis B, hepatitis C, etc.), it will never be known with any great certainty who is infected and who is not infected. Even if all in-patients were serologically screened for markers of HIV infection on admission, this procedure could not reliably detect all those who are asymptomatically infected (see Chapter 19). The only certainty that exists is that for the rest of our professional lives, more and more individuals will become infected and an ever increasing number of these individuals will require health care.

Body substance isolation (BSI) focuses on reducing the risk to patients of the transfer of micro-organisms in health care settings by the hands of health care workers[4]. It also protects health care workers from becoming infected with the potential pathogens which infect their patients. This system is based upon the premise that the blood, mucous membranes and moist body surfaces of both patients and health care workers are always colonized by or infected with a variety of infectious micro-organisms. By the consistent use of gloves by health care workers (generic glove precautions) whenever they anticipate contact with these areas, the potential for bi-directional transmission is significantly reduced.

The universal precautions system embraces the concept that the blood and certain body fluids of all patients are considered potentially infectious for bloodborne pathogens. The body fluids to which universal precautions apply are:

- Blood
- Cerebrospinal fluid
- Peritoneal fluid
- Pericardial fluid
- Pleural fluid
- Synovial fluid
- Amniotic fluid
- Semen
- Vaginal and cervical secretions
- Any other body fluids containing visible blood
- Saliva in association with dentistry, unfixed tissues and organs.

Blood is the single most important source of potential HIV infection in health care settings. The body fluids/excretions to which universal precautions **do not** apply (unless containing visible blood) in relation to the occupational transmission of HIV in health care settings are:

- Faeces*
- Urine*
- Nasal secretions*
- Sweat

- Tears
- Vomitus*
- Saliva.*

*May contain other potential pathogens

However, since some of these fluids and excretions represent a potential source for nosocomial and community-acquired infections with other pathogens, nurses should not be handling faeces, urine, nasal secretions, saliva or vomitus without wearing gloves.

The incorporation of one of these systems (preferably body substance isolation) into current, routine nursing practice is essential.

Virus fragility

There is nothing indestructible about HIV. It can easily be destroyed by a variety of physical and chemical means.

Decontamination methods

Decontamination methods are listed in Table 12.1. To assure the effectiveness of any decontamination process, equipment and instruments must first be thoroughly cleaned (preferably in the Central Sterile Supplies Department – CSSD).

Any decontamination method intended to sterilize instruments will, of course, destroy HIV. Sterilization by **heat** is the most consistently efficient method used and the following procedures are recommended. In hospitals, all sterilizable (non-disposable) instruments are sterilized by saturated steam under pressure in an **autoclave** at 2.2 bar, 134°C, maintained for a minimum of 3 minutes.

Table 12.1 Decontamination methods

Sterilization	Destroys all forms of microbial life, including high numbers of bacterial spores
High-level disinfection	Destroys all forms of microbial life except high number of bacterial spores
Intermediate-level disinfection	Destroys *Mycobacterium tuberculosis*, vegetative bacteria, most viruses and fungi but does not kill bacterial spores
Low-level disinfection	Destroys most bacteria, some viruses, some fungi, but not *M. tuberculosis* or bacterial spores

Alternative autoclave temperatures and hold times are 121°C for 15 minutes or 115°C for 30 minutes. **Hot air sterilization** can also be used as long as the centre of the load achieves and maintains a temperature of either 180°C for 30 minutes or 160°C for 1 hour. **Ethylene oxide gas (EOG)** may be used to sterilize delicate instruments. For EOG to be effective, instruments must be both clean and dry as excessive moisture can create residue which can be hazardous.

Several methods used in high, intermediate and low-level disinfection processes will also easily inactivate HIV. The most useful are boiling and chemical disinfectants.

Boiling

HIV can be inactivated by boiling at 100°C for 5 minutes.

Chemical disinfectants

Most disinfectants, if used according to the manufacturer's instructions, are easily able to destroy HIV. The most common chemical disinfectants used which are effective in inactivating HIV are:

Alkaline glutaraldehyde (2 per cent) This is used for non-corrosive disinfection of delicate instruments, e.g. fibre-optic endoscopes. To be effective, the instruments must be thoroughly cleaned prior to disinfection and the gluteraldehyde must be freshly activated. Instruments which will enter sterile body cavities are immersed in glutaraldehyde for a minimum of 3 hours. Other instruments need only be immersed for 30 minutes (unless *M. tuberculosis* is a suspected contaminant, in which case, the instrument is immersed for a minimum of 60 minutes; see Chapter 7).

Fresh aqueous solutions of sodium hypochlorite (bleach) or sodium dichloroisocyanurate These are commonly used as general surface disinfectants. **Strong solutions** of sodium hypochlorite (i.e. 10 000 parts per million (ppm) of available chlorine) are used for blood or body fluid spillages. This is equivalent to household bleach diluted 1 part bleach to 10 parts water. Community nurses who use household bleach to make up a sodium hypochlorite solution should be aware that the strength of individual brands of bleach may vary and that hypochlorite may deteriorate with age. **Weak solutions** of sodium hypochlorite (i.e. 1000 ppm of available chlorine) are used for general disinfection when surfaces are *not* contaminated with visible blood or body fluids. Granular sodium dichloroisocyanurate (e.g. Presept®) is ideal for blood or body fluid spillages. Both sodium hypochlorite and sodium dichloroisocyanurate are left in contact with the surface being disinfected for 2 minutes.

Other chemical disinfectants which inactivate HIV include hydrogen peroxide, chlorhexidine gluconate and povidone-iodine solutions. Although alcohols can inactivate HIV, they are slow acting and are therefore not recommended. If used, instruments must be thoroughly cleaned and then immersed in either 70 per cent isopropanol alcohol or industrial methylated spirits for a minimum of 1 hour.

Universal precautions in nursing practice

The adoption of universal precautions in clinical nursing practice requires the implementation of the practice points described in Table 12.2. Specific infection control practice points relevant to the nursing care of all patients, including those known to be infected with HIV (or other bloodborne pathogens), are described below.

Ward accommodation

There is no infection control justification for allocating single room accommodation to patients with HIV infection simply because they are infected with HIV. Quite clearly, with the large number of individuals in the community currently infected with this virus, hospitals will not have single room accommodation for all patients who have AIDS, let alone for all patients who may be seropositive for anti-HIV. There is no reason why patients with AIDS and HIV-related conditions cannot be nursed on an open ward with complete safety. The nursing assessment of each patient will dictate whether or not a single room is required. Table 12.3 summarizes the indications when a single room is useful. As many patients with AIDS will have nursing care issues outlined there, it is clear that a single room *will* frequently be required. However, there is a difference between a patient admitted with Kaposi's sarcoma for a biopsy (who does not require a single room) and a seriously ill patient admitted with a host of opportunistic infections.

Patients not admitted to single rooms can move about freely on the ward and, other than for universal precautions, do not require any restrictions. The major disadvantage of admitting a patient into a single room is the further sense of isolation and rejection felt by most patients with HIV-related conditions. As is usual, all nursing care must be planned with the patient. Careful explanation of IC

Table 12.2 Universal precautions

1. Hands must be washed before and after all patient contact procedures.
   Nurses who have cuts or abrasions must ensure these are covered with a
   waterproof dressing
2. Good-quality, non-sterile, disposable latex gloves and plastic aprons are
   worn when handling blood, body fluids, excretions or secretions from any
   patient, including patients with HIV-related illness. Gloves are also worn
   when touching non-intact skin or handling equipment soiled with blood and
   body fluids. Gloves are changed after contact with each patient
3. Masks and protective eyewear (or face shields) and long-sleeved gowns
   are worn during procedures which may generate droplets of blood or
   other body fluids or when there is gross environmental contamination of
   blood, body fluids, excretions or secretions. Clearly this will be required in
   midwifery and operating departments
4. Hands must be washed immediately (preferably with a povidone-iodine
   scrub, e.g. Betadine or a chlorhexidine gluconate solution, e.g. Hibiscrub
   or Hibiclens) if contaminated with blood, body fluids, excretions or
   secretions from any patient, including patients with known HIV infection
5. Special care is required when handling needles and other sharps.
   Needles must not be bent or recapped after use and must be discarded
   immediately into a puncture-resistant, waterproof container (e.g.
   SharpsBins – A.C. Daniels & Co. Ltd)
6. Local policy may still require that all specimens from patients with known
   HIV infection are sent to the laboratory with a hazard warning on them
   (e.g. Biohazard, Risk of infection). With the universal implementation of
   universal precautions for all patients, this should no longer be necessary
7. Spillages of blood and other body fluids should be covered with granules
   of NaDCC (sodium dichloroisocyanurate), such as Presept granules, left
   for a few minutes and then carefully wiped up with disposable paper
   towels or scooped up with a scooper. The area is then washed with hot,
   soapy water and allowed to dry

precautions must be given to the patient. If a patient is admitted
to a single room, this does not necessarily mean that the patient is
confined to that room. For example, patients with diarrhoea may
be allowed full ward activities, as appropriate. All patients in single
room accommodation must be frequently reassessed. The plan of
care for each shift must allow time for nurses to talk to patients,
rather than just entering the room when there is something to do.
Efforts must be made to ensure that domestic and catering staff
are aware of the IC precautions (**not** the diagnosis!), that meals
are delivered and the room cleaned. The final responsibility for
the patient's environment is a nursing responsibility.

Table 12.3   Indications for single room accommodation

1. Patients who have an opportunistic infection which normally requires a single room (e.g. pulmonary tuberculosis or salmonella infection)
2. Patients who are bleeding, likely to bleed (e.g. those with thrombocytopenia, candidal oesophagitis) or who have open or draining wounds
3. Grossly incontinent patients or those with severe diarrhoea
4. Neurological manifestations of HIV infection (e.g. confusion) which make it difficult for the patient to cooperate and maintain good standards of hygiene.
5. Patients with conditions associated with excessive, productive coughing
6. Seriously ill patients who require high dependency nursing care
7. Terminally ill patients
8. Psychological or social reasons

Protective clothing

When a patient is admitted to a single room, health care workers do not need to wear any protective clothing when entering the room just to talk to the patient, deliver meals, post, newspapers, etc. When entering a room to deliver direct nursing care such as assisting a patient to bathe, dealing with bed-pans, urinals or specimens, recording routine observations, changing dressings or dealing with incontinence, the only protective clothing necessary is a disposable plastic apron and a pair of disposable latex gloves.

Gowns are not usually required, unless the patient is grossly incontinent. Additional protective clothing is sometimes indicated, such as when dealing with spillages, assisting with invasive procedures (e.g. bronchoscopy), or managing a patient care situation in which there is likely to be a gross environmental contamination with blood or body fluids (e.g. a patient with haematemesis) or extensive draining wounds. In these circumstances, the following protective clothing is indicated: water repellent gowns, latex gloves, a mask and protective eyewear.

Most patients with HIV infection are also excretors of CMV and a mask and eye protection are appropriate in caring for patients who are coughing excessively, although the ability of patients to excrete significant amounts of CMV by coughing is not known. Some patients with AIDS have pulmonary tuberculosis and, in this condition, a mask is required. It may be more appropriate for the patient to wear a mask, for instance, when being transported to another department for investigations or treatment, in which case it is unnecessary for health care workers to do so also.

Appropriate disposable gloves are usually those made out of rubber latex, *not* plastic examination gloves. Research has shown that rubber latex gloves are vastly superior to plastic vinyl gloves and, consequently, only latex gloves should be used[5,6]. There is significant variability in the quality and watertightness of all gloves; they should be changed regularly during long procedures and hands washed thoroughly after glove removal. Suitable face masks are high filtration types used in surgery or particulate respirators, not flimsy, tissue thin paper masks. Eye protection devices should not resemble underwater goggles. Simple plastic or normal-looking glasses with plain glass lenses are available. If health care workers already wear glasses, they do not need to wear additional eye protection. In general, if a face mask is required, eye protection should be worn.

Catering staff do not need to wear any protective clothing to deliver meals. Housekeeping and domestic staff need only wear a plastic apron and a pair of disposable gloves when cleaning the room. Physiotherapists should wear gloves, plastic apron, eye protection and a face mask when giving chest physiotherapy. Social workers and other members of the hospital staff need not wear any protective clothing. Medical staff follow the same IC guidelines as those described for nursing personnel.

In general, visitors require no protective clothing, unless they are assisting in patient care activities with nursing personnel, who will advise them appropriately. Visitors with infections, or who are themselves immunocompromised, may need to take additional precautions and can be advised appropriately by nursing staff.

In patients who have pulmonary involvement, the nurse in charge will be able to advise other health care workers and visitors when a face mask is required.

As pneumonia caused by *Pneumocystis carinii* is one of the most common opportunistic diseases seen in patients with AIDS, it is worth stressing that this particular condition is not infectious to health care workers and others who have a normal immune response.

Injections and sharps

Probably the **only** time the nurse faces a significant potential risk of infection with HIV is when giving injections, caring for intravenous infusion sites or dealing with blood-contaminated sharp instruments, especially needles. Disposable syringes and needles must be used and gloves are worn when giving injections or caring for infusion sites and when handling any contaminated sharp instruments. Needle-locking syringes or one-piece needle–syringe units should be used.

Needles must not be re-inserted into their original sheaths or bent after use. It is generally unnecessary to detach the needle from the syringe after use and needles and syringes should be promptly discarded as one unit, into a rigid, puncture-proof plastic container, which is kept by (or taken to) the patient's bedside. When the 'sharps container' is three-quarters full, it is sealed, labelled appropriately (e.g. 'Risk of Infection' or 'BioHazard') and sent for incineration. The one exception is that when either venesectionists or medical staff take blood, they must remove the needle from the syringe before ejecting it into the specimen container to prevent a microscopic aerosol spray. Sharps containers must not be constructed of cardboard and must meet DHSS specifications. The range of sharps disposal bins manufactured by A.C. Daniels & Co. Ltd. are currently the best sharps containers on the market in the UK. This is because the wall thickness of their SharpsBins® is far in excess of British Standards requirements (BS 7320). In addition, they are easily assembled, simple to use and have a clearly visible 'fill line'[7].

Bed pans and urinals

Most patients will be able to use toilet facilities in their room. It is not necessary to pour disinfectants into the toilet after use; routine cleaning by housekeeping or domestic staff (wearing gloves!) is all that is required. If bed pans or urinals are used, they should be emptied as per the usual ward procedure by nursing staff (wearing plastic aprons and gloves). Clearly each patient requires his or her own individual bed pan and urinal, which may be emptied into the patient's toilet, taking care not to splash the contents, and then rinsed. It is not necessary to soak the bed pan or urinal after use in any disinfectant. They should be stored dry in the patient's room. Bed pans and urinals may also be emptied into a 'bed pan washer', making sure that the door is securely closed before turning on the machine.

Disposable bed pans and urinals that require crushing for disposal (e.g. papier mâché products manufactured by Vernaid) offer added advantages over re-usable bed pans and urinals in convenience, safety and patient satisfaction and, in the long term, are more cost effective. Disposal machines must be in good working order and serviced regularly. Many patients with AIDS will have profuse diarrhoea and if they are not able to use their own toilet, a bedside commode is preferable to using a bed pan in bed.

Linen

If visibly contaminated with blood, body fluids, excretions or secretions from any patient, including patients with known HIV-related conditions, linen is double-bagged. It is first placed in a soluble plastic bag (preferably an 'alginate-stitched' or polyvinyl alcohol bag), which is then placed into a **red** nylon bag. In the National Health Service (UK), all linen placed in red nylon bags is infected linen and no other labelling is required. Hospital laundries have their own procedure for dealing with infected linen, which, since HIV is sensitive to heat and detergents, is usually washed separately in hot, soapy water at a temperature of 71°C for 25 minutes. If the temperature is increased, the duration of the wash may be decreased. A disinfectant, such as hypochlorite, is often added.

Rubbish

Used dressings, paper towels, tubing and other rubbish visibly contaminated with blood, body fluids, excretions or secretions, from any patient, including patients with known HIV-related conditions, is placed in a heavy-duty plastic bag, sealed and sent for incineration. In the National Health Service (UK), contaminated rubbish placed in **yellow** plastic bags is always incinerated. Additional labelling is not required. When disposing of intravenous tubing, great care must be taken by nursing personnel to ensure that needles and other sharps have first been removed. This may require careful cutting off of both sharp ends. Patients who are not in a single room may dispose of their rubbish (e.g. newspapers) in the ordinary way, as long as it is not contaminated by blood or other body fluids. In the National Health Service (UK), non-infectious rubbish is disposed of in **black** plastic bags.

Crockery and cutlery

Patients with HIV infection do not generally require disposable crockery and cutlery. In those situations where the patient has a severe mouth infection, pulmonary tuberculosis or an enteric infection, it is preferable that they use their own normal crockery and cutlery, which can be kept in the patient's room. Often the patient, or the patient's visitors, can assist in washing these few dishes and silver or it can be done by nursing personnel. Rarely are disposable crockery and cutlery needed.

Instruments

Used instruments should be placed in a plastic bag or a special plastic box before being returned to the Central Sterile Supply Department (CSSD) for resterilizing. Instruments which cannot be autoclaved (e.g. endoscopic instruments), should be carefully washed with a detergent to remove all blood and body fluids and then placed in glutaraldehyde 2 per cent for 3 hours, then rinsed and stored dried. Although HIV can be easily inactivated by most disinfectants, as patients with AIDS frequently have several opportunistic infections, disinfectants which are mycobacteriocidal are used for disinfecting all instruments which cannot be autoclaved. The hospital's specific procedure for using these disinfectants (or the manufacturer's instructions) must be meticulously followed. The advice of the Control of Infection Nurse should be sought if there is any confusion about how these agents should be used.

Contaminated surfaces

Surfaces which may have been contaminated during procedures (e.g. dressing trolleys, tables and bench surfaces), should be wiped with a *weak* solution of hypochlorite (1000 ppm of available chlorine – e.g. household bleach diluted 1 part bleach to 100 parts of water) or freshly prepared glutaraldehyde 2 per cent (NB hypochlorite is corrosive to metal surfaces and fabrics). Grossly contaminated surfaces should be cleaned with either glutaraldehyde 2 per cent or a *strong* solution of hypochlorite (10 000 ppm – a 1 in 10 dilution of household bleach) which should, where possible, be left in contact with the contaminated surface for 30 minutes, prior to being wiped up with disposable paper towels.

An improved method of dealing with spillages of blood or body fluids is to sprinkle granules of NaDCC (dichloroisocyanurate), for example Presept granules, over the spillage and, after a few minutes, wipe up with disposable paper towels or scoop up with a scooper. Spillages of urine are never treated with hypochlorite, household bleach or NaDCC as a chemical reaction will occur, releasing noxious fumes.

Handwashing

Hands must be washed before and after all patient contact, thus avoiding the introduction of new potential pathogens to an already immunocompromised patient and to prevent transmitting opportunistic micro-organisms to other patients. Iodophors (complexes of iodine and solubilizers) such as povidone-iodine (Betadine®, Videne®) are appropriate as these halogenated soaps have been shown to eradicate HIV[8,9], and are effective against a wide range of potential pathogens. Chlorhexidine-based disinfectants (e.g. Hibiscrub®, Hibiclens®) will also readily inactivate HIV.[10] The use of gloves does not eliminate the need for good handwashing techniques.

Table 12.4 summarizes the standard IC precautions that are used with patients who have AIDS or are known to be infected with HIV. **These same IC precautions apply to all patients, regardless of what is known or not known regarding their status for HIV infection.** When a patient is admitted, after a nursing history is taken and the original patient care assessment is completed, the nursing care plan will reflect an adaptation of the above general IC guidelines for each individual patient. All patients with AIDS are not the same. It is not appropriate to have a rigid procedure for AIDS patients, which is implemented without modification each time a patient with this condition is admitted.

Table 12.4 Standard IC precautions – AIDS and ARC

Precaution	Procedure	Rationale
Single room	Used for patients with severe diarrhoea, excessive coughing, some opportunistic infections, seriously or terminally ill, bleeding or anticipated bleeding, enteric infections, or for psychological or social reasons	To protect the immunocompromised patient from nosocomial infections, and to protect health care workers and other patients from infection with HIV and associated opportunistic pathogens
Plastic aprons and gloves	Used when delivering direct patient care, handling specimens, or domestic cleaning	As above
Gowns, masks and eye protection	Only used in dealing with gross contamination or assisting with invasive procedures,	To protect health care workers from infection with HIV or other associated opportunistic

Table 12.4 *continued*

Precaution	Procedure	Rationale
	or when the patient is coughing excessively, or at any time in which aerosol contamination is anticipated. Masks without eye protection, either worn by the patient outside the room, or by health care workers inside the room, are required during the early treatment phase for patients with pulmonary tuberculosis	pathogens (e.g. *Mycobacterium tuberculosis*, CMV) To protect health care workers from acquisition of *M. tuberculosis* infection
Handwashing	Hands are washed prior to, and after all patient care activities If gloves are worn, hands must still be carefully washed prior to gloving, and after gloves are removed	To protect the immunocompromised patient from nosocomial infection and to protect health care workers from acquisition of HIV and associated opportunistic pathogens
	Povidone-iodine 7.5% in a non-ionic detergent base (Betadine or Videne surgical scrub) or chlorhexidine gluconate 4% containing isopropyl alcohol 4% detergent (Hibiscrub or Hibiclens) are preferred	To prevent transmission of potential pathogens to other patients
Needles, injections, and other sharps	Needles are not recapped, bent, or	Meticulous care is required in dealing

Table 12.4 *continued*

Precaution	Procedure	Rationale
	broken after use and are disposed of immediately in a rigid, plastic, puncture-resistant and waterproof 'sharps container'	with sharps to prevent needlestick injuries with possible HIV acquisition by health care workers
	Sharps container is taken to bedside or left in patient's room	Needles are not broken or snapped off in order to avoid a microscopic aerosol of infected material
	Special care is required for disposing of intravenous infusion sets	If sharp ends are not carefully cut off there is a risk that they will puncture side of plastic disposal bags, and injure ancillary staff
	Used instruments are placed in waterproof plastic bag or plastic box and returned to CSSD for autoclaving	To prevent leakage of blood or body fluids while being transported to the CSSD
Linen (visibly contaminated with blood or body fluids, excretions or secretions)	Double-bagged. First placed in red plastic alginate bag, which in turn is placed in a red nylon bag, and then closed securely and sent to the laundry	To prevent contamination of housekeeping personnel when transporting linen to laundry, and to protect laundry personnel from contamination by infected linen
	Gloves are worn when handling infected linen	
Contaminated material	All infected rubbish, including dressings, drainage tubing and intravenous fluid administration sets (with sharp ends cut off at both ends!) are placed in a heavy-	To protect housekeeping and portering personnel from contamination

Scrupulous care must be taken to ensure no sharps are placed in |

Table 12.4 *continued*

Precaution	Procedure	Rationale
	duty yellow plastic bag, securely closed, and sent for incineration	rubbish bags
Crockery and cutlery	May use ordinary dishes and silverware	Disposable crockery and cutlery rarely needed
	A patient who has an enteric or mouth infection, or has pulmonary tuberculosis, may keep individual dishes and silver in room	To prevent risk of transmitting opportunistic pathogens to other patients
Specimens	Gloves must be worn when handling all specimens	To prevent contamination with infected blood and body fluids, affecting everyone who is handling specimens
	Specimen container and specimen request form may be labelled with a suitable warning sticker (e.g. 'BioHazard' or 'Risk of infection') and transported to the laboratory in an impervious plastic bag	To alert laboratory personnel of special risk To prevent leakage during transport to laboratory
Ward privileges	If ambulatory, patient may have full ward privileges (e.g. may go to TV room, hospital shop, etc.)	To prevent isolation
	Patients with diarrhoea should use their own toilet	To prevent contamination
	Visitors are to be encouraged	

Because of the vast numbers of individuals in the community who are currently infected with this retrovirus and are unaware of it, nurses will often be caring for patients in which the infection is unidentified. Therefore it is essential to adopt sensible IC procedures for **all** patients. Special care must now be taken to avoid contamination with blood and body fluids from every patient. Strict attention must be paid to good handwashing techniques, wearing gloves when dealing with all blood and body fluids. Diligent care when dealing with needles and other sharps has now become even more obligatory in nursing care. With the advent of AIDS, the days of nurses adopting a casual approach to blood and body fluids from any patient are gone forever. If a nurse or other health care worker has a parenteral (e.g. needlestick or cut) or mucous membrane (e.g. splash to the eye or mouth) exposure to blood or other body fluids, the instructions in Table 12.5 should be followed.

Nurses or other health care workers who have cuts, abrasions or any type of skin lesion, should ensure that these are covered with a

Table 12.5 Procedure for treating parenteral or mucous membrane exposure to blood/body fluids

---

1. Parenteral exposure:
   - Injury should be encouraged to bleed by local venous occlusion
   - This is followed by washing the inoculation site for 5 minutes in running water, using povidone-iodine 7.5% in a detergent base (Betadine or Videne surgical scrub), or a 4% chlorhexidine gluconate with 4% isopropyl alcohol detergent (e.g. Hibiscrub, Hibiclens) or any soap or detergent if the above are not available
2. Mucous membrane exposure:
   - Splashes in the mouth: the mouth should be washed out, using running water
   - Splashes into the eye: the eye should be well irrigated with either running water or sodium chloride 0.9%
3. The accident should immediately be reported to the senior nurse in charge and an 'Incident Report' should be made out, fully documenting the accident
4. The nurse should be seen in the Occupational Health Department, or by his or her own physician, who will advise on serological screening for anti-HIV
5. Serological screening for anti-HIV: A baseline specimen of blood should be taken and either tested for anti-HIV, or stored frozen. Further specimens of blood are tested at 3 and 6 month intervals following exposure
6. The nurse should be examined and health status documented every 6 months for 1 year following the accident. This also provides an opportunity to offer reassurance

---

waterproof dressing, and that gloves are worn when caring for any patient in whom it is anticipated that exposure to blood or other body fluids may occur.

Summary

It is difficult to legislate in policy specific infection control procedures that apply to the variables of clinical nursing practice. **Universal precautions** require a change in attitude, an acceptance of the concept that whatever IC procedure is appropriate for a patient or client known to be infected with HIV is also appropriate for every patient, in every clinical situation, all the time. Nursing staff have to be involved in the creation and ownership of new IC policies which incorporate **universal precautions**. These policies must then be supported by senior nurse managers who are ultimately responsible for ensuring that a procedural basis for a safe working environment is established. The days of having separate IC policies and procedures for patients known to be infected with HIV has long past.

References

1. Centers for Disease Control (1987). Recommendations for Prevention of HIV Transmission in Health Care Settings. *Morbidity and Mortality Weekly Report (MMWR)*, 21 August, **36**(2S), 3S–18S.
2. Centers for Disease Control (1988). Update: Universal Precautions for Prevention of Transmission of Human Immunodeficiency Virus, Hepatitis B Virus and other Bloodborne Pathogens in Health Care Settings. *Morbidity and Mortality Weekly Report (MMWR)*, 24 June, **37**, 377–88.
3. UK Health Departments (1990). *Guidance for Clinical Health Care Workers: Protection Against Infection with HIV and Hepatitis Viruses: Recommendations of the Expert Advisory Group on AIDS.* HMSO, London.
4. Jackson, M.M. and Lynch, P. (1991). An attempt to make an issue less murky: A comparison of four systems for infection precautions. *Infection Control and Hospital Epidemiology*, July, **12**, 448–50.
5. Korniewitcz, D.M., Laughon, B.E., Cyr, W.H. *et al.* (1990). Leakage of virus through used vinyl and latex examination gloves. *Journal of Clinical Microbiology* **28**(4), 787–8.
6. Kotilainen, H.R., Brinker, J.P., Avato, J.L. *et al.* (1989). Latex and vinyl examination gloves: quality control procedures and implications for health care workers. *Archives of Internal Medicine* **149**(12), 2749–53.
7. Hopkins, V. (1994). Personal communication. A.C. Daniels & Co. Ltd, 130 Western Rd, Tring, Herts., HP23 4BU, UK.

8. Martin, L.D., McDougal, S. and Loskoski, S.L. (1985). Disinfection and inactivation of the human T-lymphotropic virus type III/lymphadenopathy-associated virus. *Journal of Infectious Diseases* **152**, 400–3.

9. Asanka, M. and Kurimura, T. (1987). Inactivation of human immunodeficiency virus (HIV) by povidone-iodine. *Yonago Acta Medica* **30**(2), 89–92.

10. Montefiori, D.C., Robinson Jr., W.E., Modliszewski, A. *et al.* (1990). Effective inactivation of human immunodeficiency virus with chlorhexidine antiseptics containing detergents and alcohol. *Journal of Hospital Infection* **15**(3), 279–82.

Further reading

Ayliffe, G.A.J., Coates, D. and Hoffman, P.N. (1993). *Chemical Disinfection in Hospitals*. Public Health Laboratory Service, London (ISBN 0-901144-34-7).

Crow, S. (1989). *Asepsis, The Right Touch (Something Old is Now New)*. The Everett Companies, USA (ISBN 0-944419-15-1).

Henderson, D.K. (1994). HIV transmission in the health care setting. In *Textbook of AIDS Medicine*, eds Broder, S., Merigan, T.C. Jr. and Bolognesi, D., William & Wilkins, Baltimore (ISBN 0-683-01072-7).

Pugliese, G., Lynch, P. and Jackson, M.M. (1991). *Universal Precautions: Policies, Procedures, and Resources*. American Hospital Association Company, American Hospital Publishing, Chicago (ISBN 1-55648-055-5).

Wilson, J. and Breedon, P. (1990). Universal precautions – A new approach to infection control. *Nursing Times*, 12 September, **86**(37), 67–8.

13

The Risk of Occupational Exposure to HIV

Now, well into the second decade of our experience with this disease, the known means of viral transmission are generally understood. The risk of occupational exposure and transmission of HIV in health care settings can be described in relation to: the reality (epidemiology) of occupationally acquired HIV infection; strategies designed to manage this risk; the management of occupational exposure to HIV; and strategies for managing the HIV-infected health care worker.

The reality of the risk

Occupational exposure to HIV among health care workers is not a rare event. In the USA it is estimated that at least 50 000 occupational exposures to HIV have occurred since the beginning of the epidemic[1]. Although the statistical probability of becoming infected following occupational exposure is low, the emotional impact on those exposed is significant. In addition, in the USA, over 100 health care providers may have become infected with HIV in the health care setting[2]. In the UK, in the period 1985–92, 176 significant occupational exposures to HIV were reported to the PHLS Communicable Disease Surveillance Centre. Since the beginning of the epidemic, at least four health care workers have become infected in the UK as a result of occupational exposure and there are six other health care workers (two surgeons and four nurses) with possible occupationally acquired HIV infection, probably infected when working in Africa or in the USA.[3].

The number of health care workers who have been occupationally exposed and infected with this virus throughout the world is not known, but in some institutions, especially in the developing world, the numbers may be significant[4]. The risk of health care workers acquiring HIV infection from patients depends on:

• the prevalence of the virus in the population served;

- the length of time the health care worker has practised;
- exposure-specific factors;
- biological factors; and
- the likelihood of transmission from each accidental exposure.

HIV prevalence

There are geographical variations in the numbers of HIV infections reported. The North Thames and South Thames regions (London) in England have the largest numbers of both AIDS cases and HIV infections in the UK. The Thames regions (and Scotland) also report the highest cumulative number of AIDS cases and HIV-1 infections per million resident population in the UK[5]. Health care providers are more likely to come into contact with patients infected with HIV in large city hospitals, clinics and community services rather than in other parts of the country.

The length of time the health care worker has practised

The frequency of blood or body fluid contamination for various groups of health care workers, e.g. surgeons, has been estimated. For example, in one study focused on general surgery, cutaneous contamination was documented in about 6 per cent of operative procedures[6]. In another study[7] focused on obstetric procedures, body fluid contamination occurred approximately 42 per cent of the time and, in this same study, 23 per cent of staff were shown to have broken skin on their hands and arms! The estimated frequency of exposure can be extrapolated to calculations focusing on the life-time risks of HIV acquisition to various categories of health care workers. In general, the longer the health care worker practises and the greater the frequency with which risk-associated procedures are performed, the greater the risk of being exposed to HIV in the occupational setting.

The circumstances under which the procedures are performed will also influence the degree of risk. For example, emergency procedures are more likely to involve a degree of risk than an elective procedure carried out in a controlled environment.

Exposure-specific factors

The type of exposure is important. Two types of exposures are defined for surveillance purposes in the UK; **percutaneous exposure** and **mucocutaneous exposure**. Percutaneous exposure is one in which the skin is cut or penetrated by a needle or other sharp object (e.g.

scalpel blade, trochar, tooth, bone spicule). Mucocutaneous exposure is one which involves the eye(s), inside of the nose or mouth, or an area of non-intact skin of the person exposed. Percutaneous exposure carries the greatest risk. In addition, percutaneous exposures which involve fresh blood and hollow needles are significantly associated with increased risk of infection[3].

The characteristics of the exposure, e.g. type of wound, depth of injury, type of instrument, amount of blood contamination may also be associated with likelihood of infection. The type of body fluid is also important, blood being the single most important risk. Exposure to concentrated virus in laboratories where serological test kits are manufactured also carries significant risk.

Biological factors

The **volume of the inoculum** may be important and in general, the greater the volume of the inoculum, the greater the risk. However, not only is the size of the inoculum important, but also the **concentration of virus in the inoculum**. Blood has a higher HIV concentration than non-bloody body fluids. In addition, the **strain of the virus** to which the health care worker is exposed is significant. Some strains of HIV are more virulent than others and some are resistant to antiretroviral drugs, such as zidovudine (AZT), which may affect the efficacy of post-exposure prophylaxis[3]. The disease stage of the source patient may also be important, with those at end-stage presenting the greatest risk. This may be due to the titre of virus in their blood, the relative resistance of HIV to zidovudine at that stage of their illness, circulating cell-free virus, etc., or it may simply be associated with the fact that patients at end-stage illness have more contact with health care providers and are the focal point of more exposure-prone procedures.

The likelihood of HIV transmission from accidental exposure

The observed seroconversion rate following percutaneous exposure to HIV-infected blood varies and ranges in large studies from 0.18 per cent[8] to 0.56 per cent[9]. In smaller samples, the range is higher, from 2 per cent in the UK[3] to 5.8 per cent in South Africa[4]. The generally accepted estimated risk of seroconversion after percutaneous exposure to HIV is approximately 1 in 300 or 0.33 per cent[10], although it may be higher depending on the subcategory of percutaneous exposure, e.g. venepuncture, intramuscular injection, etc. This risk has remained relatively stable during the first decade of the epidemic[11] and it must be compared with the risk of exposure to other bloodborne pathogens. For example, the risk of infection among susceptible health care workers following percutaneous exposure to hepatitis B virus from a patient who is 'e' antigen positive is approximately 30 per cent (150 in 500).

Tuberculosis

Since the early 1980s, notifications of cases of active tuberculosis have risen, especially in the USA and especially in the age range 25–40 years. This resurgence is principally due to the prevalence of HIV infection in this group, and homelessness[12]. The World Health Organization estimates that there will be more than 90 million new cases of TB in the 1990s and that 30 million people will die from TB with a doubling of the mortality rates in Africa and Asia. This increase is principally due to poor quality control programmes, exacerbated by demographic factors (accounting for 75 per cent of the predicted increase), but the escalation of HIV infection will account for 25 per cent of the projected increase[13]. In addition, it is estimated that, worldwide, by early 1992, at least 4.6 million people were co-infected with HIV and *M. tuberculosis*[14].

In the USA, Africa and Asia, the emergence of a significant increase in cases of **multi-drug resistant tuberculosis** is alarming. TB is typically seen early in HIV infection, well before other AIDS-defining opportunistic diseases. In addition, drug-resistant TB in an individual who is infected with HIV is associated with a high mortality rate. *M. tuberculosis* is usually transmitted from one person to another by the respiratory route and infection control precautions are implemented which involve protecting both health care workers and other patients from nosocomial infection. **Anyone who is immunocompromised, including health care workers who are infected with HIV, are uniquely susceptible to infection with** *M. tuberculosis*.

In the USA, especially in New York City, large numbers of patients co-infected with HIV and drug-resistant tuberculosis are now being cared for. Although an increase in cases of active TB in the UK has been seen, so far this increase has come from individuals who have recently immigrated, or whose families immigrated to the UK from the Indian subcontinent, where the prevalence and incidence of TB is high[15]. However, other groups in the UK who are at an increased risk of developing active TB include the elderly, the homeless and those who are infected with HIV[16].

There exists a real risk to health care providers of *M. tuberculosis* infection in health care settings where patients with active tuberculosis are cared for, especially in that window period prior to diagnosis and treatment. This risk becomes more significant if the health care provider is immunocompromised and the emergence of multi-drug resistant tuberculosis compounds the hazard. A detailed discussion of infection control procedures in relation to preventing nosocomial mycobacterial infections can be found in Chapter 7 and in Appendix 3.

Strategies designed to reduce the risk

Models for effective infection control have continued to evolve since the beginning of the epidemic. AIDS, more than any other disease, highlighted the need for a rational and effective approach to infection control. However, the role of serological testing for HIV infection continues to be discussed within the context of developing 'tiers' of infection control, i.e. one tier focused on known or suspected HIV-infected patients and requiring more stringent infection control precautions than those which are required for patients not thought to be infected with HIV, i.e. a two-tier system. Testing is crucial to this model and it is worth reviewing exactly what an HIV antibody test result means.

HIV testing

A confirmed, positive HIV antibody test result indicates exposure and current infection. It cannot define the disease stage or response to treatment, although other serological markers (e.g. p24 levels, etc.) may be useful in doing this. A negative HIV antibody test usually means that an individual is not infected with HIV. However, from an infection control point of view it is meaningless. There are several reasons why a person can test negative but still be infected. The two most important reasons are that it takes anywhere from 8 to 24 weeks for a person to seroconvert, i.e. test positive, following exposure and infection. In addition, if a person is tested and is not infected at the time of the test, their result will be negative. However, they could be exposed and infected with the virus at any time after the test. There is no blood test which can guarantee that a person is not infected.

Models of infection control

A two-tier system of infection control is flawed in logic in that health care workers will always be caring for patients sometimes infected with HIV whose infection status is unknown to both them and their carers. Consequently, more reasoned models of infection control have been developed, including **universal precautions**[11,17] and **body substance isolation**[18]. Both of these models require the use of appropriate barriers whenever contact with potentially infectious bodily fluids is anticipated. In the USA, the implementation of one or other of these two models is now legally mandated by the US Department of Labor's Occupational Health and Safety Administration (OSHA)[19]. A risk assessment takes place in relation to the procedure, not the patient. Whatever barrier precaution is deemed appropriate in a procedure for a patient with known HIV infection, that same precaution is applied each time that procedure is used for all patients, without exception. A detailed discussion of infection control models can be found in Chapter 12.

Policies, procedures and staff education

Clearly all health care facilities must have current infection control policies and procedures and must equally monitor their implementation. These policies should form the basis of ongoing staff education initiatives which must commence with orientation/induction programmes.

Management of occupational exposure to HIV

In addition, an agreed protocol must be developed for the management of occupational exposure to bloodborne pathogens. A systematic approach is required which includes the following components[1,20,21]:

- Different levels of potential risks must be categorized and stratified and specifications for follow-up for each defined.
- Employees must be made aware of the protocols through in-service educational programmes. Employers should make available to health care workers a system for promptly initiating evaluation, counselling and follow-up after a reported occupational exposure that may place the health care worker at risk of acquiring HIV infection.

  Mechanisms must be in place which will ensure the protection of both patient and employee confidentiality.

- Health care workers must be educated and supported to report exposures immediately after they occur, because certain interventions that may be appropriate (e.g. prophylaxis against hepatitis B virus) must be initiated promptly to be effective.
- When an exposure occurs, the circumstances should be recorded in the health care worker's confidential medical records. Relevant information includes:
  - date and time of exposure;
  - job duty being performed by the health care worker at the time of exposure;
  - details of exposure, including amount of fluid or material, type of fluid or material, and severity of exposure, e.g. for a percutaneous exposure, depth of injury and whether fluid was injected; for a skin or mucocutaneous exposure, the extent and duration of contact and condition of the skin (e.g. chapped, abraded, intact);
  - description of source of exposure, including, if known, whether the source material contained HIV or hepatitis B virus; and
  - details about counselling, post-exposure management, and follow-up.
- The procedure for post-exposure first aid must be included in the protocols. Accepted procedures[1] emphasize the need for the decontamination of the exposure site as soon as patient safety permits. The area is washed well with soap and water and, if the exposure site requires suturing, it is irrigated thoroughly prior to closure. The use of antiseptics and techniques to make the wound bleed following exposure seem sensible although there is no evidence to suggest they have made a critical difference. Exposed mucous membranes should be flushed with clean water or, if the eyes are involved, irrigated with sterile, normal saline.
- After an occupational exposure, both the exposed worker and the source individual should be evaluated to determine the possible need for the exposed worker to receive prophylaxis against hepatitis B. Because of the potentially severe consequences of hepatitis B virus infection, hepatitis B vaccine, which is both safe and highly effective, should be offered to any susceptible health care worker who has an occupational exposure and has not previously been vaccinated with hepatitis B vaccine. Hepatitis B immune globulin may also be indicated, particularly if the source patient or material is found to be positive for hepatitis B surface antigen (HBsAg).
- A policy must be included which encourages serological testing of the source patient and the exposed employee. This policy

must address the issues of informed consent and must outline pre- and post-test counselling support for both the patient and employee. Serological follow-up and medical surveillance must be encouraged and the employee instructed to contact the occupational health service, or their own physician, if they develop any symptoms suggestive of acute primary HIV infection (see Chapter 6).

- Counselling and information to prevent possible transmission to the employee's sexual partner should form an essential part of the protocol.
- An institutional policy should be developed in order to guide the prescribing of antiretroviral drugs, e.g. zidovudine (AZT), zalcitabine (ddC), didanosine (ddI), as part of post-exposure prophylaxis. There is no scientific evidence to date to suggest that zidovudine (AZT) or any other antiretroviral drug will protect against infection when given following occupational exposure. However, health care workers may very well expect chemoprophylaxis and the institution's position must be thought out well in advance of the stresses surrounding the actual incident.

Post-exposure chemoprophylaxis

Following occupational exposure to blood or body fluids, the issues surrounding the use of chemoprophylaxis with antiretroviral drugs needs to be discussed with the exposed health care worker. It can reasonably be anticipated that the following concerns will be identified during this discussion:

- Is chemoprophylaxis available?
- What are the protocols for prophylaxis, i.e. when does drug administration commence, how frequently are drugs taken and what is the duration of prophylaxis?
- What are the side-effects of the antiretroviral drug being offered?
- Can it be safely taken by women if they are pregnant or may become pregnant during the course of prophylaxis?
- Will it work, i.e. will it protect against HIV infection?
- Is a blood test for HIV antibodies required?
- How long is the follow-up period after completing the course of drugs?

Availability

A well-thought-out policy must be in place to guide the prescribing of antiretroviral drugs for chemoprophylaxis. There must be ownership of this policy and its existence well-known and understood by all health care employees. The policy should address: the theoretical rationale for post-exposure prophylaxis; outline the risk of occupationally acquired HIV infection due to exposure; describe the limitations of current knowledge of the efficacy of antiretroviral drugs when used as post-exposure prophylaxis; describe current knowledge of the toxicity of antiretroviral drugs in uninfected individuals who take the drug after occupational exposures; and, the need for post-exposure follow-up (including HIV serological testing), regardless of whether antiretroviral drugs are taken. If the policy supports the use of antiretroviral drugs for chemoprophylaxis, then it is axiomatic that those drugs must be available immediately on notification that an incident has occurred and chemoprophylaxis is to be offered. Issues surrounding informed consent, confidentiality and counselling must be addressed in the policy, as well as the issue of cost, i.e. who is to pay for the drugs.

If chemoprophylaxis is to be taken, prophylaxis should commence as soon as possible following exposure.

The HIV-infected health care worker

The risk of HIV transmission from an infected health care worker to a patient during routine patient care activities is so small that it cannot be accurately measured. However, the potential for HIV transmission does exist during exposure-prone invasive procedures, i.e. those associated with risk for exposure of a patient's blood stream to blood or body fluids from a health care worker. To date, only one case of probable infection to patients from an HIV-infected dentist has been documented[22,23]. The events surrounding the incidents, which led to six patients being infected, will probably never be known with any degree of certainty. However, they were likely to have been extraordinary and unlikely to be repeated.

Other viruses, such as hepatitis B virus and herpes simplex virus have been transmitted to patients by infected health care workers during exposure-prone procedures[24] and the fact remains that transmission of HIV from an infected health care worker to a patient is possible, although unlikely. Consequently, professional advice has been published[24–26].

All professional guidelines stress the primacy of the patient's interest, which recognizes that nothing should ever be done by health care professionals which could put their patients at risk, no matter how low that risk is. Accordingly, guidelines in the UK (and the USA) recommend that health care workers who believe that they may have been infected with HIV seek medical advice and diagnostic antibody testing, if appropriate. If health care workers are infected, they must seek medical and occupational advice. In general, they should not perform exposure-prone procedures and must remain under regular medical and occupational health supervision. If exposure-prone procedures have been performed, infected health care workers should inform their local Director of Public Health (DPH), or, in Scotland, the Chief Administrative Medical Officer, on a confidential basis, who will then decide on the appropriateness of conducting any 'look-back' exercises. Employers must ensure the confidentiality of their employees' health status and be able to offer appropriate clinical re-assignments. They must be able to respond effectively to any form of discrimination and ensure that they offer meaningful in-service education, focused on the issues of HIV infection and universal infection control precautions.

HIV-infected health care workers must not practise in clinical environments where patients with tuberculosis or other contagious illnesses are being nursed. Consequently, it is not safe for HIV-infected health care workers to be assigned to dedicated HIV units, as they risk being exposed to TB and a whole range of infectious illnesses which, because of their own immunocompromised state, they are uniquely susceptible to.

Summary

We have almost 15 years of experience in caring for patients infected with HIV. In our early years, in the twilight of our ignorance, the cause of AIDS was unknown, as was the potential risk to health care professionals in caring for patients with this disease. In the clear daylight of the second decade of our collective experience, we now know that patients with HIV infection can be cared for safely. The key to our continuing success in developing and offering competent and compassionate care lies in in-service education and in adapting our clinical practice in the light of the known means of viral transmission. Dilemmas remain – they have always been there. Continuing discussion and adopting more flexible postures will facilitate a confident and mature, professional rationale for our convictions.

References

1. Gerberding, J.L. (1994). Managing occupational exposures to HIV. In *Textbook of AIDS Medicine*, eds Broder, S., Merigan, T.C. Jr. and Bolognesi, D., Williams & Wilkins, Baltimore, MD, pp. 841–4.
2. Centers for Disease Control (1992). Surveillance for occupationally acquired HIV infection – United States 1981–1992. *Morbidity and Mortality Weekly Report (MMWR)*, **41**, 823–5.
3. PHLS Communicable Disease Surveillance Centre (1993). Health care workers and HIV: surveillance of occupationally acquired infection in the United Kingdom. *Communicable Disease Report*, 8 October, **3**(11), R147–R153.
4. Tait, D.R., Pudifin, D.J., Gathiram, V. *et al.* (1992). HIV seroconversion in health care workers, Natal, South Africa. *Abstracts*, Eighth International Conference on AIDS, Amsterdam, July, abstract PoC 4141.
5. PHLS Communicable Disease Surveillance Centre (1994). AIDS and HIV-1 infection in the United Kingdom: monthly report. *Communicable Disease Report* **4**(15), 69–72.
6. Gerberding, J.L., Littell, C., Tarkington, A. *et al.* (1990). Risk of exposure of surgical personnel to patients' blood during surgery at San Francisco General Hospital. *New England Journal of Medicine* **332**, 1788–93.
7. Kabukoba, J.J. and Young, P. (1992). Midwifery and body fluid contamination. *British Medical Journal* **305**, 26.
8. Ippolito, G., Puro, V., De Carli, G. and the Italian Study Group on Occupational Risk of HIV Infection (1993). *Abstracts*, Ninth International Conference on AIDS, Berlin, June, abstract PO-C18–3021.
9. Henderson, D.K., Fahey, B.J., Willy, M. *et al.* (1990). Risk for occupational transmission of human immunodeficiency virus type 1 (HIV-1) associated with clinical exposures: a prospective evaluation. *Annals of Internal Medicine* **113**, 740–6.
10. Heptonstall, J., Porter, K. and Gill, O.N. (1993). Occupational transmission of HIV. Summary of published reports. *PHLS Internal* Report, September.
11. Centers for Disease Control (1987). Recommendations for Prevention of HIV Transmission in Health-care Settings. *Morbidity and Mortality Weekly Report (MMWR)*, **36**(Suppl. 2S): 1S-19S.
12. Barnes, P.F., Block, A.B., Davidson, P.T. *et al.* (1991). Review article – Current concepts: Tuberculosis in patients with human immunodeficiency virus infection. *New England Journal of Medicine*, 6 June, **324**(23), 1644–50.
13. WHO (1994) Press Releases, WHO/6 (21 January 1994), WHO/9 (26 January 1994). World Health Organization, Geneva.
14. Mann, J., Tarantola, D.J.M. and Netter, Thomas W. (eds) (1992). *AIDS in the World: A Global Report*. Harvard University Press, London, pp. 148–63.
15. Watson, John M. (1993). Editorial: Tuberculosis in Britain today.

British Medical Journal, 23 January, **306**(6872), 221–2.

16. PHLS Communicable Disease Surveillance Centre (1993). Tuberculosis in England and Wales, *Communicable Disease Report*, **3**, 85.
17. Centers for Disease Control (1988). Update: universal precautions for prevention of transmission of human immunodeficiency virus, hepatitis B virus, and other bloodborne pathogens in health care settings. *Morbidity and Mortality Weekly Report (MMWR)* **37** 337–82, 387–8.
18. Lynch, P., Jackson, M.M., Cummings, J. *et al.* (1987). Rethinking the role of isolation practices in the prevention of nosocomial infections. *Annals of Internal Medicine* **107**, 243–6.
19. US Department of Labor – OSHA (1991). Occupational exposure to bloodborne pathogens; final rule. *Federal Register* **56**, 64175–82.
20. Henderson, D.K. (1994). HIV transmission in the health care environment. In *Textbook of AIDS Medicine*, eds Broder, S., Merigan, T.C. Jr. and Bolognesi, D., Williams & Wilkins, Baltimore, MD, pp. 831–40.
21. Centers for Disease Control (1990). Recommendations and Reports: Public Health Service Statement on Management of Occupational Exposure to Human Immunodeficiency Virus, Including Considerations Regarding Zidovudine Postexposure Use. *Morbidity and Mortality Weekly Report (MMWR)*, 26 June, **39**(RR-1), 1–14.
22. Centers for Disease Control (1990). Possible transmission of human immunodeficiency virus to a patient during an invasive dental procedure, *Morbidity and Mortality Weekly Report (MMWR)* **39**, 489–93.
23. Centers for Disease Control (1991). Update: transmission of HIV infection during an invasive dental procedure – Florida. *Morbidity and Mortality Weekly Report (MMWR)* **40**, 21–33.
24. Centers for Disease Control (1991). Recommendations for Preventing Transmission of Human Immunodeficiency Virus and Hepatitis B Virus to Patients During Exposure-Prone Invasive Procedures. *Morbidity and Mortality Weekly Report (MMWR)* **40**, RR-8.
25. UK Health Departments (1994). *AIDS/HIV-Infected Health Care Workers: Guidance on the Management of Infected Health Care Workers*, Recommendations of the Expert Advisory Group on AIDS. HMSO, London.
26. United Kingdom Central Council for Nursing, Midwifery and Health Visiting (1994). 1. Acquired immune deficiency syndrome and human immunodeficiency virus infection (AIDS and HIV infection), 2. Anonymous testing for the prevalence of the human immunodeficiency virus (HIV). *Registrar's Letter* **4**, 1–7; 1–3.

Further reading

Centers for Disease Control (1991). Recommendations for Preventing Transmission of Human Immunodeficiency Virus and Hepatitis B Virus to Patients During Exposure-Prone Invasive Procedures. *Morbidity and Mortality Weekly Report (MMWR)* **40**, RR-8.

Gerberding, J.L. (1992). HIV transmission to providers and their patients. In *The Medical Management of AIDS*, 3rd edn, W.B. Saunders, London (ISBN 0-7216-6752-X), Chapter 4.

Gerberding, J.L. (1994). Managing occupational exposures to HIV. In *Textbook of AIDS Medicine*, eds Broder, S., Merigan, T.C. Jr. and Bolognesi, D., Williams & Wilkins, Baltimore, MD (ISBN 0-683-01072-7).

Henderson, D.K. (1994). HIV transmission in the health care environment. In *Textbook of AIDS Medicine*, eds Broder, S., Merigan, T.C. Jr. and Bolognesi, D., Williams & Wilkins, Baltimore, MD (ISBN 0-683-01072-7).

United Kingdom Central Council for Nursing, Midwifery and Health Visiting (1994). 1. Acquired immune deficiency syndrome and human immunodeficiency virus infection (AIDS and HIV infection), 2. Anonymous testing for the prevalence of the human immunodeficiency virus (HIV). *Registrar's Letter* **4**.

UK Health Departments (1994). *AIDS/HIV-Infected Health Care Workers: Guidance on the Management of Infected Health Care Workers*, Recommendations of the Expert Advisory Group on AIDS. HMSO, London.

14

The Individualized Care of Patients with HIV Disease

Patients admitted for investigation or treatment of HIV infection and associated opportunistic disease may be in a rapidly changing clinical situation. Therefore nursing care must be assessed, planned and evaluated on a daily basis. This requires a comprehensive understanding by the nurse of the rationale which underpins strategic nursing care.

Strategic nursing care is that care which is developed and implemented by registered nurses, designed to meet the immediate needs of patients, solve identified actual problems and prevent recognized potential problems from being realized. Because of their training and experience, their comprehensive understanding of the nursing issues involved, and their teaching and management skills, registered nurses are able to assess and plan the individualized nursing care most appropriate for each patient, leading and supervising the nursing team implementing this care. Care delivered must be evaluated frequently (often on a shift-by-shift basis) and modified according to the patient's response to nursing intervention. The registered nurse is ideally placed to act as the patient's advocate and to liaise effectively between the patient and other members of the health care team.

Strategic nursing care embraces the concept of a problem-solving approach to the individualized care of each patient. However, it is more than a nursing process style of care. It includes assessment and planning of nursing care on a hospital-wide basis, taking into consideration all the real and possible issues governing the implementation of care and includes both logistical, educational and managerial aspects, which, if not anticipated, may preclude the delivery of individualized, high quality care. In this chapter we are going to explore planned care for individual patients; further chapters will discuss the issues and back-up nursing support required to deliver this care effectively.

Strategic nursing care: a model for patients with HIV-related disease

Behavioural models of nursing, as conceived by Henderson[1], Roper *et al.*[2] and Orem[3], are valuable tools by which individualized nursing care of patients with HIV-related disease can be planned and implemented efficiently and effectively. These models describe needs and self-care requisites necessary for normal, healthy living. The use of these models allows for the speedy identification by the nurse of unmet needs and deficits in self-care requisites. A nursing assessment includes the recognition of unmet needs and actual problems. It further identifies potential problems associated with the patient's condition (social, psychological, physical and medical), specific illness, hospitalization and medical treatment. Identifying and documenting needs, self-care requisites, actual problems and potential problems facilitates planning appropriate nursing intervention and allows the effectiveness of this intervention to be evaluated.

In discussing the strategic nursing care of patients with HIV-related disease, an eclectic approach to behavioural models of nursing has been used. The overall objective of planned nursing care is to 'assist the individual, sick or well, in the performance of those activities contributing to health or its recovery (or to peaceful death) that he would perform unaided if he had the necessary strength, will or knowledge. And to do this in such a way as to help him gain independence as rapidly as possible'[4].

Needs

In common with all individuals, patients with HIV-related disease have needs which they or others must meet for health to be maintained. The following list, adapted from Henderson's 'Components of basic nursing'[4] and Roper's 'Activities of living'[2] itemizes the needs which may be examined during the nursing assessment:

1. The need for adequate respiration
2. The need for adequate hydration
3. The need for adequate nutrition
4. The need for urinary and faecal elimination
5. The need to control body temperature
6. The need for movement and mobilization
7. The need for a safe environment
8. The need for personal cleansing and dressing
9. The need for expression and communication

10. The need for working and playing
11. The need for adequate rest and sleep
12. The need to maintain psychological equilibrium
13. The need to worship according to own faith
14. The need to express sexuality
15. Needs associated with dying.

By examining these requisites or needs, problems may be identified. These may be either current problems (actual problems) or problems that may be anticipated due to the patient's need deprivation, medical condition or treatment (potential problems).

1. The need for adequate respiration

Potential problems	**Origin of problem**
Dyspnoea, cough, tachypnoea, cyanosis	Pneumonia (*Pneumocystis carinii*, CMV other opportunistic pathogens) Neoplastic involvement from Kaposi's sarcoma or anaemia

Objectives of care

1. To maintain optimal respiratory function.
2. To alleviate cough.
3. To keep patient well oxygenated.

Nursing intervention

Assessment
Vital signs (blood pressure/pulse/respiratory rate/body temperature), arterial blood gases (ABG), colour, respiratory effort, chest sounds, sputum production and mental status should be noted and documented as a baseline assessment.

Position
The patient should be placed in a position which facilitates good respiratory function. Sitting the patient upright, leaning forward and well supported is frequently useful in that it allows the accessory muscles (sternomastoid, pectoralis major, platysma and latissimus dorsi) to assist respiratory effort.

Oxygen
Depending on the patient's clinical condition and arterial blood gases (ABG), the physician may prescribe supplemental oxygen to be administered. In general, the lowest concentration of oxygen needed

to overcome hypoxaemia will be ordered. Concentrations of inspired oxygen less than 40 per cent are well tolerated for long periods of time and may be administered by Ventimasks (Vickers Limited Medical Group) or Edinburgh masks (British Oxygen Co. Ltd). Double nasal cannulae may be preferred as they are comfortable and do not interfere with eating, drinking and the wearing of spectacles, although the inspired oxygen concentration provided is unpredictable. An oxygen flow rate of 2 litres per minute will provide approximately a 30 per cent concentration. High concentrations of supplemental oxygen are sometimes required. They can be administered by Polymasks (British Oxygen Co. Ltd) or MC masks (Medical and Industrial Equipment Ltd), both of which deliver approximately a 60 per cent concentration at a flow rate of 4–6 litres per minute. Oxygen administered by these masks requires humidification. Oxygen concentrations of greater than 60 per cent, which have significant toxic effects on the alveolar capillary endothelium and bronchi, should not be used for long periods unless absolutely necessary for the patient's survival. Oxygen therapy should be continuous rather than intermittent, aiming to maintain a constant arterial partial pressure of oxygen between 60 and 80 mmHg.

Patient education
Patients should be taught deep-breathing and coughing exercises. The employment of an incentive spirometer is useful for deep-breathing exercises.

Chest physiotherapy
Extensive chest physiotherapy will be required to assist in establishing and maintaining clear lung fields. Postural drainage is frequently required.

Suction
Patients with severe respiratory embarrassment will require suction. Disposable gloves, plastic apron, high filtration mask and eye protection are necessary when suctioning patients as explosive coughing releases a potentially contaminated aerosol spray.

Medications
Medications are administered as prescribed and potential side-effects should be anticipated. These include:

Medication	Possible side-effects
Pentamidine isethionate	Hypoglycaemia (or more rarely,
NB: test urine twice daily for	hyperglycaemia)
sugar and acetone.	Hypotension
Monitor daily	Abscesses at injection
blood glucose	sites – skin rashes

estimates (normal: 2.5 – 4.7 mmol/l) (45–85 mg/100 ml)	Tachycardia Pruritus Thrombocytopenia
Aerosolized pentamidine Trimethoprim sulfphamethoxazole (co-trimoxazole) Others: DFMO (difluore- methylomithine), sulfadoxine and pyrimethamine and Dapsone	Cough and bronchospasm Drug fever Rash Leucopenia Nausea and vomiting; various haematological disorders – rash, nephrotoxicity; neurological disorders

Other medications may be prescribed, including **expectorants** (bromhexine HCL or mixtures containing either syrup of ipecacuanha, guaiphenesin or saturated solution of potassium iodide), **cough suppressants** (mixtures containing either dextromethorphan, codeine phosphate or pholcodine), and other **antibiotics**.

Reassurance
Patients with respiratory distress require frequent reassurance from the nurse. They are often anxious, tending to panic if they feel they cannot breathe. The 'nurse call system' should be placed within easy reach of the patient.

Mouth care
Oxygen is drying to mucous membranes and frequent mouth care will be required. Patients should rinse their mouth out with water or a pleasantly flavoured mouthwash solution every hour.

Nasal care
If nasal cannulae are used, it is useful if the anterior nares are lightly coated with a protective ointment, such as Vaseline or glycerine.

Evaluation
Patients should be reassessed frequently and changes in

vital signs and body temperature;
colour;
sputum production;
chest sounds; and
arterial blood gases

documented. Changes in respiratory status must be reported to the physician immediately. The patient must also be frequently reassessed for signs of new chest infections. Frequent measurements of arterial blood pressure must be made while patients are receiving pentamidine isethionate.

2. The need for adequate hydration

Potential problems	Origin of problem
Dehydration	Inadequate intake of oral fluids: dysphasia secondary to *Candida albicans* infection or KS lesions, lethargy, confusion or coma Fluid loss: diarrhoea, nausea, vomiting, GI suctioning, fever and diaphoresis, hyperpnoea
Electrolyte imbalance	Diarrhoea, nausea, vomiting, GI suctioning

Objectives of care

1. To correct dehydration and electrolyte imbalance.
2. To maintain optimal hydration and electrolyte homeostasis.

Nursing intervention

Assessment
The patient should be weighed daily (at the same time each day) and an exact record of fluid intake and output maintained. Skin turgor should be assessed on a daily basis.

Oral fluids
The patient should be encouraged to drink frequent, small amounts of oral fluids as tolerated. For all patients, especially those with fever, a plentiful supply of fresh iced water should be kept on the patient's bedside locker.

Intravenous rehydration
The physician will prescribe a regime of intravenous fluids. These fluids must be infused at the correct flow rate, as ordered by the physician.

Electrolyte replacement
Electrolytes will be added to intravenous infusions according to the physician's prescription. Patients with potassium imbalance may be continuously assessed by using a cardiac monitor.

Mouth care
Dehydrated patients require frequent (2-hourly) mouth care.

Evaluation
Effective rehydration and electrolyte replacement will result in normal skin turgor, blood pressure, heart rate and absence of signs of mental confusion or vertigo (if due to dehydration).
   Plasma electrolyte levels should be carefully monitored and results outside normal parameters reported to the physician immediately.

Normal electrolyte parameters:
Potassium: 3.8–5.0 mmol/l (mEq/l)
Sodium: 135–145 mmol/l (mEq/l)
Chloride: 100–106 mmol/l (mEq/l)

3. The need for adequate nutrition

Actual problem	**Origin of problem**
Weight loss	Catabolism associated with AIDS

Potential problems	
Further severe weight loss and malnutrition	Increased catabolism, fever, diarrhoea, nausea and vomiting Profound anorexia Dysphagia – KS lesions in GI tract, malabsorption

Objectives of care

1. To keep patient well nourished.
2. To prevent further weight loss.
3. To enhance weight gain.

Nursing intervention

Assessment
Weigh patient and take history of previous dietary patterns, including likes, dislikes and any known food allergies. Note the current dietary habit of the patient as many patients with AIDS will be on special diets, often as 'alternative' forms of treatment (e.g. macrobiotic diets). The dietitian should be informed of the patient's admission and, after interviewing the patient, will be able to advise on a nutritional regime.

Oral nutrition
The patient may tolerate small, frequent meals better than the traditional three meals a day. Every effort should be made to present the patient with food he or she likes. This can be brought in by visitors

if it is not readily available in the hospital. Yogurts and meal substitutes (Carnation, Ensure Plus) are often well tolerated. If allowed by the physician, a small amount of sherry prior to meals may stimulate appetite. Prescribed anti-emetics should be given an hour before meals. Usually the dietitian will advise the nurse on any special diets ordered for the patient. Some patients may wish to follow their own special diet, such as a macrobiotic diet. This may present a conflict as current medical opinion does not feel this diet is useful in a catabolic condition. This can be discussed with the patient but, in the end, the patient's wishes must be respected. They may feel their diet is their only remaining hope.

Enteral tube feeding
Enteral feeding is often employed in AIDS patients who are seriously ill and cannot be maintained on oral nutrition. A nasogastric tube is passed, usually being left *in situ*. Isotonic lactose-free formulae are often employed, the solution generally being administered at between 50 and 100 ml an hour, depending on the patient's tolerance of it. Diarrhoea is a severe reaction to enteral feeding but may be controlled by reducing the rate of administration. An alternative regime is to pass a nasogastric tube, leaving it *in situ* for a morning or an afternoon and only feeding the patient during this time, making up nutritional requirements with either oral or parenteral feeds.

Parenteral nutrition
Solutions of protein, lipids and carbohydrates may be infused intravenously. Trace elements, electrolytes and vitamins may be added. Short-term peripheral parenteral nutrition can be employed, although it is more usual for parenteral nutrition to be administered via a central line. There are risks associated with **total parenteral nutrition (TPN)**. Patients frequently become hyperglycaemic due to the carbohydrate load. Insulin may be added to the solution to control this. All patients on TPN should have 4-hourly urinalysis for sugar and ketone bodies as well as daily blood glucose estimates. Great care must be taken of the infusion site and line as they frequently become infected. When TPN is discontinued, it must be done gradually and the patient carefully observed for signs of hypoglycaemia.

Medications
Anti-emetics are almost universally prescribed for patients with AIDS who have nausea and vomiting. Probably the most frequently used anti-emetic is metoclopramide (Maxolon®), which can be given either orally or by intramuscular or intravenous injection. Anti-emetic suppositories such as prochlorperazine maleate (Stemetil®) may be

useful with some patients. **Antidiarrhoeals** may be effective with some patients. However they are notoriously ineffective in many patients with AIDS who have severe diarrhoea. The most common antidiarrhoeals used include diphenoxylate Hcl with atropine sulphate (Lomotil) and loperamide Hcl (Imodium). Codeine phosphate may also be used.

Most patients with AIDS will have **vitamin supplements** prescribed. Many will be on their own regime of 'mega-dose' vitamin therapy. As fat-soluble vitamins (A, D, E and K) are toxic in high doses, the physician must be aware of any medication the patient has brought in with him or her and is taking in hospital. This includes vitamin preparations.

Evaluation
If nutritional support is successful, the patient should show a weight gain or, at least, a cessation of weight loss. Unfortunately, weight loss and malnutrition are generally profound, persistent and progressive. The patient must be weighed weekly and recordings of fluid intake and output maintained. Abdominal girth is measured weekly. The patient's abdomen is marked clearly so that all nursing personnel measure the girth consistently. Bowel sounds should be assessed 4-hourly when on enteral feeding.

The nutritional support required in HIV disease is discussed further in Chapter 15.

4. The need for urinary and faecal elimination

Potential problems	Origin of problems
Diarrhoea	Opportunistic infections (e.g. cryptosporidiosis, CMV amoebiasis, *Isospora belli*), KS lesions in the GI tract, or of idiopathic origin
Oliguria	Dehydration
Incontinence	Confusion, loss of mobility, terminal illness

Objectives of care

1. To control or minimize effects of diarrhoea and incontinence.
2. To achieve effective implementation of enteric IC precautions, if indicated.
3. To facilitate correction of water imbalance.

Nursing intervention

Assessment
Frequency of bowel movements should be documented and fluid intake and output recorded.

Toilet facilities
Patients with diarrhoea should be nursed in a single room which has private toilet facilities. If the patient is not ambulatory, a bedside commode is preferable to using a bed pan in bed. Bed pans may be carefully emptied (to avoid splashing) in the patient's toilet, or the contents disposed of in the bed pan washer.

Skin care
The skin must be kept clean and dry. It is essential that facilities are made available for patients to wash their hands after using the toilet. If the patient is incontinent, protective or barrier creams may be useful in preventing excoriation of the skin (e.g. Sprilon® spray – Pharmacia GB Ltd. or Vitamin A + D Ointment – Emollient® – E. Fougera & Co.).

Hydration
Patients with severe diarrhoea may become quickly dehydrated and the patient must be encouraged to drink adequate amounts of fluids to replace those lost due to diarrhoea. Intravenous rehydration may be necessary in some patients.

Nursing care of the incontinent patient
Urinary incontinence may be managed by leaving an urinal carefully placed between the patient's legs. Alternatively, external catheters, such as the Texas® latex penile sheath (Cory Brothers Ltd) or Uro-Flow® non-allergenic penile sheaths, with hypo-allergenic, adhesive, distensible foam liners (Downs Surgical Ltd) may be used. Patients with faecal incontinence should be nursed on clean, dry incontinence pads, which are placed on a linen drawsheet over a plastic sheet. All patients who are incontinent must be checked hourly.

Diet
The dietitian may be consulted in order to assess if a change in the patient's diet may assist in controlling faecal incontinence.

Pressure area care
Patients who are incontinent are at an increased risk of developing pressure sores. Pressure area care, including turning the patient on alternative sides, should be undertaken every 2 hours. It is useful to re-assess the patient daily using the **Norton scale**[5].

Infection control
Nurses must wear rubber latex disposable gloves (of the correct size) and plastic aprons when disposing of urine or faeces and when caring for incontinent patients. Contaminated linen is double-bagged in a soluble plastic bag, which is then placed in a red nylon bag, sealed and sent to the laundry. Careful handwashing, prior to and after caring for patients is exceptionally important with patients who have enteric infections. Wearing gloves does not decrease the need for good handwashing technique. If patients have enteric infections they should have their own set of crockery and cutlery, which may be kept in the patient's room. This can be washed by the nurse after use. This is preferable to presenting food to a patient with gastro-intestinal symptoms on unattractive disposable paper plates and asking the patient to use plastic knives, spoons and forks.

Evaluation
Effective nursing intervention will prevent dehydration secondary to severe diarrhoea, skin excoriation and pressure area breakdown. It will also help to minimize the psychological effects of severe diarrhoea and/or incontinence.

5. The need to control body temperature

Potential problem
Fever and night sweats

Origin of problem
Opportunistic infections

Objectives of care

1. To assist in maintaining normal body temperature (36–37.5°C).
2. To keep the patient comfortable.

Nursing intervention

Assessment
Patients with HIV disease should have their vital signs and body temperature recorded 4-hourly. The occurrence of night sweats is common in both conditions and should be documented in the nursing notes.

Medication
The physician may prescribe medication to reduce body temperature, such as aspirin or paracetamol BP (acetaminophen USP). These should be administered as ordered.

Comfort
The patient should be kept clean, dry and well hydrated. Prolonged fever increases metabolic processes. The patient should be encouraged to eat a nutritious diet. Glucose drinks, such as Lucozade, may be beneficial to some patients, although they may exacerbate diarrhoea in others. Bed clothes and linen should be light, dry and clean. If hyperpyrexia occurs, sponging with tepid water may prove useful. Iced drinks must be available for the patient with fever.

Evaluation
Pyrexia and intermittent fevers should be detected promptly and medication administered as per the physician's orders.

6. The need for movement and mobilization

Potential problems
Muscle atrophy
Decubitus ulcers
Deep vein thrombosis

Origin of problem
Restricted mobility
Weakness and bed rest
Catabolism
Peripheral neuropathy

Objectives of care

1. To prevent the formation of decubitus ulcers and deep vein thrombosis.
2. To minimize muscle wasting.
3. To achieve full mobilization and independence within the limits of the patient's abilities.

Nursing intervention

Assessment
The patient's level of independence and ability to ambulate, along with any signs of muscle wasting, pressure sores or venous thrombosis will be assessed daily.

Physiotherapy
Patients not confined to bed should be walked frequently and encouraged to be as independent as possible. Patients on bed rest must have active and passive lower limb exercises and their position changed every 2 hours. A pull-rope, attached to the end of the bed, or a trapeze bar on a bed frame may prove useful with many patients.

Pressure area care
Patients on bed rest or semi bed rest must have 2-hourly pressure area care. Gentle massage with a lanolin-based cream (TLC cream or baby lotion) is soothing to the patient and allows an opportunity for the nurse to inspect pressure sites. Patients with restricted mobility should be commenced on a Norton scoring scale[5] as illustrated in Fig. 14.1. Patients with a total score of 14 or less are prone to develop pressure sores and patients with a total score below 12 are more likely than not to develop pressure sores.

It is also useful to commence a patient on a 'Relief of pressure chart'[2] as illustrated in Fig. 14.2.

Nursing care must be organized in order to turn the patient every two hours and lifting must be skilful in order to prevent shearing force to the skin. The skin must be kept dry, cool and clean. Dehydration, malnutrition and anaemia are all predisposing factors to the development of pressure sores. When possible, these must be corrected.

Evaluation
Effective nursing care will promote mobilization and independence and result in absence of pressure sores, venous thrombosis and excessive muscle wasting.

7. The need for a safe environment

Potential problems	**Origin of problem**
Nosocomial infection	Immunodeficiency
Accidents	Weakness
	Confusion
	Hospital environment and equipment
	CMV retinitis

Objectives of care

1. To prevent nosocomial infection.
2. To maintain a safe environment.

Nursing intervention

Assessment
An assessment of the patient's mental status includes determining his or her ability to understand and cooperate in the planned care. The patient's physical condition is assessed, including sight, a history of vertigo, seizures, falls and general state of debilitation.

Norton's scoring scale		
Patient's name:	Date:	

Physical condition:
Good 4
Fair 3
Poor 2   Score: _____
V. bad 1

Mental condition:
Alert 4
Apathetic 3
Confused 2   Score: _____
Stuporous 1

Activity:
Ambulant 4
Walk/help 3
Chairbound 2   Score: _____
Bedfast 1

Mobility:
Full 4
Sl. limited 3
V. limited 2   Score: _____
Immobile 1

Incontinent:
Not 4
Occasionally 3
Usually/ur. 2   Score: _____
Doubly 1

* * * Total score:

Fig. 14.1 Norton's scoring scale

Relief of pressure chart				
Date	Time	Position of patient	Relief of pressure achieved by	Nurse's signature
12/11	0800	Lying on back	Turned on left side	W. Jones.
"	1000	LYING ON LEFT SIDE	TURNED ON RIGHT SIDE	E. Karn
"	1200	Lying on right side	Turned on to back	J. hand.
"	1400	Lying on back	Turned on left side	A. Hilton

Fig. 14.2 Relief of pressure chart

Infection control
Infection control (IC) procedures will be implemented as per Chapter 12 on this aspect of nursing care. All patients with immunodeficiency are at increased risk of nosocomial (i.e. hospital-acquired) infection, although patients with HIV disease are more in danger of previously acquired, latent infection. As patients with HIV disease are at increased risk from new infections, it is essential that when in hospital they are not exposed to the added risk of nosocomial infections.

Safety
The following aspects must be taken into account when care is planned in order to maintain a safe environment:

- **Oxygen** When oxygen is in use, cigarette smoking is not allowed and 'Hazard' notices are prominently displayed in the patient's room. If spanners (wrenches) are needed for oxygen tanks, 'non-sparking' wrenches must be used. Heating pads and other electrical appliances are not used.
- **Equipment** All equipment must be carefully put away after use so that it does not present a hazard to patients who are ambulatory. It is essential that a clear pathway is maintained between the patient's bed and the toilet.
- **Miscellaneous** Floors are kept clean and dry. If patients are confused or sedated, bedside rails are kept in the upright position when the patient is in bed and the bed is kept in the low position. The 'nurse-call system' is always kept within easy reach of the patient.

Evaluation
Effective planned care will reduce potential safety hazards and prevent the patient from acquiring nosocomial infections.

8. The need for personal cleansing and dressing

Potential problems	**Origin of problem**
Poor oral hygiene	Dehydration
Inadequate body hygiene	Infection
	Lethargy
	Confusion
	Incontinence
	Immobility

Objectives of care

1. To maintain good oral hygiene.
2. To preserve the integrity and cleanliness of the integumentary system.

Nursing intervention

Mouth care

Ambulatory patients should be encouraged to brush their teeth with a soft toothbrush after each meal and taught how to use dental floss or dental tape to keep the teeth clean. Glycerine and lemon swabs may be used. Mouthwash solution is useful for patients who have a dry mouth or halitosis. Candidiasis ('thrush') is a common opportunist infection in patients with HIV disease, requiring treatment with antifungal preparations, such as topical applications of nystatin oral suspension or amphotericin lozenges. In patients with HIV disease, systemic antifungal medication may be needed. Fluconazole (Diflucan), either orally or intravenously is commonly used. Candidal oesophagitis may occur as well as disseminated candidiasis in some patients with AIDS.

Body hygiene

The patient should have a daily bath or shower. If confined to bed, a daily bed-bath is required. Patients who are ambulatory should be encouraged to dress in clean outdoor clothes for part of the day. Patients who have fever and/or night sweats may need assistance in washing after an episode of sweating, requiring careful drying and a change of night clothes and bed linen. Talcum powder after washing is often soothing.

Pressure area care

Two-hourly pressure area care is required for patients confined to bed, as described previously.

Infection control

Patients who have skin lesions and cannot use the shower, should have an antibacterial agent, such as Triclosan 2 per cent (Ster-Zac bath concentrate – Hough Hoseason & Co. Ltd), in their bath to prevent secondary infection. Personal clothing which becomes contaminated can safely be disinfected by washing in a washing machine with ordinary detergents, on the hot cycle. Patients should have their own toothbrush and razor. These should not be shared with anyone else. An electric razor may be useful, especially if the patient has a bleeding disorder.

Evaluation
The patient remains clean and dry and the integument intact. Candidiasis is controlled.

9. The need for expression and communication

Potential problems	Origin of problem
Impaired cognition	Neurological consequences of
Disorientation	infection with HIV or CNS
	opportunistic disease
Isolation	Fear of AIDS by family, friends, health care workers
	Excessive IC precautions

Objectives of care

1. To minimize the effects of neurological dysfunction.
2. To prevent the deleterious effects of social isolation.

Nursing intervention

Assessment
Establish the status of the patient's orientation to time, place and events. Document visitors the patient wishes to see (and any he or she does not wish to see).

Visitors
Caring for the patient's visitors is often a delicate task, especially if they do not know the patient's diagnosis or sexual orientation. No information on any aspect of the patient's condition may be given to any visitors without the patient's express consent. With the patient's permission, visitors should be encouraged. The special friend(s) or lover of a homosexual patient often assumes the role of the patient's next of kin, which must be respected. As always, all visitors to the hospital must be treated with respect and consistent courtesy. An officious or abrupt manner displayed by health care workers to visitors can do immeasurable damage to their willingness to visit the patient and is demoralizing to the patient. It is also an

unpardonable professional transgression. If possible, visitors should be allowed throughout the day.

Some patients with AIDS will have been abandoned by both friends and family. With the patient's permission, it is possible to contact voluntary support groups (e.g. the Terrence Higgins Trust) who can arrange for members from their organization to visit the patient. The hospital's voluntary services may also be able to provide this service.

Communication aids
The patient should have easy access to a telephone, stamps and stationery. If in a single room, it may be possible for the patient to have a television set. The patient should have a bedside radio (with earphones), newspapers and magazines. The 'nurse-call system' must always be within easy reach of the patient. There should be a clock and a calendar in the patient's room.

Time for talking/listening/touching
Nursing care plans must take into account the fact that patients need to talk to their nurses. Listening, holding a patient's hand and just quietly being with the patient is a necessary aspect of nursing art.

Infection control
Appropriate IC precautions, as described previously, are necessary for patients who are immunocompromised or infectious. However, excessive IC precautions represent another barrier between the patient and other human beings and must be avoided. When appropriate, the patient should be encouraged to enjoy full ward privileges and to mix with other patients.

Reality orientation
Patients who are confused must be gently reminded of their environment, day and date and reassured that they are safe. They must not be spoken to as if they were children. It is generally useful if first names are used when speaking to the patient unless he or she has objected to this. There is nothing wrong in nurses using their own first names when talking to patients. Patients often relate better to health care workers when allowed to use their first names rather than using 'Nurse Adams' or 'Miss Williamson'.

Evaluation
A plan of care which is designed to allow patients both space and time

to communicate with their families, friends and health care workers will reduce the sense of loneliness, rejection and isolation felt by many patients with AIDS.

10. The need for working and playing

Potential problems	Origin of problem
Economic hardship	Loss of employment
Mental deterioration	Boredom, CNS involvement, loneliness

Objectives of care

1. To provide access to appropriate financial resources.
2. To minimize effects of boredom and loneliness.

Nursing intervention

Assessment
Effects of absence from usual employment are assessed and the nursing history documents the patient's neurological status and the presence of any sensory deficits or physical disablement. The history should include information relating to the patient's past leisure time activities, hobbies and interests. It is important to assess whether the patient expects visits from family and significant others (lover, friends) or has been abandoned.

Financial problems
It is probable that all patients with long-term illness, including AIDS, will eventually need to claim various State benefits to which they are entitled. As the social security system is confusing and complex, the patient should be interviewed by a social worker as soon as possible.

In the UK, individuals with HIV disease can obtain information on benefits and entitlements from specialist welfare advisers at a variety of non-governmental organizations, including the Terrence Higgins Trust (071 831 0330), Immunity (071 388 6776), Landmark (081 678 6686) and LEAN (081 519 9545). In addition, advice is available from the Department of Social Security freephone (0800 666 555). The prompt issue of medical and sickness certificates while the patient is in hospital is important and should not be left until the patient asks for them. The social worker may also be able to assist patients who have been dismissed by their employers as a result of illness.

Leisure time activities
It is important that patients have access to television viewing and a radio. The library services of the hospital should be introduced and arrangements made for the patient to purchase newspapers and magazines. An occupational therapy assessment may be indicated for some patients. Special interests and hobbies should be encouraged.

Visitors
Visiting times must be flexible and visitors encouraged. If the patient has no visitors, with his or her permission, the volunteer services or a voluntary organization may be able to arrange visitors for the patient. The largest voluntary organization in the UK for patients with AIDS is the Terrence Higgins Trust and they can be contacted by telephone on (London) 071 831 0330 or 071 242 1010. It is also important for the patient to have visits from health care workers, especially if they are being nursed in single rooms. Time must be made available to visit and talk to the patient rather than entering the room to 'do' something.

Evaluation
The patient receives all necessary assistance to deal with claiming benefit entitlements, planning leisure-time activities and arranging for visitors.

11. The need for adequate rest and sleep

Potential problem   **Origin of problem**
Insomnia   Pain, discomfort or anxiety

Objective of care

To ensure that the patient has uninterrupted periods of sleep.

Nursing intervention

Assessment
The patient's usual sleeping environment (e.g. own or shared bed) and habits are ascertained. This includes noting the time the patient usually goes to bed, periods of wakefulness during the night and usual time of rising. Any current complaints of pain or signs of anxiety are noted.

Comfort
Noise is a frequent cause of complaint from all patients in hospital. Every effort must be made to eliminate unnecessary noise, especially during the night. This specifically includes loud talking or laughter at the nurses' station. Drinks containing caffeine (tea, coffee, colas) should be avoided after the evening meal and a hot milk drink (e.g. Horlicks) may be useful in helping to settle the patient. If the physician allows, an alcoholic drink may be beneficial. The patient should be assisted to void before retiring and the bed linen should be straightened. Pressure area care and a back rub are also useful in helping the patient relax before retiring. With seriously ill patients, requiring intensive nursing during the night, care should be planned so that all required care is given at one time, allowing the patient 2-hour periods of uninterrupted sleep. Most patients in hospital benefit from an afternoon 'rest period' shortly after lunch. Visitors should be asked not to visit during this time.

Medication
Analgesics or night sedation may be prescribed by the medical staff. Night sedation is ineffective if pain is present. Often appropriate analgesia is sufficient to allow the patient to fall asleep. The benzodiazepine group of drugs are the most useful type of hypnotics used and include nitrazepam and flurazepam. Chloral hydrate capsules, methyprylone and chlormethiazole edisylate are sometimes useful if benzodiazepines prove ineffective. Barbiturates should be avoided. Anxiety may have to be treated with anxiolytic medication such as diazepam, chlordiazepoxide or lorazepam. Early morning wakening may be a sign of clinical depression, which requires specific treatment with antidepressant medications, such as amitriptyline Hcl, doxepin Hcl or trimipramine maleate.

Evaluation
With well-planned nursing care, patients should obtain adequate rest and sleep while in hospital.

12. The need to maintain psychological equilibrium

Actual problem
Anxiety

Origin of problem
Stress associated with progressive, terminal illness, fear of loss of confidentiality

Potential problems
Ineffective coping

Loss of control

Social isolation	Withdrawal of social supports Isolation in hospital
Loss of self-esteem	Guilt, altered body image, stigma of AIDS, perception of self as contagious to others
Depression	Helplessness, grief associated with loss of – personal relationships – self-esteem – physical potency – control – sexuality – effective role in life

Objectives of care

1. To allow patient to ventilate feelings and emotions.
2. To alleviate predisposing factors to psychological dysfunction.
3. To offer support.
4. To facilitate referrals to appropriate support personnel/agencies.

Nursing intervention

Assessment
During the first few days of admission, the level of anxiety present can be ascertained. Loss of adequate coping mechanisms and signs or symptoms of clinical depression must be noted. The patient's general affect may change from day to day (or from shift to shift). This must be assessed and documented in order to plan effective nursing intervention.

Anxiety
Anxiety is neither inappropriate nor uncommon in a life-threatening illness such as AIDS. Manifestations of anxiety occur on several levels, ranging from mild tension to sympathetic nervous system overflow and panic. Most patients will require assistance in handling excessive anxiety.

Level 1 (Mild) The patient is alert, enquiring, relatively relaxed and defence mechanisms are working well. In this level, patients are receptive to information.
Level 2 (Moderate) Increased alertness and heightened emotional state. The patient is more receptive to sensory information than

factual information and is able to learn relaxation techniques. In this level, patients are able to solve most problems on their own.

Level 3 (Severe) Sympathetic nervous system overflow is present with typical fight-or-flight responses. With severe anxiety, patients are no longer able to solve problems on their own, needing the advocate skills of the nurse. Physical signs and symptoms of anxiety are often present such as tachycardia, restlessness, irritability and a feeling of 'butterflies in the stomach'. The patient is frightened.

Level 4 (Panic) The patient is overwhelmed by fear – unable to concentrate, having more pronounced physical signs of sympathetic overactivity, such as insomnia, tachycardia, profuse perspiration (especially on the palms and forehead), frequency of micturition and defaecation, rapid breathing and vertigo.

Patients do not progress from level 1 through to level 4, but fluctuate from one level to another. Stressful events occurring during illness may precipitate more severe levels of anxiety. Stressors in AIDS include:

- Progressive debilitation
- Sensational media interest
- Rejection: family, lover, friends, employer
- Infection control precautions ('isolation')
- Discrimination
- Termination of treatment
- Required rapid changes in lifestyle
- Progressive changes in body image
- Threatened (or actual) loss of confidentiality
- Growing awareness of prognosis.

Intervention designed to alleviate excessive anxiety includes discussing with patients their fears, rationally highlighting their identifiable strengths to cope with stressors, and encouraging socialization and leisure-time activities. Most hospitals have clinical psychologists on their staff who can offer more skilled assistance to the patient in alleviating anxiety and teaching relaxation techniques. Severe anxiety or panic generally requires anxiolytic medication, such as benzodiazepines (discussed previously). These drugs are more useful for short-term management of acute anxiety rather than long-term use.

Depression

Clinical depression is common in AIDS, and its early recognition allows prompt treatment. Patients may despair, complain of sleep disturbances (early morning wakening, difficulty in falling asleep), lose the ability to concentrate, show a loss of interest, energy and further anorexia. Ideas of self-reproach are associated with feelings of despair, hopelessness and guilt. Delusions (false, fixed beliefs) of being punished for being homosexual are common. Loss of sexual interest and impotence is frequent. Suicidal feelings may be articulated, suicide being a significant risk. Mental retardation, as seen in depression, in patients with AIDS often acts as a brake on suicidal acts but it cannot be relied upon. In general, antidepressant medication is required for all but the mildest incidents of depression.

Although there are various types of antidepressants, the **tricyclic** group of antidepressants are the safest and most commonly prescribed. These include amitriptyline, trimipramine, clomipramine and imipramine. **Tetracyclic antidepressants** are also used, e.g. mianserin hydrocloride (Norval®, Bolvidon®), maprotiline (Ludiomil®) and have less cardiovascular and anti-cholinergic side-effects. Another group of antidepressants, known as **monoamine oxidase inhibitors (MAOI)** such as phenelzine, mebanazine and tranylcypromine, are less often prescribed.

If a patient is prescribed antidepressant medication, it is imperative that the nurse is aware to which group the drug belongs. MAOIs require specific dietary restrictions as foods rich in tyramine (cheese, Bovril, Oxo, Marmite, chianti and some types of beer) may interact with these drugs and provoke a hypertensive crisis with the risk of subarachnoid haemorrhage. MAOIs also interact with pethidine (meperidine Hcl USP), opiates, phenothiazines and alcohol. In the 2–3 weeks before antidepressants become effective, the risk of suicide remains real. Antidepressants are generally very effective. Some antidepressants tend to be sedating while others tend to be stimulating. Treatment may have to continue for several months if a relapse is to be prevented.

Patient support groups
A useful way to help patients deal with the various psychological dysfunctions which may occur in AIDS is to form support groups for those with this diagnosis. These groups are best led by a clinical psychologist who specializes in this condition or by a psychiatric nurse specialist, who has had special training in leading these groups. Following discharge, support groups can be attended on an out-patient basis.

Individual counselling and psychotherapy
In all stages of HIV infection, from seroconversion to fully expressed AIDS and eventual death, individual counselling and psychotherapy will be needed. Although all physicians caring for patients with AIDS will have good counselling and basic psychotherapy skills, the advice and assistance of clinical psychologists will be needed.

Family and significant others
It is not only the patient who requires psychological and emotional support. Family, husbands and wives, lovers and friends all display various levels of anxiety. Enormous demands are commonly made upon nursing staff and the highest degree of skill and sensitivity is required.

Central nervous system disease
HIV can directly cause CNS damage, patients exhibiting signs of a slowly progressive dementia. Gross cognitive changes may occur. The patient will become confused and disoriented. Motor (lower limb weakness) and sensory (blindness) changes may occur. Opportunistic diseases (toxoplasmosis, encephalitis secondary to various opportunistic pathogens, etc.) may also occur, causing a variety of signs and symptoms, all affecting the patient's ability to maintain psychological equilibrium. Some of these diseases are treatable; many are not.

Evaluation
Psychological dysfunction should be recognized early and nursing intervention and medical treatment implemented to alleviate and contain the mental distress which the patient is suffering. Patients will be able to learn to use effective relaxation techniques. Nursing personnel will liaise closely with other care givers.

13. The need to worship according to faith

Potential problem   **Origin of problem**
Religious deprivation   Isolation, guilt

Objective of care

To facilitate access between patient and chaplain or religious adviser.

Nursing intervention

Assessment
The patient's religious faith and any special religious needs should be ascertained. The patient should be asked if he or she would like the hospital chaplain to visit.

Facilitating worship
Chaplains and other religious advisers must, at the patient's wish, have complete access. Often patients can be taken to the hospital

chapel for religious services. It is essential that patients have the opportunity of attending confession and of receiving the holy sacraments. The Sacrament of the Anointing of the Sick (i.e. Extreme Unction or Last Rites) is extremely important and this event should be entered in the patient's nursing notes. The sacrament of Holy Communion is important to members of the Church of England and the Roman Catholic Church. At the patient's request, chaplains can make available religious literature and a Bible. The opportunity to participate in religious worship is a tremendous comfort to many patients with AIDS. Patients should not be visited by religious advisers whom they have not requested to see.

Evaluation
The patient will have opportunities to worship and be comforted by religious beliefs.

14.   The need to express sexuality

Actual problem
Need to modify sexual
behaviour

Origin of problem
Infectious nature of HIV
infection

Potential problems
Loss of libido
Development of unsafe
sexual behaviour
patterns
Grief associated with loss
of sexuality

Progressive illness
Guilt
Internalized
homophobia
Changing body image, loss of
sexual partner

Objectives of care

1.   To help patients adjust to changing sexual status.
2.   To provide patients with information on safer sex.

Nursing intervention

Assessment
Ascertain patient's attitude towards sexual expression and current problems. Determine patient's knowledge of safer sex techniques.

Patient education
Many patients have immense feelings of guilt over past sexual behaviour which may have predisposed them to infection with HIV. Christ

and Wiener[6] have described five behaviour patterns some patients adopt in response to this guilt:

1. celibacy;
2. denial or rejection of facts leading to continued high levels of sexual activity;
3. celibacy with close friends while engaging in multiple anonymous sexual contacts;
4. increased use of drugs and alcohol; and
5. development of small groups of sexual contacts.

Some patients with AIDS have described feelings of internalized homophobia, i.e. an internalization of society's prejudicial attitudes towards homosexuals. This may lead to a belief that homosexuality caused their disease or anger and blame directed at their sexual partner(s).

Reality orientation may reinforce factual information regarding AIDS and its transmission. Some patients need reminding that AIDS is caused by a virus, not by homosexuality, and that, although homosexuals were especially vulnerable to attack by the virus in the first years of the epidemic, **all** sexually active individuals outside of monogamous relationships are at risk. AIDS is a human disease, not a homosexual disease. As the vast majority of individuals infected with HIV were infected several years ago before the various 'high-risk' sexual activities were identified, no one individual or groups of individuals are to blame for its current pandemic status.

In the current state of knowledge, 'high risk' sexual behaviour is well established. All persons have a responsibility to modify their sexual behaviour accordingly. This includes patients with HIV disease. It also includes all sexually active individuals outside of monogamous relationships. Table 14.1 lists current advice for 'safer sex'.

Leaflets explicitly describing safer sex practices are available from both the Health Education Authority (Mabledon Place, London WCIH 9TX, Telephone 071 383 3833) and the Terrence Higgins Trust (52–54 Gray's Inn Road, London WCIX 8JU, Telephone 071 831 0330). In the United States, this information is available from many organizations including: the San Francisco AIDS Foundation, 333 Valencia St, San Francisco, California 94103, Telephone (415) 864 5855 and GMHC, 129 West 20th St., New York, New York 12231, Telephone (212) 807 6664. These may be ordered and stocked on wards or units where patients with AIDS may be admitted, and used in patient education programmes. It may be useful to give some patients the telephone numbers of groups which offer 'safer sex' advice. In the UK, the Terrence Higgins Trust runs an AIDS 'Help-Line' every day on (London) 071 242 1010. In the United States, the Gay Men's Health Crisis (GMHC) have an AIDS 'Hot-Line' on (New York) 212-807 6655. This allows individuals an opportunity independently to obtain information and advice from a source they trust and reinforces patient education efforts in hospital.

If patients are given the right information, most will make the necessary changes in their lifestyle to respond responsibly to the presence of this threat in the community. Some patients with AIDS may have significant psychological dysfunction preventing them from reacting appropriately to health education efforts. In these cases, the nurse should discuss with the attending physician the advantages of a referral to a clinical psychologist who is more skilled in assisting patients adjust to the dynamics of AIDS.

Table 14.1   Safer sex guidelines

---

1. **High-risk sexual activity**
   Unprotected anal or vaginal sexual intercourse, either active (insertive) or passive (receptive)
   Oral–anal ('rimming') sexual contact. Although it is uncertain if HIV could be transmitted via this activity, new evidence (see Chapter 3) suggests it may be involved in the transmission of a 'Kaposi's sarcoma agent'. It certainly is involved in the transmission of enteric infections and the active partner is most at risk
   Sharing sex toys (e.g. dildos) and traumatic sexual activity, e.g. manual–anal ('fisting') and sado-masochistic sexual activities (if blood is drawn)

2. **Medium/low-risk sexual activity**
   Protected anal or vaginal sexual intercourse. 'Protected' refers to the male, insertive party wearing a good quality, intact, rubber latex condom, preferably one pre-lubricated with nonoxynol-9
   Performing oral sex on a man who ejaculates into your mouth may be medium- or high-risk sexual activity

3. **Low-risk sexual activity**
   Performing oral sex on a woman
   Performing oral sex on a man, avoiding ejaculation into the mouth

4. **No risk sexual activity**
   Mutual masturbation
   Erotic touching, caressing and massage
   Kissing and non-genital licking

N.B. Clearly if neither partner is infected with HIV, all of the above activities would be safe from a HIV transmission point of view

Evaluation
Adequate support and educative efforts will enable the patient to adjust to his changing sexuality and modify future sexual behaviour to protect himself and others.

15. Needs associated with dying

Actual problems	**Origin of problem**
Fear, anxiety and loneliness	Impending death, manner of death, loss of power and control
Potential problems	
Physical problems associated with dying from AIDS	Pathophysiology of HIV disease
Inability to adjust to impending death	Fear

Objectives of care

1. To alleviate or control physical problems associated with dying from AIDS.
2. To support and reassure the patient through the various psychological stages associated with death.

Nursing intervention

Assessment
Physical problems associated with AIDS affect the dying patient and include:

Pain	Incontinence
Dyspnoea	Cough
Nausea/vomiting	Pressure sores
Immobility	Dysphagia
Open lesions/wounds	Confusion
Fever	Dehydration.

In assessing the dying patient, the presence of the above should be noted and care planned accordingly, as discussed previously in this chapter. It is important to ascertain the extent of the patient's knowledge about their own impending death. It is rare that a patient, seriously ill with AIDS, is unaware that he or she is dying. If assessment indicates that the patient is, this fact should be made known to the physician, who has the primary responsibility of discussing the patient's prognosis with him or her. If (or when) the patient's level of anxiety permits, practical aspects of his or her death may be gently discussed. This may include referral to a legal adviser for patients who have not made a will. It is extremely important that the nursing notes indicate who is to be informed when the patient dies. This information should come from the patient. It would be tragic simply to inform the family, when the most significant relationship may be the patient's lover.

Wills
Patients should be encouraged to make a final and legal will. Patients requiring assistance with this should be directed to the administrative department of the hospital or to the social worker. Under **no** circumstances should nurses help draw up wills or witness them.

Psychological stages of dying
Although it is true that no two individuals react in the same way to impending death, there seem to be commonalities in their reactions. Dr Elisabeth Kubler-Ross has elegantly described these[7] as the five 'stages of dying':

1. **Denial** 'No, not me.' This is a typical reaction when a patient learns that he or she is terminally ill. Denial is important and necessary. It helps cushion the impact of the patient's awareness that death is inevitable.
2. **Rage and anger** 'Why me?' The patient resents the fact that others will remain healthy and alive while he or she must die. God is a special target for anger since He is regarded as imposing, arbitrarily, the death sentence. To those who are shocked at her claim that such anger is not only permissible but inevitable, Dr Ross replies succinctly, 'God can take it'.
3. **Bargaining** 'Yes me, but . . .' Patients accept the fact of death but strike bargains for more time. Mostly they bargain with God – 'even among people who never talked with God before.' Sometimes they bargain with the physician. They promise to be good or to do something in exchange for another week or month or year of life. Notes Dr Ross: 'What they promise is totally irrelevant, because they don't keep their promises anyway'.
4. **Depression** 'Yes me.' First, the person mourns past losses, things not done, wrongs committed. Then he or she enters a state of 'preparatory grief', getting ready for the arrival of death. The patient grows quiet, does not want visitors. 'When a dying patient doesn't want to see you any more,' says Dr Ross, 'this is

a sign he has finished his unfinished business with you and it is a blessing. He can now let go peacefully'.

5. **Acceptance** 'My time is very close now and it's all right.' Dr Ross describes this final stage as 'not a happy stage, but neither is it unhappy. It's devoid of feelings but it's not resignation, it's really a victory'.

In reality, patients go back and forth, from one stage to another, not necessarily in consecutive order. However, this model provides a good guide for the nurse in trying to understand the different phases of coming to terms with a terminal illness. In Stage 4, nurses can be helpful in reminding patients of the achievements of their lives, the impact that all human beings have by living a life however short. If the patient has not been abandoned, loved ones have time to express their love and respect, reassuring the patient that he or she will be remembered.

Last offices

Usual last offices are carried out. The patient is washed and the room tidied. Loved ones are allowed to see the body before further procedures are carried out. The nurse must be accessible during this time as often their grief is close to unbearable. After the body has been viewed, it is placed in a shroud and then gently placed in a heavy-duty plastic body bag. Nurses must wear disposable gloves and a plastic apron when carrying out last offices. Once the body has been placed in the body bag, no further IC precautions are required.

Summary

The individualized care of patients with AIDS and HIV-related illnesses requires skill, competence and confidence. These are based on a factual understanding of the pathophysiology of HIV infection and a comprehensive knowledge of modern models of nursing care, designed to offer all clients, regardless of race, age, creed, sex, sexual orientation or disease, the highest quality of compassionate, non-judgemental nursing care. Anything less is disreputable to the profession and discreditable to the nurse.

References

1. Henderson, V. (1964). The nature of nursing. *American Journal of Nursing* **64**(8), 62–8.

264   *The Individualized Care of Patients*

2. Roper, N., Logan, W.W. and Tierney, A.J. (1980). *The Elements of Nursing.* Churchill Livingstone, London.
3. Orem, D.E. (1980). *Nursing: Concepts of Practice,* 2nd edn. McGraw-Hill, New York.
4. Henderson, V. (1964). *Basic Principles of Nursing Care.* International Council of Nurses, Geneva.
5. Norton, D., McLaren, R. and Exton-Smith, A. (1975). *An Investigation of Geriatric Nursing Problems in Hospital.* Churchill Livingstone, Edinburgh.
6. Christ, G.H. and Wiener, L.S. (1985). Psychosocial issues in AIDS. In *AIDS: Etiology, Diagnosis, Treatment and Prevention,* eds DeVita, V.T. Jr., Hellman, S. and Rosenberg, S.A., J.B. Lippincott, New York, p. 283.
7. Kubler-Ross, E. (1969). *On Death and Dying.* Macmillan, New York.

Further Reading

Brunner, L.S. and Suddarth, D.S. (eds) (1992). *The Textbook of Adult Nursing.* Chapman & Hall, London (ISBN 0-412-43980-8).
Durham, J.D. and Cohen, F.L. (1987) The Person with AIDS: Nursing Perspective. Springer, New York (ISBN 0-8261-56304).
Flaskerud, J.H. and Ungvarski, P. (eds) (1992). *HIV/AIDS: A Guide to Nursing Care,* 2nd edn. W.B. Saunders, Philadelphia (ISBN 0-7216-3718-3).
Hinchliff, S.M., Norman, S.E. and Schober, J.E. (eds) (1993). *Nursing Practice & Health Care,* 2nd edn. Edward Arnold, London (ISBN 0-340-55788-5).
Meisenhelder, J.B. and LaCharite, C.L. (eds) (1989). *Comfort in Caring: Nursing the Person with HIV Infection.* Scott, Foresman & Co., Glenview IL (ISBN 0-673-52004-8).
Neuberger, Julia (1987). *Caring for Dying People of Different Faiths.* The Lisa Sainsbury Foundation Series, Austen Cornish, London.
Sims, R. and Moss V.A. (1995). *Palliative Care for People with AIDS,* 2nd edn. Edward Arnold, London (ISBN 0-340-61371-8).

15

Nutrition and HIV Disease

Weight loss and thinness are common in all stages of HIV disease. In Africa, weight loss and emaciation, associated with diarrhoea ('slim disease'), is one of the most frequent manifestations of HIV disease[1]. In the Western world, weight loss is also common and an 'HIV wasting syndrome' has been an AIDS defining indicator disease since 1987[2]. A progressive, involuntary weight loss typically appears in the early stages of HIV disease and increases in severity as the disease progresses. In addition, metabolic changes and deficiencies of specific nutrients, vitamins and minerals are frequently associated with HIV disease, especially in late stage illness[3]. HIV disease has a significant impact on the nutritional status of the individual, ultimately resulting in various types of malnutrition in most individuals infected with HIV. In turn, malnutrition has an equally deleterious impact on immune function, morbidity and mortality in persons with HIV disease. Iatrogenic factors, e.g. drugs used in the treatment of HIV disease, may also adversely influence nutritional status and the efficacy of drug therapies currently used in HIV disease may be affected by the underlying nutritional status of the individual (see Fig. 15.1).

Nutrition refers to the processes involved in taking in, assimilating and utilizing nutrients. Nutrients include both **macronutrients** (carbohydrates, proteins, fats) and **micronutrients** (vitamins, minerals and trace elements). Nutritional processes include ingestion, digestion, absorption, metabolism and effective utilization of nutrients. Nutrients are needed for tissue growth and repair and for maintenance of functional systems in the body. Each individual process may be impaired during HIV disease. A variety of external factors, e.g. economic, socio-cultural, behavioural, etc., may also influence nutritional status.

Malnutrition results from a change in any of the above processes or factors and may result in either **over-** or **undernutrition**. The primary causes of undernutrition are well-defined and are associated with deficiencies of one or more nutrients, due to (a) inadequate ingestion, (b) absorption, (c) utilization, and/or (d) increased excretion, and (e) requirements[4].

Different types of malnutrition in chronic disease are characterized in terms of both metabolic and nutritional changes (Table 15.1). All the following forms of malnutrition can be seen in HIV disease:

Protein-energy malnutrition (PEM)   This may be seen in patients in all stages of HIV disease, resulting in involuntary weight loss or wasting[5]. PEM is similar to starvation and lean body mass is preserved relative to fat by adaptive mechanisms, e.g. decreased

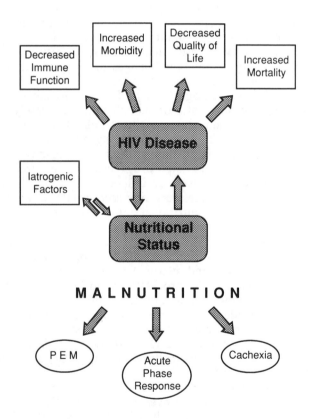

Fig. 15.1   Relationship between HIV disease and nutritional status

Table 15.1 Different types of malnutrition[3]

Type	Cause and characterization
Protein-energy malnutrition (PEM)	Starvation – the body's needs for protein, energy fuels, or both, cannot be met by diet[7]. Primary cause may be inadequate intake or secondary to malabsorption, decreased utilization or changes in metabolism, resulting in weight loss and wasting
Acute phase response	Metabolic changes which occur as a result of tissue injury, infection, stress, or inflammation and characterized by weight loss and changes (i.e. decreases) in the circulating levels of various plasma proteins, e.g. albumin[8]
Cachexia	A clinical syndrome involving a mixture of metabolic abnormalities that lead to a marked and sudden weight loss through accelerated wasting of host *tissue mass, failure of adequate nutrient intake, absorption and utilization.*[6] *Cachexia is often a feature of late HIV disease*

basal metabolic rate or resting energy expenditure[3].

Acute phase response This is a type of malnutrition seen in both acute and chronic illnesses, including HIV disease. Patients experience weight loss and loss of lean body mass. It occurs during acute episodes of opportunistic infections or periods of stress.

Cachexia This is frequently linked with end-stage HIV disease and is characterized by a profound and sudden depletion of lean body mass, especially muscle, and a variety of metabolic disorders. The changes associated with cachexia cannot usually be reversed by nutritional interventions[6].

Mechanisms of malnutrition in HIV disease

A variety of mechanisms of malnutrition in HIV disease have been defined[3], including reduced food intake, drug–nutrient interactions, malabsorption, and altered metabolism (Fig. 15.2), and one or more of these components may be involved.

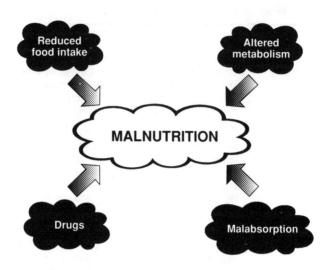

Fig. 15.2 Mechanisms of malnutrition

Reduced food intake

Several factors may lead to a reduced dietary intake during HIV disease. **Anorexia** (loss of appetite) may result from the disease process itself, mediated by a variety of cytokines (as discussed in Chapter 4), including tumour necrosis factor (TNF), interleukin-1 and interferons. These cytokines are frequently elevated in patients with HIV disease[9] and have been associated with anorexia[10]. **Pain** and **dysphagia** (difficulty in swallowing), secondary to a number of opportunistic conditions or lesions, e.g. buccal candidiasis, various herpesvirus infections, Kaposi's sarcoma, aphthous ulcerations, etc., may all contribute to a reduced dietary intake. **Nausea** and **vomiting**, caused by infections or tumours, or by drug treatment, is a frequent cause of a reduced food intake, as is **diarrhoea.** Decreased neurological function, especially the AIDS dementia complex, can affect food intake due to changes in both cognition and behaviour. Psychosocial causes, e.g. intentional weight loss, stress associated with bereavement, loss of employment, etc., have also been identified as significant factors in weight loss due to a reduced food intake in some individuals with HIV disease[11].

Drug–nutrient interactions

Many drugs used for treatment or prophylaxis in HIV disease potentially affect the processes of nutrition[12,13]. Side-effects of these drugs may include **gastro-intestinal symptoms**, e.g. amphotericin B, sulphadiazine, etoposide, can all cause **nausea, anorexia** and **vomiting**. Other drugs, e.g. trimethoprim-sulphamethoxazole and pentamidine, can cause a variety of **micronutrient imbalances**, such as glucose intolerance, folate deficiency, etc. and are noxious to various organs (pancreas, liver, kidneys) which play a major role in digestion. Antiretroviral drugs, such as zidovudine (AZT), are extremely toxic agents and can have a profound effect on nutritional status. In addition, zidovudine causes **myopathy** (muscle weakness), **anaemia** and **gastro-intestinal symptoms**. Antibiotics may disrupt the normal flora of the gastro-intestinal tract, increasing the risk of both diarrhoea and further gastro-intestinal opportunistic infections.

Malabsorption

Malabsorption commonly occurs as a result of various gastro-intestinal infections, which cause **inflammation** and **diarrhoea**. Common gastro-intestinal infections seen in patients with HIV disease include *Cryptosporidium* spp., *Isospora belli*, *Microsporidium*, *Salmonella* spp., and environmental mycobacteria, e.g. *M. avium-intracellulare* (MAC). Opportunistic infections associated with diarrhoea are the most frequent cause of malabsorption and weight loss in patients with HIV disease[11]. Kaposi's sarcoma can also occur in the gastro-intestinal tract, causing diarrhoea and subsequent malabsorption. Antacids, H_2 antagonists, e.g. cimetidine and other drugs which alter the pH and secretory function of the gastro-intestinal tract, may contribute to malabsorption.

Altered metabolism

Opportunistic infections result in **fever** and **hypermetabolic states** in which excessive calories are burned, leading to rapid wasting (acute phase response). Stress can also produce hypermetabolism. Various cytokines, e.g. tumour necrosis factor (TNF), interleukin-1 and the interferons influence metabolic processes. As these cytokines are often inappropriately produced during HIV disease, they may alter normal metabolic regulations, including fat (lipid) metabolism, leading to weight loss and cachexia.

The effects of malnutrition on HIV disease

Malnutrition is either directly or indirectly the cause of significant patient problems frequently encountered in HIV disease. These problems are described in Table 15.2 and may result in a debilitated patient, unable to function optimally and at risk of losing his/her independence. An essential element in patient care is the prevention of malnutrition and restoration of nutritional adequacy to malnourished patients.

Table 15.2   Consequences of malnutrition in HIV disease

Malnutrition in HIV disease:
Further depresses an already compromised immune system, increasing both frequency and severity of opportunistic events[14]
Increases morbidity, which in turn:
    Lessens effectiveness of drug treatments
    Decreases ability to withstand opportunistic events
    Prolongs periods of hospitalization
    Increases cost of treatment
    Decreases many indicators of quality of life:
        Increases dependency on others and decreases self-care ability
        Reduces muscle strength, energy and mobility
        Alters body image
        Increases despondency and decreases general enjoyment of life
Increases mortality:
    Nutritional status is the most important determinant of both survival and mortality[15,16]

Assessment

Nutritional evaluation should be carried out early, soon after HIV disease is diagnosed. Elements of a comprehensive assessment would include those items in Table 15.3. A multi-disciplinary approach to both assessment and intervention is needed. However, an early referral to a dietitian is essential.

Ideal body weight can be estimated using the formulae in Table 15.4[15], remembering that weight in pounds is converted to kilograms, i.e. one kilogram equls 2.2046 pounds (lbs). Nutritional assessment data which indicate nutritional depletion might include those items shown in Table 15.5.

Table 15.3 Nutritional assessment/evaluation

History
Normal weight; recent weight loss
Usual diet composition; current use of supplements
Average caloric intake
Anorexia, nausea, vomiting and/or diarrhoea
Systemic and local pain
Depression
Current chemotherapy
Economic status in relation to being able to buy food
Patient's ability to prepare food

Physical assessment – anthropometrics
Body weight and height
Estimated ideal body weight (see Table 15.4)
Per cent body weight change over time
Measurements of
   Triceps skinfold
   Mid-arm muscle circumference
Body temperature and heart rate

Laboratory investigations (as ordered by physician)
24-hour nitrogen balance determination
Serum albumin (and pre-albumin) and transferrin levels
Total protein
Haemoglobin and haematocrit
White cell and total lymphocyte count

Risk factors

Important risk factors for malnutrition in HIV disease are **anorexia** (most frequent), **diarrhoea** and **fever** (most severe), although many patients have combined risk factors[17]. As opportunistic infections, especially those associated with diarrhoea, are a frequent cause of weight loss in patients with HIV disease, any unexplained weight loss should alert nurses to the possibility of covert infection[11]. Weight loss of 10 per cent or more can have a significant impact on the patient's functional status and survival prospects[12,18].

Malnutrition can occur in patients with a seemingly adequate caloric intake who do not have significant weight loss and, consequently, decisions to intervene nutritionally must be based upon the results of a valid assessment by a dietitian[19]. The physician, in liaison with the dietitian, may order a variety of laboratory investigations, especially serum albumin, an important tool used to monitor malnutrition.

Table 15.4   Estimating ideal body weight

Men	106 lb (48.1 kg) for first 5 feet in height 6 lb (2.7 kg) for each inch over 5 feet
Women	100 lb (45.4 kg) for first 5 feet in height 5 lb (2.3 kg) for each inch over 5 feet
Example	The ideal weight for a man measuring 5 feet, 8 inches in height would be 106 lb + 48 lb (6 lb × 8 inches) = 154 lb (or 70 kg)

Table 15.5   Data indicative of nutritional depletion

Recent weight loss	> 10%
Serum albumin	< 35 g/l
Serum transferrin	< 2 g/l
Triceps skinfold thickness:	
Males	< 10 mm
Females	< 13 mm
Upper-arm circumference:	
Males	< 23 cm
Females	< 22 cm
Lymphopenia	present
Skin anergy	present

Nutritional interventions

Early assessment allows for early intervention. Intervention areas include dietary counselling and patient education; drug therapy; oral supplements; enteral feeding and total parenteral nutrition.

Dietary counselling and patient education

Patients need to have a good understanding of the nutritional implications of HIV disease and the importance of maintaining body weight by eating a balanced diet, especially high-protein, calorifically dense foods. They need to have the opportunity to periodically consult a dietitian. This will allow an opportunity for ongoing monitoring and space to discuss alternative diets which patients may be contemplating. Patient education might also focus on sensible measures which may promote a healthier lifestyle, e.g. stress management and the need for regular exercise, and practical aspects of nutrition, especially food safety. Food safety is particularly important in HIV-infected individuals who, as a result of a progressive decrease in the effectiveness of their immune system, are more prone to food-borne illnesses as a consequence of eating contaminated food. These illnesses often present with nausea and vomiting, fever, diarrhoea, abdominal pain (cramping) and headache. They are often difficult to treat and can be extremely serious (even fatal) in an individual who is immunocompromised. Patient education can help patients to 'eat defensively', avoiding the potential for food poisoning. The following recommendations can be made:

- **Shopping** Buy perishable foods (those which require refrigeration or freezing) last and check that the 'sell-by date' of all foods is current. Ensure that safety seals on tins and jars are intact and that tins are not dented or otherwise damaged.

- **Fridges and freezers** Ensure that refrigerators are kept between 0 and 5°C and that freezers are kept at 0 to −18°C. Refrigerator and freezer thermometers are inexpensive and should be used.

- **Food storage** Store cooked and uncooked (raw) foods **separately** in the refrigerator. All raw meats should be stored in plastic bags and kept in the lower part of the refrigerator to prevent possible contamination of other foods by drippings.

- **Frozen foods** Some frozen foods, e.g. vegetables, fish fingers, etc., can be cooked from frozen. Those foods which need defrosting should be thawed out in the refrigerator (or microwave oven on the defrost setting), **not** at room temperature.

- **Handwashing** Wash hands thoroughly in warm, soapy water and rinse well, prior to and after handling all food, especially raw meats! Cover any cuts or lesions with a waterproof bandage or wear a disposable plastic glove (available from supermarkets for catering use). Use paper towels or cloth towels once only!

- **Chopping (cutting) boards** Use a separate chopping board for raw meats. Chopping boards made from hard plastic or marble are easier to clean and disinfect than are those made from wood. Disinfect chopping boards daily with a weak solution of bleach (or put in dishwasher, if appropriate).

- **Meats, poultry, fish, eggs** Ensure that they are all **well cooked** and are consumed soon after cooking and not left at room temperature.

- **Raw foods** Do not eat raw eggs or softboiled eggs or omelettes (unless they are well cooked). Do not eat homemade mayonnaise. Avoid pâtés, raw or partially cooked poultry, meats (e.g. steak tartare), fish (e.g. sushi, partially cooked or steamed clams, oysters, prawns, etc.).

- **Left-overs** These are safe if they are kept in the refrigerator for no longer than 3 days. Heat thoroughly (75°C) before eating and do not reheat more than once. It is often better to put leftovers in a plastic bag and put them in a freezer.

- **Milk, cheese and yoghurt** Eat only those products which have been **pasteurized**. Avoid eating blue vein cheeses, e.g. Stilton.

- **Vegetables and fruits** Wash thoroughly before use. A good idea is to wash them in cooled, boiled water or a disinfecting solution, e.g. 1 gallon of water and 20 drops of 2 per cent iodine (available at any chemist or drugstore). Let produce stand in the solution for about 10–15 minutes and rinse well.

- **Drinking water** Do not use tap water or even **bottled water**. Tap water should be used after it has been boiled, cooled and then stored in the refrigerator. It should be prepared daily.

- **Eating out** Be careful! Avoid eating salads (choose hot soups instead) and be careful of drinking water.

Both dietitians and nurses will be able to suggest ways to manage nutritionally related symptoms or side-effects, such as lack of appetite, mouth soreness, dysphagia, nausea and diarrhoea. Practical advice is available in the form of patient education booklets, both in the UK[20] and the USA[21], and copies can be easily obtained for patient distribution.

Drug therapy

Drugs used to control nausea, vomiting and diarrhoea, or as appetite stimulants, are commonly used to help improve the patient's nutritional status.

Antidiarrhoea drugs

Patients should be encouraged not to use antidiarrhoea drugs which are available over the counter without first consulting their medical practitioner. These drugs are often contraindicated for treating diarrhoea which is caused by enteric pathogens until the infection has been treated. The most common antidiarrhoea drugs used are antimotility agents, such as **co-phenotrope** (Lomotil), **loperamide**

hydrochloride (Imodium, Arret®, Diocalm Ultra®) and **codeine phosphate**. Absorbents and bulk-forming drugs, e.g. kaolin, are not useful for acute diarrhoea. **Octreotide** (Sanostatin®) is sometimes used for severe diarrhoea, especially *Cryptosporidium*-induced secretory diarrhoea[22]. For the prevention and treatment of fluid and electrolyte imbalance in patients with acute diarrhoea, especially those who are frail and undernourished, **oral rehydration therapy (ORT)** may be helpful. Nurses can teach patients how to make up a sugar and salt ORT solution, or advise them on using proprietary preparations, e.g. Dioralyte®, Rehidrat®, etc.

Anti-emetic drugs

Several drugs are available which are useful in managing nausea and vomiting. Some of the more commonly used agents include **metoclopramide** (Maxolon), **domperidone** (Motilium®), and **prochlorperazine** (Stemetil®). Some of these drugs are also available in an injectable form and as suppositories or in buccal preparations. Side-effects include extrapyramidal reactions (especially in children and young adults) which are manifested by Parkinson-like dystonic muscular spasms. This is an important and distressing side-effect which can be successfully terminated by the administration of an antimuscarinic drug, e.g. **benzhexol hydrochloride** (Artane®), **procyclidine hydrochloride** (Kemadrin®), once recognized.

Many patients use **cannabis** (Marijuana) to control nausea. However, it is an illegal substance in the UK and cannot be prescribed. Its use, however, is widespread and it probably has no significant side-effects, other than being mildly hallucinogenic in some individuals. A desire to increase the dose and withdrawal symptoms are unusual[23].

Appetite stimulants

The appetite may be stimulated by small doses of **alcohol**, e.g. sherry or wine, by **cannabis** and by a variety of 'tonics', which probably owe their alleged efficacy to the power of suggestion rather than any inherent property of the preparation. **Megestrol acetate** (Megace®) is used for the treatment of anorexia, weight loss and cachexia in patients with HIV disease. It is supplied as an oral suspension (40 mg/ml) and the usual prescribed dose is 400–800 mg/10–20 ml per day. Side-effects are generally mild but varied. However, occasional, more serious side-effects include venous thrombosis and impotence. Nurses should consult the product insert for detailed information on side-effects. Megace is not given to pregnant women.

Oral supplements

Oral supplements are often used at an early stage in patients with HIV disease to help maintain weight, reverse nutritional deficiencies and promote anabolism (growth and repair of body tissue).

Supplements of micronutrients

Malnourished patients with HIV disease develop a variety of micronutrient deficiencies which further depress their immune system and adversely affect both their ability to recover from opportunistic events and their response to chemotherapy[22]. Possible deficiencies include minerals, vitamins (A, C, E, B group) and trace elements (iron, copper, zinc, iodine, selenium, magnesium, etc.). In addition, any infection, including HIV infection, speeds up the production of **oxidants**, which are **free radical molecules** produced by various cellular-enzymatic reactions in the body. Free radicals both damage and reduce the ability of tissues to resist infection and tumours. Increased free radical activity may also trigger programmed cell death (apoptosis), as discussed in Chapter 5, causing a further depletion of CD4+ T lymphocytes.

Consequently, oral supplementation of micronutrients may be useful, especially ensuring adequate intake of **beta-carotene** (precursor to vitamin A), **zinc** and various **anti-oxidants**, such as vitamins C and E. Trace elements thought to be important in effective immune system function include **zinc** and **selenium**. Finally, increasing the levels of **essential polyunsaturated fatty acids (EFA)**, e.g. **omega-6** (linoleic acid, derived from vegetable oils such as corn, safflower, sunflower and soybean oils) and **omega-3**, which is present in coldwater fish oils and includes **EPA** (eicosapentaenoic acid) and **DHA** (docosahexaenoic acid), may improve immune function.

It would seem sensible for most patients to take a comprehensive, over-the-counter **multiple vitamin and mineral preparation**, ensure an adequate supply of **anti-oxidants** and ensure an adequate intake of essential polyunsaturated fats by taking a **fish oil** and **linoleic acid** (e.g. **soya lecithin**) capsule each day.

Enteral feeding

A regular diet may be supplemented with calorie-counted high-energy and protein-rich foods eaten as snacks between meals. However, supplementation is generally better accomplished by using commercial products and, as a wide variety of nutritionally complete foods are available, a dietitian's advice is essential.

Enteral supplementation or total nutrition

These formulae may be given via a soft, small-calibre nasogastric or nasoduodenal tube or through an endoscopically or surgically placed gastrostomy or jejunostomy tube. They may be given as additions to a regular diet or as total nutrition.

The choice of oral or enteral supplements, or products used for enteral nutrition, will be based on what the patient is able to tolerate. Different types of formulae include:

Milk-based polymeric formula Polymeric formulae provide protein and other nutrients intact or in a partially hydrolysed form. Polymeric formulae require normal gut function for maximum digestion and absorption. If patients can tolerate lactose, milk-based products are less expensive, easily available and often more palatable than lactose-free polymeric formulae.

Lactose-free polymeric formula When lactose causes diarrhoea, lactose-free polymeric formulae are given and milk drinks avoided. Calcium supplementation may be required in lactose-free diets.

Elemental formula Unlike polymeric formulae, the protein in elemental formulae is provided in the form of peptides or free amino acids (peptide-based formulae are sometimes referred to as **semi-elemental**). These formulae require less effective gut functioning before absorption and are commonly used in patients with malabsorption and diarrhoea.

Each commercially prepared enteral formula varies in relation to the composition of carbohydrates and fats, the caloric and protein content and its osmolality. The specific content of each formula is listed in the *Monthly Index of Medical Specialities* (*MIMS*) (UK), the *British National Formulary* and the *Physicians' Desk Reference* (*PDR*) (USA), but the following general comments can be made:

Carbohydrates Carbohydrates may include lactose (if tolerated), or, in lactose-free diets, carbohydrates are supplied in the form of maltodextrin, modified starch, sucrose, corn syrup and/or hydrolysed cornstarch.

Fats Two types of fats are included in enteral formulae: **long-chain triglycerides (LCT)** and **medium-chain triglycerides (MCT)**. Fat is an excellent source of calories, however, LCTs are not well-tolerated by patients with impaired gut function and cause mucosal irritation, further compromising nutrient absorption. MCTs are better tolerated and, consequently, are more commonly used in enteral formulae. In addition, the **total fat content** is important. High fat content, e.g. > 15 per cent, can promote immunosuppression and fat intolerance is frequent in patients with small bowel involvement[14]. Consequently, low-fat enteral formulae (i.e. fat content < 5 per cent) are usually used. As MCTs do not contain linoleic acid, supplements of EFAs, especially omega-6 should be given.

Caloric/protein content Most enteral formulae are designed to deliver 1.0–1.5 kcal (and 0.02–0.04 g of protein) per ml. Special enteral formulae usually deliver 1.5–2.0 kcal (and 0.06–0.08 g of protein) per ml[22].

Osmolality The concentration of osmotically active particles in solution determines its infusion rate. **Isosmolar** formulae are routinely given to patients with relatively intact gut function and are infused at full strength at an initial rate of approximately 40 ml/hour. **Hyperosmolar** formulae are given to patients with gut dysfunction and are initially infused at ¼ strength. As tolerance develops, the strength of hyperosmolar diets may be advanced to ½, ¾, and eventually to full-strength. Both types of formulae are infused at an initial rate of 40 ml/hour, the eventual infusion rate being (up to 100–125 ml/hour) dependent upon the patient's tolerance and calculated total caloric and protein requirements[22].

Caring for patients with feeding tubes

Following insertion of a nasogastric or nasoduodenal tube, an abdominal X-ray is ordered to ensure that the tube has been properly positioned. Continuous feeding is achieved by use of a volumetric pump and the formula, strength and rate of infusion will be prescribed by the physician. The head of the bed is elevated 30° or more while the infusion is being administered. The tube should be aspirated and the amount of content ('residuals') noted every 2 hours. If more than 150 ml, the infusion should be discontinued for 2 hours. After this time, residuals should be re-checked and if < 150 ml, the infusion is re-started, otherwise the physician must be consulted. The tube is flushed every 4 hours with 20 ml of sterile water. Intake and output records are maintained and the patient's weight is recorded (in kilograms) weekly on the vital signs chart. The patient's urine should be tested for sugar and acetone each shift and if the urinary sugar is 4+, a serum glucose test should be done immediately. A normal laboratory value for (fasting) serum glucose is 3.9–5.6 mmol/l (or 70–110 mg/dl). If the serum glucose level is > 6 mmol/l (or > 160 mg/dl), the physician must be notified for treatment orders. The patient must be observed for an increase in temperature, increasing abdominal distention, nausea, vomiting or diarrhoea. Extra supplements of minerals (e.g. zinc, calcium, phosphate, magnesium) may be ordered and vitamin supplements may also be prescribed. Regular blood tests, e.g. full blood count and biochemical assays, are used to monitor the patient.

Parenteral nutrition

Intravenous nutrition may be given as **supplemental parenteral nutrition**, or, where it is the sole source of nutrition, as **total parenteral nutrition (TPN)**. Parenteral nutrition requires the intravenous infusion of solutions containing glucose, fat, amino acids, electrolytes, trace elements and vitamins. Because of the high concentration of glucose (10–50 per cent) and protein in these solutions, which cause venous thrombosis, they are normally administered via a central venous catheter. The objectives of TPN in severely malnourished patients with HIV disease include slow, continued gains in weight, lean body mass and quality of life. TPN is initiated in hospital and can be continued in an out-patient or community setting[15,24].

Central venous catheter

Catheter insertion requires full aseptic conditions and is never appropriately done as an emergency procedure. It is not inserted on the wards but either in the operating theatre (operating room) or in a specialized area, e.g. angiography department, where full surgical precautions can be observed. Various catheters are available, e.g. Teflon, silicone and polyurethane, some of which (e.g. Hickman Catheter®) incorporate a Dacron cuff for siting at the distal exit of the skin tunnel, where it provokes a sterile inflammatory process, causing the surrounding tissues to adhere to and anchor the cuff into position.

Central Venous Access
The catheter is placed in the superior or inferior vena cava or right atrium, or a large vein leading to these vessels. Catheter may also be inserted via the internal jugular vein, femoral vein or the cephalic vein. However, both neck and antecubital fossa insertion sites are uncomfortable and difficult to manage. Inserting a catheter in the groin (femoral vein) increases the risk of infection. Consequently, most physicians will choose to insert the catheter **infraclavicularly** into the **subclavian vein**, positioning the tip of the catheter in the

mid-portion of the **superior vena cava**. Triple-lumen catheters are associated with increased risk of infection and are not generally used in patients requiring long-term parenteral nutrition.

A single-lumen catheter (e.g. Hickman®, Silastic Broviac®, etc.) is burrowed through the subcutaneous tissue in the anterior chest wall and exits away from the site of subclavian vein puncture. Some silicone catheters (Port-a-Cath®, Mediport®) have a portal which is placed under the skin and sutured to the chest wall. Access to the portal is via a special Huber point needle which may remain in place for up to 1 week. If the brachial vein in the antecubital fossa or the femoral vein is used, a special 'long line' will be required.

The catheter is inserted under local anaesthesia with the patient sedated and in the head-down position (unless contraindicated) as a precaution against the risk of air embolism during the negative-pressure phase of respiration[25] and to permit dilatation of the neck and shoulder vessels. During the procedure, the nurse instructs the patient to turn his/her face away from the insertion area to prevent possible contamination of the insertion site. The patient will need to be supported during the procedure to permit hyperextension of the shoulder. This can be facilitated by placing a rolled sheet or towel vertically along the spinal column. The insertion site should be shaved, if necessary, and an appropriate skin disinfectant used, e.g. chlorhexidine 0.5 per cent in 70 per cent spirit. During the insertion, the physician may instruct the patient to bear down with his/her mouth closed (**Valsalva's manoeuvre**) to increase intrathoracic pressure and distend the neck veins. The nurse must help the patient to remain still during the procedure. Following insertion (and after re-positioning of the catheter), a chest X-ray is taken to confirm correct catheter placement before TPN commences. In-line filters are not used as the particles to be infused are too large to go through a filter. A special occlusive dressing covers the insertion site.

Caring for a patient receiving TPN via a central venous catheter

Following commencement of TPN, the appropriate ongoing assessment, nursing interventions and evaluation, are as shown in Table 15.6. Hospital and home-care units should have current protocols for caring for patients having TPN and these should be reviewed on a regular basis. TPN solutions will be prepared, either commercially or in pharmacy under a laminar flow hood and are normally supplied in a 3–litre bag, sufficient for one 24-hour period. Pharmacy departments will normally supply the infusion with the administration set attached. The nurse must prime the tubing and connect it to the TPN catheter. The inside and outside of the hub of the catheter and the end of the administration set are sprayed with a disinfectant, e.g. isopropyl alcohol 70 per cent, and allowed to dry before the connection is made. The hub will be set in an iodine-impregnated foam pad[26].

Table 15.6 Nursing protocols: TPN

1. Infuse TPN solution and 20% fat emulsion as per physician's orders, using an alarmed volumetric pump and check infusion rate every hour. Standard infusion rates are:

   TPN solution
   Day 1   40 ml/hour
   Day 2   80 ml/hour   } by volumetric pump
   Day 3   80–125 ml/hour

   Fat emulsion solution
   Infuse 500 ml of 20% fat emulsion over 6–8 hours at least three times per week by volumetric pump

   Do not make any rapid changes to infusion rate. Adjustments to rate must not exceed 10% of the original rate
2. Monitor vital signs 4 hourly and notify the physician if the oral temperature is > 38°C
3. Record fluid intake and output
4. Weigh daily (at the same time) and record weight in kilograms on patient's observation flow sheet. When stable, weigh twice weekly
5. Initiate 24-hour urine collections for estimation of urea nitrogen and electrolyte excretion twice weekly, e.g. commencing at 6:00 a.m. every Monday and Thursday
6. Test blood glucose concentration four times a day, using test strips (e.g. BM-Test 1-44®, Dextrostix®, etc.) and a meter. If these are not available, test urine for sugar and acetone four times daily and record on patient's observation flow sheet. If urine sugar is 4+, request a STAT serum glucose test. If the serum glucose is > 6 mmol/l (or >160 mg/dl), contact the physician for further orders
7. The insertion site is covered with a sterile, semi-occlusive transparent dressing, e.g. Op-site ® or sterile gauze, according to the TPN protocol. Inspect site daily for signs of inflammation and lack of integrity of dressing
8. When necessary, change dressing according to TPN protocol, using full aseptic technique. Standard protocols include cleaning the entry site with 0.5% chlorhexidine in 70% spirit then dressed with Op-site[26]. Send a swab from the site to the Microbiology Department for culture and sensitivity
9. Ensure a pair of atraumatic clamps are kept at the bedside for emergency use
10. No medications or blood products are given via the parenteral nutrition catheter. The TPN catheter is not used for CVP measurements or withdrawing blood samples. The only time a blood sample from the

catheter may be required is if catheter infection is suspected

11. Change the administration set every 24 (or 48–72) hours as per TPN protocol, only using administration sets with a Luer lock fitting
12. If TPN is temporarily stopped, the catheter should be flushed with 5–10 ml of normal saline when the feed is discontinued and again, prior to recommencing TPN
13. A single bag of TPN solution must not be infused over a longer period than 24 hours. If any feed remains after this time, it is discarded
14. Ensure standard TPN laboratory examinations are drawn weekly according to TPN protocols for comprehensive biochemical monitoring. Test for[22,27]:

Daily	Glucose, electrolytes and blood urea nitrogen (when patient is stable, change from daily monitoring to twice weekly)
Baseline then twice weekly	Serum albumin, transferrin, liver function studies, serum creatinine, haemoglobin, haemocrit, white blood cell count, calcium, phosphate and magnesium levels
Baseline then weekly	Prothrombin time, micronutrient tests, e.g. copper, zinc, transferrin, triglyceride, prealbumin, retinol binding protein

Standard composition of TPN

A standard TPN solution contains protein, carbohydrates, electrolytes, micronutrients (vitamins, minerals and trace elements).

Protein   Protein is utilized by the body in the form of **nitrogen (N_2)** and is needed for tissue (especially muscle) growth and repair. Protein is the only source of N_2 and each 6.25 g of whole protein contains 1 g of N_2 (10 g N_2 = 62.5 g protein). Most adult patients with HIV disease require 2.0–2.5 g/kg of protein daily[22] which is given as mixtures of essential and non-essential synthetic l-amino acids.

Carbohydrate   This is given for energy and heat production and is measured in kilocalories (kcal). A sufficient amount of non-protein carbohydrate calories ('protein sparing') must be given to ensure that the amino acids are used for tissue growth and repair and not energy. Glucose (dextrose) is the preferred source of carbohydrate and is used in various strengths, from 10 to 50 per cent. The usual energy requirement for adults with HIV disease[22] is 35–40 kcal/kg, e.g. approximately 2500–3000 kcal daily.

Fat   Fat is also given for protein-sparing energy and has the advantage of a high energy to fluid volume ratio, neutral pH, iso-osmolarity with plasma and provides essential fatty acids. Patients undergoing standard TPN therapy should receive 3 to 5 per cent of their daily caloric intake in the form of fat. This may be achieved by routinely administering 500 ml of a 20 per cent fat emulsion (usually derived from soya bean oil) containing 2 kcal/ml over 6–8 hours at least 3 times a week[22]. Several days of adaptation may be needed to attain maximal utilization of fat emulsions. Reactions to a 20 per cent fat emulsion include episodes of pyrexia and, rarely, anaphylactic responses[23]. Additives are never mixed with fat emulsions unless their compatibility has been approved by a pharmacist.

Micronutrients Micronutrients, e.g. vitamins, minerals and trace elements, and **electrolytes**, e.g. sodium, chloride, potassium, etc. are added by pharmacy to the daily infusion as prescribed.

Complications of central TPN therapy

A variety of complications are associated with central TPN administration. Complications can be technical, infectious or metabolic.

Technical complications
Important technical complications include catheter misplacement, pneumothorax, thrombosis, catheter embolism and, importantly, **air embolism**.

Air embolism can be fatal and may occur when the patient is in the upright or semi-upright position and the integrity of the subclavian venous catheter infusion system is disrupted (disconnected)[22]. This event is characterized by the sudden onset in the patient of severe respiratory distress, associated with both cardiac and neurologic deficits. Treatment involves the immediate positioning of the patient in the 'Durant position' (lying on the left side with the head down and the feet elevated) and prompt syringe aspiration of blood and air from the subclavian catheter. Prevention relies on ensuring the integrity of the catheter system, i.e. secure fixation of all catheter connections and using only Leur Lock (never 'male–female') catheter connections.

Infectious complications
Infectious complications include insertion-site infection, primary catheter infection and secondary infections.

Localized **insertion-site infection** is easily detected as the surrounding skin becomes erythematous and tender and the catheter tract may exude purulent drainage. **Primary catheter infection** is more difficult to detect. However, the key diagnostic triad of catheter infection (in order of occurrence) is [22]:

1. a 'plateau' temperature pattern (38.0–38.5°C) for 12–24 hours;
2. unexplained hyperglycaemia (> 6 mmol/l or 160 mg/dl);
3. leucocytosis (> 10 000 WBC/hpf).

Both insertion-site and primary catheter infections, when diagnosed, require that the TPN catheter be removed (and the tip sent to the microbiology department for culture and sensitivity). A new central TPN catheter must be inserted at a new site. The physician will prescribe appropriate antibiotic therapy for the infection.

Metabolic complications
A range of metabolic complications are associated with TPN therapy, including high and low serum levels of glucose, sodium, potassium, phosphates, chloride, calcium, etc.

Hyperglycaemia is the most frequent metabolic complication of TPN therapy, even in non-diabetic patients. Insulin may be prescribed to be given concurrently with the TPN solution and it is usually given separately by a syringe-pump. The blood glucose level should be maintained at ≥ 6 mmol/l (160 mg/dl). Insulin may be added to the TPN solution but no more than 40 units of insulin should be added to 1 litre of solution. If insulin is added to the TPN solution, it is added as 10 unit increments (i.e. 10 units in each litre of TPN solution) and the blood glucose level is maintained by giving additional insulin intravenously until control is achieved by the insulin in the TPN solution.

Hypoglycaemia (blood glucose level < 3.9 mmol/l or < 70 mg/dl) often occurs when the TPN solution is suddenly discontinued. Hypoglycaemia is usually prevented by 'tapering off' TPN therapy, ensuring that oral carbohydrate intake is sufficient before discontinuing TPN. If hypoglycaemia occurs, it is generally treated by infusions of 10 per cent dextrose in normal saline.

During TPN therapy, the patient should be as ambulatory as possible and if being discharged, intensive patient education programmes can prepare the patient to take a large share of the responsibility for successful home treatment.

Peripheral parenteral nutrition (PPN)

Short-term (not more than 5–7 days) peripheral parenteral nutrition may be given through an 18-gauge intravenous cannula inserted into a peripheral vein but the parenteral nutrition solution has a lower concentration of glucose. A standard litre of PPN solution contains 500 ml 20 per cent dextrose in water and 500 ml 10 per cent amino acids, plus vitamins, minerals and trace elements. In addition, a daily infusion of 500 ml of 20 per cent fat emulsion is given. The cannula is re-sited every 48–72 hours and the insertion site is routinely dressed with a transparent polyurethane film dressing, e.g. Op-Site®.

References

1. Colebunders, R., Mann, J.M., Francis, H. *et al.* (1987). Evaluation of a clinical case definition of acquired immunodeficiency syndrome in Africa. *Lancet*, 28 February, i(8531), 492–4.
2. Centers for Disease Control (1987). Revision of the CDC surveillance case definition for acquired immunodeficiency syndrome: a report by the Council of State and Territorial Epidemiologists, AIDS Program. *Morbidity and Mortality Weekly Report (MMWR)*, 14 August, 36(Suppl. 1), 1–15S.
3. Raiten, Daniel J. (1990). *Nutrition and HIV Infection: A Review and Evaluation of the Extant Knowledge of the Relationship between Nutrition and HIV Infection.* LSRO, Federation of American Societies for Experimental Biology, Bethesda, MD.
4. Herbert, V. (1973). The five possible causes of all nutrient deficiency: illustrated by deficiencies of vitamin B12 and folic acid. *American Journal of Clinical Nutrition* 26, 77–88.
5. Kotler, D.P. (1989). Malnutrition in HIV infection and AIDS. *AIDS* 3(Suppl. 1), S175–S180.
6. Kern, K.A., Norton, J.A. (1988). Cancer cachexis. *Journal of Parenteral and Enteral Nutrition* 12, 286–98.
7. Torun, B., Viteri, F.E. (1988). Protein-energy malnutrition. In *Modern Nutrition in Health and Disease*, 7th edn, eds Shils, M.E. and Young, V.R., Lea & Febiger, Philadelphia, pp. 746–73.
8. Fleck, A. (1988). Acute phase response: implications for nutrition and recovery. *Nutrition* 4, 109–17.
9. Lähdevirta, J., Maury, C.P.J., Teppo, A.M. *et al.* (1988). Elevated levels of circulating cachectin/tumor necrosis factor in patients with acquired immunodeficiency syndrome. *American Journal of Medicine* 85, 289–91.
10. Grunfeld, C. and Palladino, M.A. Jr. (1990). Tumor necrosis factor; immunologic, antitumor, metabolic and cardiovascular activities. *Advances in Internal Medicine* 35, 45–71.
11. Summerbell, D.C., Perett, J.P. and Gazzard, B.C. (1993). Causes of weight loss in human immunodeficiency virus infection. *International Journal of STD & AIDS*, July/August, 4, 234–6.
12. Fields Newman, C. and Horn, B. (1988). Drug–nutrient interactions. In *AIDS Guidebook.* The Cutting Edge Consulting, Freemont, CA (cited in Raiten, Daniel J. (1990)). *Nutrition and HIV Infection: A Review and Evaluation of the Extant Knowledge of the Relationship between Nutrition and HIV Infection*, LSRO, Federation of American Societies for Experimental Biology, Bethesda, MD.
13. Ghiron, L., Dwyer, J. and Stollman, L.B. (1989). Nutrition support of

the HIV-positive, ARC and AIDS patient. *Clinical Nutrition* **8**, 103–13.

14. Andrassy, Richard J. (1990). Nutrition and immunocompromise: An overview. *AIDS Patient Care*, December, **4**(Suppl. 1), S9–S12.
15. Ellis, W., Basinger, G., Paul, J. *et al.* (1994). The use of home total parenteral nutrition in a patient with AIDS. *AIDS Patient Care*, February, **8**(1), 6–10.
16. O'Sullivan, P., Linke, R.A. and Dalton, S. (1985). Evaluation of body weight and nutritional status among AIDS patients. *Journal of the American Dietetic Association* **85**, 1483–4.
17. Schwenk, A., Bürger, B., Wessel, D. *et al.* (1993). Clinical risk factors for malnutrition in HIV-1 infected patients. *AIDS* **7**(9), 1213–19.
18. Mascioli, Edward (1993).Nutrition and HIV infection. *AIDS Clinical Care*, November, **5**(11), 85–7.
19. McQuiggan, Maggie (1990). Enteral nutrition for the hospitalized HIV patient. *AIDS Patient Care*, December, **4**(Suppl. 1), S13–S16.
20. Ross, Hazel (1993). *Nutrition & HIV Infection*. The AIDS Education and Research Trust (AVERT), UK (see below for ordering details).
21. Physicians Association for AIDS Care (1993). *HIV Disease: Nutrition Guidelines: Practical Steps for a Healthier Life*. Stadlanders Pharmacy, USA (see below for ordering details).
22. Hickey, Michael S. (1992). *Handbook of Enteral, Parenteral and ARC/AIDS Nutritional Therapy*. Mosby Year Book, USA.
23. British Medical Association and the Royal Pharmaceutical Society of Great Britain (1994). *British National Formulary*, March, No. 27.
24. Mughal, M. and Irving, M. (1986). Home parenteral nutrition in the United Kingdom and Ireland. *The Lancet*, **ii**, 383–7.
25. Taylor, Mary (1994). Total parenteral nutrition (Parts 1 & 2). *Nursing Standard* **8**(23), 25–8 and **8**(24), 37–9.
26. Pritchard, A.P. and David, J.A. (eds) (1988). *The Royal Marsden Hospital Manual of Clinical Nursing Procedures*, 2nd. edn. Harper & Row, London.
27. Howard, Lyn J. (1991). Parenteral and enteral nutrition and therapy. In *Harrison's Principles of Internal Medicine*, Vol 1, 12th (International) edn, eds Wilson, J.D., Braunwald, E., Isselbacher, K.J. *et al.*, Part 4(75). McGraw-Hill, London, pp. 427–34.

Further Reading

Hickey, Michael S. (1992). *Handbook of Enteral, Parenteral and ARC/AIDS Nutritional Therapy*. Mosby Year Book, USA (ISBN 1-5566-4341-1)
Raiten, Daniel J. (1990). *Nutrition and HIV Infection: A Review and Evaluation of the Extant Knowledge of the Relationship between Nutrition and HIV Infection*. LSRO, Federation of American Societies for Experimental Biology, Bethesda, MD.
Taylor, Mary (1994). Total parenteral nutrition (Parts 1 & 2). *Nursing Standard* **8**(23), 25–8 and **8**(24), 37–9.

Patient education booklets

UK

Ross, Hazel (1993). *Nutrition & HIV Infection.* The AIDS Education and Research Trust (AVERT), UK (Telephone: UK 0403 210202 or write to 'AVERT', 11 Denne Parade, Horsham, West Sussex RH12 1JD, England, for a free copy).

USA

Physicians Association for AIDS Care (1993). *HIV Disease: Nutrition Guidelines: Practical Steps for a Healthier Life.* Stadlanders Pharmacy, USA (Telephone: USA 1-800-238-7828, or write to PAAC, 101 West Grande Ave., Suite 200, Chicago, IL 60610, for a free copy).

16

Discharge Planning and Community Care

Almost all patients with AIDS will require community nursing services at some point in their illness. Successful community nursing care is in part dependent upon good discharge planning procedures when clients are in hospital. The following discusses discharge planning in the UK; however, the principles of safely discharging a patient to home applies in most countries.

Discharge planning

Effective discharge planning requires strategic planning by hospitals and health authorities and just as there is often an admissions policy, there must be a discharge policy. Table 16.1 can serve as a model for this policy[1].

On admission, the nursing assessment must include the relevant social history of the patient. This should include an assessment of the requisites for health described in Chapter 14 which can then be reassessed and documented upon discharge. A standard format can be used to detail the social history aspects of the nursing assessment if it is carefully designed so that it can be individualized for each patient. The Social History Form in Appendix 5 outlines some of the essential information that a social history must elicit. This form can also serve as a permanent record of the patient's discharge plans.

Procedures for safe discharge should be established and should include guidance for hospital nursing personnel, community nursing personnel and for local authority staff. The following is a suggested model for effecting the safe discharge of patients with AIDS and HIV-related conditions.

Table 16.1 Discharge policy

Aims
1. The safe discharge of all adults to situations where:
   (a) Their treatment and recovery will be continuous with that given in hospital
   (b) Their immediate needs for warmth, food and relief from pain are met
   (c) They have shelter and are safe from molestation
2. The implementation of procedures for safe discharges for adults, and the monitoring of practices and progress
3. Close cooperation with local authority (municipal) services
4. Coordination of effort between hospital and community-based health care professionals
5. Establishing effective lines of communication with all parties involved

Objectives commensurate with these aims are to ensure that:
1. Each individual patient receives the care and attention necessary without having to compete with others
2. Where a patient is found to need nursing care, he or she will not be discharged unless there is suitable provision
3. All vulnerable patients (and those living alone) have someone to see them into their home
4. Planning for discharge starts as soon as possible (preferably before admission)
5. The handover of the care of the patient from hospital to the community should provide for continuous cover for the patient

Planning process
1. Weekly planning meetings are held by the ward team to coordinate and take responsibility for the recovery and safe discharge of all patients. It is essential that relevant community nursing staff attend these meetings
2. The planning meeting will assess the ability of the patient to manage the situation which will be encountered on discharge and advise the responsible physician accordingly
3. The planning meeting will decide which pre-discharge preparations are required and the ward sister (head nurse) is responsible for seeing that these preparations are put into effect and for setting a target date for the patient's discharge
4. The responsibility for successful discharge shall fall to the nurse in charge of the ward at the time of the patient's discharge. This nurse will have the authority to cancel the discharge if the arrangements agreed by the planning meeting are not yet completed
5. The discharge is not effective until the persons/agencies in the community have taken over any of the caring duties deemed necessary, and until that time, responsibility for the patient's continuing care shall remain with the hospital

6. Responsibility for medical cover must be transferred to the patient's general practitioner (family doctor) in advance of the patient's discharge
7. It is the responsibility of the ward sister to see that all parties concerned have been informed of the patient's discharge by the end of the discharge day

Hospital nursing personnel

1. A Social History Form can be initiated in the out-patients department or the accident and emergency department by the nurse effecting the admission. It remains the responsibility of the nurse admitting the patient to the ward to complete the form as far as possible during the initial nursing assessment.
2. The nurse in charge of the ward is responsible for ensuring that the Social History Form has been initiated by the end of the first day of admission.
3. As soon as it becomes clear that either local authority or community nursing services are currently being provided on a regular basis, these agencies are notified of the admission. This should occur within 24 hours of admission or, if at the weekend, as soon as the offices open.
4. The Hospital Admissions Office must send notification of the patient's admission to their GP (general practitioner) or health centre as soon as possible, on the day after admission.
5. For patients living alone at the time of admission, the nurse in charge should ensure that:
   (a) a set of house keys has been located and kept either with the patient or in a safe place;
   (b) arrangements are made through friends/neighbours/ relatives to look after the accommodation, that any pets are cared for, and if not, then the social services are notified immediately;
   (c) any documents or valuables are itemized and kept with the patient or in the security department.
6. Any information coming in about a patient from a relative/ friend/neighbour is taken and recorded by nursing staff. All relevant information on the social circumstances of the patient should be collected, and sought if not offered, from relevant agencies by the time of the first planning meeting after admission.
7. At the planning meeting, a provisional plan is made for:
   (a) likely treatment;
   (b) likely length of stay;

    (c) the direction of discharge (e.g. own home, convalescence, extended care facility);

    (d) the patient's need for care at point of discharge;

    (e) any agencies which might offer care.

8. The plan is reviewed at each planning meeting subsequently and, as the patient returns to fitness, action is delegated to alert and involve relatives/friends of the patient and agencies as appropriate.

    The patient's consent is required prior to notifying any outside agencies of any of the patient's medical details. In the event that the patient does not consent, then it should be carefully explained to the patient that community services cannot be adequately arranged.

    Representatives of all community agencies involved should be invited to planning meetings.

9. The decision on an appropriate avenue for discharge is made by the planning team in consultation with the patient and their family and friends.

10. All action necessary to prepare the patient and the home environment is instigated by the planning meeting. The views of the community agencies/family and friends should be given by the social work member of the team if the representatives are not able to attend themselves, or if not, by others who have met them. It is the responsibility of the social worker to see that these views are represented in some way at the planning meetings.

11. For patients being discharged to convalescence or extended care facilities, the date is set by the receiving facility. It must be clear that the hospital will re-admit the patient if convalescence breaks down prior to his or her return home date.

12. If the patient is to return directly home and needs support, referrals should be made at least 2 weeks in advance of any likely discharge date to the relevant agency. This should be conducted in terms of a request for assessment of the patient whilst in hospital, i.e. before the next planning meeting. At the planning meeting, a date is fixed, having regard to service provisions, and all relevant agencies are notified of the decision on the same day.

13. The date of the discharge, if it involves community services, should be fixed at least 1 week in advance, and if possible, at the penultimate planning meeting, so that the final planning meeting confirms all arrangements.

14. As soon as the date of the discharge is set, all relevant parties are notified, including transportation services, if required.

15. The decision as to who notifies whom is made at the planning meeting.

16. During the last week in hospital, the patient should be visited by representatives of any agencies providing community care, and preferably by the individual carer.
17. Prior to discharge, each patient should receive written confirmation, on one document, of the dates and times of relevant visits to them by community services.
18. Before the patient leaves the ward, it is the responsibility of the nurse in charge on that day to ensure that:
    (a) the patient has all necessary drugs and dressings and has been instructed (preferably by a pharmacist) how to use them;
    (b) the patient has all valuables and effects held by the hospital given to them or their escort;
    (c) they have access to their accommodation;
    (d) there is someone to see them inside safely (other than transportation personnel);
    (e) the patient is equipped with a written document of agencies who will be visiting him or her, with dates and times;
    (f) where relevant, a letter for the receiving nursing advisor accompanies the patient;
    (g) the patient has adequate supplies of food to last them until the next visit by someone providing a shopping service where needed;
    (h) power, heating and water supplies in the accommodation are fully operational;
    (i) the patient has enough money for essential needs to last him or her until the next day when banks/post offices are open;
    (j) all relevant agencies have been fully informed;
    (k) the patient is fully informed;
    (l) all equipment and adaptations have been provided.
19. Responsibility for the care of the patient is transferred to the escort and then to the person settling the patient into the home. That person ensures that all items in 18 above, except (j), are correct before leaving the patient.
20. The escort or the receiver of the patient should take responsibility for notifying the discharging ward immediately of any deficiencies in the provision.
21. The patient can be said to have been safely discharged only when comfortably settled, with immediate needs for food, warmth and relief from pain met, and there is a comprehensive plan for the continuing care of that individual within the community, understood by all parties.

Discharge against medical advice

Attempts should be made to dissuade patients from taking their own discharge against medical advice. The patient may agree to see a counsellor or psychiatrist prior to leaving and if so, this should be facilitated. In every case, the patient is told (and this is documented in writing) that the health authority will accept no responsibility for the consequences of patients taking their own discharge and that community services cannot be guaranteed.

Community nursing personnel

1. Where a known patient is admitted to the hospital, the district nurse should notify the ward of the service being provided, including treatment given prior to admission. Where possible, this should be done by a visit to the ward.
2. If the patient is known to live alone, social services should be notified as soon as possible if arrangements are needed to protect the patient's home. Any action taken in this way is also to be notified to the ward.
3. When a known patient is to be discharged to the care of a district nurse, the district nurse should visit the hospital during the week preceding discharge in order to discuss the continuing care needs of the patient with both the ward nursing staff and the patient.
4. All home assessments should be carried out within 24 hours of the discharge.
5. The district nurse should notify the ward of the first day the visit can be made to the patient being discharged.

Local authority staff (municipal services)

1. Where a client of the social services is actively serviced by any of these sections:

   Home helps   Social work   Community social work
   Meals service   Day centre   Residential homes

   and is known to have entered hospital, notice of the involvement is to be sent to the ward immediately.
2. Where the client lives alone, the agent of social services should ensure that arrangements have been made to protect the property.
3. The disclosure of any other personal details is only with the consent of the client.
4. The agent should telephone the ward to arrange a time to visit

and to attend the next planning meeting. The agent should also notify the hospital social worker. Agents may decide it is appropriate for a hospital social worker to convey their views at the planning meeting and can negotiate with the hospital social work department for this to be done.

5. The agent should visit the client in hospital as soon as possible and negotiate the release of information to the ward staff. This is then given to the nurse in charge.

6. During the patient's stay in hospital, any information or developments that occur in the home, including the care of any children, should be notified to the ward immediately.

7. All improvements to the home that are essential to the patient's safe return should be initiated as soon as they are identified and completed prior to the safe discharge of the client.

8. Adaptations in the home will be initiated by the hospital occupational therapy department and paid for by the local authority. Adaptations are to be completed prior to the safe discharge of the client.

9. As soon as a discharge date is foreseeable, the hospital will contact the community agencies for a service. Where the patient has not received a service within the last 3 months (including time in hospital), the agency will make an assessment of the level of need within 1 week of a request. Preferably this will entail a visit to the patient in hospital, and at the latest, a report within that week on the level of service that will be offered.

10. One week after the initial request for an assessment is made, a discharge date may be arranged depending on the findings and the views of the community.

11. Any objections or information should be communicated to the ward before or at the discharge planning meeting. For extremely dependent/handicapped clients, this may involve a separate conference at the hospital, which all agencies should endeavour to attend.

12. Where a patient goes to convalescence without being visited in hospital, the community agencies will have 2 weeks' notice of the return home date, and will assess on the first working day after return with a view to starting the service as soon as possible.

13. The patient will be visited within 24 hours of discharge by all agencies, or on the first working day where the full notice has been given.

District nursing service

Clearly, enough district nurses in a health authority are required to be able to offer a nursing visit at any time of the day or night and at weekends. Many patients with AIDS can only be cared for safely in the community if they have access to round-the-clock nursing care. A central contact point which can identify and locate any district nurse in the area, 24 hours a day, is required. This involves clerical support and a paging system.

Home carers scheme

Within the group of home help employees, a team should be set up which can provide all that a caring relative might to a patient with AIDS living in the community. This scheme would require special training for these individuals to enable them to carry out special tasks as, for example, assistance with personal hygiene.

Discharge co-ordinator

The appointment of a discharge coordinator facilitates the safe and efficient discharge of patients to home and to community services. The discharge coordinator can assist in planning an unbroken chain of individualized patient care by facilitating effective communications between patients, relatives, friends, hospital and community agencies, by participating on a practical level as well as an educational and advisory level. They can also assist in the promotion of quality assurance regarding transfers between hospital and community.

Nursing care in the community

All members of the primary health care team may be involved in the care of clients with HIV-related illness, for example general practitioner, health visitor, district nurse, family planning nurse, school nurse, practice nurse and community psychiatric nurse. Clearly their involvement in the discharge planning process is essential if continuity of care is to be realized. Clients should be encouraged to give permission for their GP (general practitioner) to be fully informed of their condition so that meaningful community nursing care can be assessed and planned with the support of the client's medical adviser. On occasion, clients refuse to give permission for their GP to be informed of their diagnosis, and although the client's wishes must be absolutely respected, this situation is fraught with real difficulties and the client should be explicitly made aware that there are potential problems involved. In these circumstances, district nurses will have to liaise with hospital medical staff in caring for these individuals. However, most GPs establish trusting relationships with their clients and it is becoming more unusual for patients to refuse permission for their GP to be informed of their medical condition.

Clients with AIDS and AIDS-related conditions can live safely with healthy members of the family in the community without any fear of HIV transmission from the client to family and friends. In advising clients with HIV infection, community nursing staff should take the following points into consideration.

Personal hygiene　Good general personal hygiene practices should be adopted. Razors, toothbrushes or other implements which could become contaminated with blood should not be shared. Sanitary towels must be disposed of in heavy-duty yellow plastic bags which can be discreetly collected and sent for incineration along with other contaminated wastes. Tampons may be flushed down the toilet. Individuals with HIV infection should wear gloves when cleaning fish bowls, bird cages, gardening and dealing with cat litter trays because of the risk of contamination with potential parasitic pathogens (e.g. *Toxoplasma gondii, Cryptococcus neoformans*).

General hygiene　Individuals with HIV infection can safely prepare cook and serve food for others, observing usual standards of good hygiene (i.e. hands washed prior to food preparation and after handling any uncooked foods). Special crockery and cutlery is not necessary and all crockery and cutlery should be washed after use in hand hot water with a detergent (a disinfectant is not needed) and left to drip dry.

Linen visibly contaminated with blood, body fluids, excretions or secretions can be safely washed in a washing machine on the hot cycle. The hot cycle on standard washing machines exceeds the Department of Health recommendations of 71°C (160°F) for not less than 3 minutes plus mixing time. The temperature and the addition of a detergent will inactivate any HIV and added disinfectants are not necessary. If the patient is too ill to do his or her own laundry, it can be done by a home help, friends or, if necessary, arrangements can be made by the district nurse to have it processed at a local authority laundry. In this case, it is first placed in a water-soluble red plastic bag which is placed in a red nylon (or heavy-duty plastic) bag. In general, district nurses make arrangements with the environmental health department in their local authority to collect the laundry. This must be done discreetly; colour-coded bags of contaminated laundry or rubbish must not be left outside the patient's home, visible to neighbours and collection personnel must be well educated so that they do not arrive wearing bizarre protective clothing (which, of course, is not necessary). If this point is not attended to, inadvertent breaches of confidentiality might result with disastrous consequences for the client.

Individuals with HIV infection can use the same toilet and bath or shower as anyone else in the household; normal domestic cleaning is adequate after use (disinfectants are not necessary).

Clearly individuals with HIV infection may use, for example, the library, pub, restaurant, cinema, as any other member of the community might. There is no possibility of HIV transmission in public swimming baths[2].

In general, individuals with HIV infection should be encouraged to continue their usual employment and they may have to be discreet regarding informing their employer and fellow workmates of their medical condition.

Patient education Health education designed to promote the primary prevention of others and secondary prevention for the client should be implemented. District nurses will need to discuss 'safer sex' practices with clients and leaflets are available from a variety of sources, for example the Terrence Higgins Trust and Health Education Authority. Individuals with HIV infection should be advised not to donate blood, tissues, organs, semen or carry donor cards. They should not breast-feed infants. Patient education is discussed in more detail in Chapter 17.

Dental treatment Ideally, clients who are infected with HIV should inform their dentist of this fact when presenting for treatment. However, this has often resulted in a refusal by a dentist to treat an infected individual. As all dentists have been advised by the Department of Health in the UK, and the CDC in the USA[3,4], to observe universal precautions on all patients, all the time, regardless of what they know or do not know regarding their serological status for anti-HIV, it probably is in the client's best interest if they do not inform their dentist of their infectivity. This is an unfortunate state of affairs, however it must be realized that dentists (and doctors) do not have the same ethical duty of care towards clients as professional nurses do, and can quite legally, refuse to treat (except in an emergency) individual patients.

The following points should be considered when assessing and planning care for clients in the community. It is essential that community nurses caring for patients with HIV infection are themselves free of any infectious illness (e.g. colds, herpes labialis) so as not to transmit any infections to the client. Good handwashing technique prior to nursing the patient and on completion of nursing care is required. Community nursing staff (and their managers) must know and understand the local operational policies and procedures for the community nursing care of clients with HIV-related illness. If no operational policies and procedures exist, they should be urgently prepared.

Equipment Community nurse managers should ensure that all equipment needed for the usual IC precautions is readily available to community nurses. This will include supplies of:

- appropriate disinfectants (e.g. Presept granules (NaDCC) or Virusorb absorbent powder (chlorine powder) and NaDCC (Presept) disinfectant tablets. Disinfectants are chiefly needed to deal with spillages, which are not common;
- plastic aprons;
- effective, high filtration face masks (e.g. Vigilon masks);
- disposable non-sterile rubber latex or good quality plastic gloves (of the correct size);
- soluble red plastic bags for contaminated linen, and red nylon linen bags;
- sharps container (e.g. Daniels Sharps Bins);
- eye protection device;
- heavy-duty yellow plastic bags for contaminated rubbish;
- paper towels;
- antiseptic soap (e.g. Betadine Surgical Scrub or Hibisol);
- incontinence pads, dressing packs, and other nursing equipment;
- specimen labels (e.g. 'BioHazard' or 'Risk of Infection').

Sharps Extreme caution must be taken when dealing with or disposing of needles and other sharp instruments. A suitable sharps container can be left in the client's home until it is two-thirds full, when it is sealed and arrangmenets are made to collect it for incineration. Small portable sharps containers are available (Daniels – Safe-T-Bin) which can be safely carried by the district nurse.

Injections Community nurses must wear disposable gloves when giving injections or during venesection. Needles must never be recapped or reinserted into their original sheaths and the needle is not disengaged from the syringe prior to disposal, but is disposed of as a single unit into the sharps container. The only exception is after the collection of blood, when the needle is carefully disengaged from the syringe (preferably with a needle holder) to avoid a microscopic aerosol contamination when the blood is injected into the specimen container. Vacuum collection devices (e.g. Vacutainers) are preferable to a syringe and needle for venesection.

Inoculation accidents and mucosal contamination with blood Follow the procedure outlined in Chapter 12.

Cuts Any cuts or open lesions on the arms or hands of nursing personnel must be covered with a waterproof, occlusive plaster (tape). Nurses with eczema should not deliver care to any client, including those with known HIV infection.

IC precautions No protective clothing or IC precautions are required to enter the client's home, for introductions (shaking his or her hand) or talking to the client.

Toilets If the client has restricted mobility and cannot use the toilet, a bedside commode or 'chemical toilet' may be useful. Bed pans and urinals are carefully emptied into the toilet (avoiding splashing), rinsed and stored dry (i.e. they are not left soaking in a disinfectant). District nurses wear disposable gloves when handling bed pans and urinals and when dealing with incontinent clients. After flushing, it is not necessary to pour disinfectants into the toilet.

Spillages Spillages of blood, or those body fluids listed in Chapter 12 from any patient, including those known to be infected with HIV, are carefully covered with a suitable disinfectant, such as Presept granules, left for 5–10 minutes and then carefully wiped up with disposable paper towels which are disposed of into a yellow plastic bag. Nurses wear gloves and a plastic apron when dealing with spillages. If spillages occur on carpets, they are carefully mopped up with paper towels, and chlorine or NaDCC disinfectants are not used. After wiping up the spillage, the area of carpet can be cleaned with a detergent and hot soapy water.
   The client should be encouraged to maintain social relationships and not to become isolated. Family and friends frequently require reassurance regarding the infectious nature of the client's condition.

Terminal care Many clients with HIV-related conditions will require terminal care at home. This is not always possible due to neurological dysfunction or lack of any non-nursing support from family or friends. However, the terminal care of clients with AIDS at home is otherwise much the same as it is for any other client. Attention to symptom control is paramount and this will require a twilight or night community nursing service.

Death at home   The usual last offices are carried out observing the same IC precautions which were in operation when the client was alive. Disposable gloves and aprons are worn by those performing last offices. Undertakers will bring a plastic cadaver bag and will put the body into it. Once the body is in the cadaver bag, transport personnel do not require any protective clothing to handle the body.

Specialist community nurses

It may be useful for health authorities to train and appoint a specialist district nurse (ideally, a community nurse teacher) to act as an expert resource for his or her colleagues. However, all community nurses must become expert in the care of clients with HIV infection and the unique issues involved in this disease. Community nurses are by the very virtue of their training clinical nurse specialists and it is not necessary to establish a further specialization within district nursing.

Summary

Operational policies must exist which allow community nurses the time to complete a home-care nursing assessment prior to the client's discharge from hospital. The actual delivery of nursing care to clients with an HIV-related illness in the home is exactly the same as that required for the nursing care of any seriously ill client. Because of the various opportunistic infections clients with AIDS may present with, additional IC precautions, beyond universal precautions, may be needed. Community nurses have an immense role to play in this epidemic – perhaps the most critical role of all. Every opportunity for health education must be embraced and, with careful discharge planning, district nurses will be able to coordinate all the services clients require. These nurses are strategically placed to make a real impact on the quality of care required and evidence to date indicates they are responding to this challenge with their usual brand of improvization, courage and compassion.

References

1. Crowther, P., Donnelly, D., Hill, P. *et al.* (1987). *Discharge from hospital.* A discussion document with reference to the Riverside (West) Health Authority, 2 February.
2. Royal Society of Medicine (1987). Public swimming pools and AIDS. *The AIDS Letter* **I**(4), 8.
3. DHSS (1986). Guidance for surgeons, anaesthetists, dentists and their teams in dealing with patients infected with HTLV-III. *Acquired Immune Deficiency Syndrome AIDS,* Booklet 3 (April), CMO (86)7, 6.
4. Centers for Disease Control (1987). Recommendations for Prevention of HIV Transmission in Health-Care Settings. *Morbidity and Mortality Weekly Report (MMWR),* 21 August, **36**(2S) 7–8S.

17

The Nurse as a Health Educator

At the end of this chapter, the reader will:

[Short-term goal] **Understand** the underlying principles and practice of patient education and **have an opportunity** to demonstrate the technical skills needed to effectively participate in primary, secondary and tertiary health promotion activities.

[Long-term goal] Be **enabled** to practise the skills of health education and fulfil the educative role of the professional nurse.

[Objectives] 1. **Describe** a systematic model of health education appropriate for use in a clinical setting.
2. **Identify** the critical elements of:
   (a) assessing learning needs;
   (b) planning an educational response;
   (c) implementing patient education encounters;
   (d) evaluating learning
3. **Demonstrate** practice techniques related to effective patient education.
4. **Discuss** obstacles to patient learning.
5. **Outline** a strategy for patient education activities in your own practice setting.

The concept of the nurse as a 'health educator' is implicit in the definition of nursing as described by Henderson[1] and explicit in the Philosophy for Nursing of the Riverside Health Authority[2]. In the UK, 'Project 2000' programmes which prepare individuals to become registered professional nurses stress the importance of ensuring that learners acquire skills in relation to the 'identification of health related learning needs of patients and clients, families and friends and to participate in health promotion'[3]. Today, in the 'age of AIDS', the role of the nurse in primary, secondary and tertiary prevention is paramount. This chapter is designed to illustrate effective patient/client education techniques which nurses can use as 'educators for health' in primary, secondary and tertiary prevention roles (Fig. 17.1).

There are various models of health education available, all having relevance and uses with different individuals, cultures and situations. Although no single model of health education is always ideal in the variety of situations found in clinical practice, probably the most useful for nurses is an eclectic 'educational model' (Fig. 17.2). This is based on the belief that health behaviour is a product of prior learning and that this behaviour can be changed by educational processes. In this model, the nurse acts as a teacher and the patient/client accepts the role of the learner. This approach has been labelled 'teaching for health' and has been extensively described by Coutts and Hardy[4]. Their model sets out the following activities designed to identify and solve health-related problems:

- Informing (giving information)
- Advising
- Helping with the acquisition of skills
- Assisting with the process of clarifying beliefs, feelings and values
- Enabling the adaptation of lifestyle

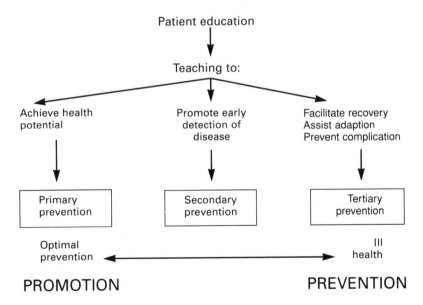

Fig. 17.1 Health education and prevention

Assess learning needs/potential
learning opportunities

Plan education programmes

Implement appropriate teaching

Evaluate effectiveness of encounter

Fig. 17.2 Educational model

- Promoting change in the structures and organizations which influence health status
- Providing a model of values and behaviour related to health.

Inherent in an educational model is the ability of the nurse to **assess** the learning needs of patients/clients and relatives and potential learning opportunities available, **plan** patient/client education programmes, **implement** appropriate teaching methods and techniques which promote health and **evaluate** the effectiveness of the patient/client educational encounters.

Assessing learning needs

In order to assess the learning needs of patients/clients and relatives, the nurse must first identity:

- prior knowledge and use of language;
- what the client needs/wants to know;
- the optimum teaching learning circumstances; and
- any barriers to learning.

Different individuals will have different learning needs, often based on their intelligence, education, social and cultural background. The patient/client's perception of what they need to know is often different to that of the nurse. The best way to establish what a patient/client needs to know is just to ask him or her. For example, 'What is your understanding of high-risk sexual behaviour?' or 'can you explain to me how your discharge medications are to be taken?' This allows the nurse an opportunity to ascertain prior knowledge and to assess the language (i.e. the words) the patient uses to communicate and to describe behaviour. This will assist in determining what learning deficits exist and inform as to how much the patient/client wants, needs (and is able) to learn.

It is essential to provide privacy and time to adequately define learning needs and to give the patient/client permission and opportunity to ask questions. It is axiomatic that the nurse must know the patient and his/her individual circumstances, have clinical confidence and competence to engage in an educational encounter in relation to the specific issue being discussed and is comfortable in using language familiar to the patient.

During this phase it is important to assess the optimum circumstances in which effective patient education encounters can be initiated. Learning can only occur when the individual is ready to learn. Barriers to learning include:

- differences between teacher and client in cultural, social and educational background and differences in primary language;
- differences between teacher and client in values, sex, sexual orientation, religion and beliefs;
- distractions due to confusion, pain, depression, fatigue or anxiety;
- contradictory messages received from other sources;
- faults in the teaching plan/technique: lack of privacy, time, competence and/or confidence of teacher;
- differences in language: nurse's language not understood by client or client's language not understood by nurse.

Planning an educational response

Planning a patient education activity takes into account the educational technique to be used, the timing of the activity and the end product (i.e. the goals) (Fig. 17.3). **Goals** are sometimes referred to as 'Aims' and are defined as **broad, general statements of goal direction, which contains reference to the worthwhileness of achieving it**[5]. Just as the assessment phase involves the patient, so too must the planning stage (to the extent his/her clinical condition permits). The goals/aims of the activity must be negotiated with the patient. This involves asking the patient what he/she wants to know, what they think they should know or offering possible learning options. In addressing learning needs, the client and the nurse should negotiate both short-term and long-term goals (i.e. what the client will be able to do or accomplish as a result, both in the short-term and in the longer term, of the educational encounter). For example, a short-term goal that might be negotiated with a client in reference to safer sexual behaviour might be that at the end of the session the client would

Negotiate: Goals (Aims), i.e. broad general statements of goal direction, which contain references to the worthwhileness of achieving it.

Short-term Goal(s) & Long-Term Goal(s), i.e. what the client **will be able to do** as a result of the teaching/learning encounter

e.g. Teaching Session: Safer Sexual Behaviour
Short-term goal: "at the end of this session, the client will *understand* the sexual means of HIV transmission"
Long-term goal: "at the end of this session(s), the client will be *enabled* to adopt a safer means of expressing his/her sexuality in order to prevent secondary infectious disease acquisition & transmission of HIV to others"

Fig. 17.3 Planning an educational response – the goals

understand the sexual means of HIV transmission. The long-term goal might be that the client would be enabled to adopt safer ways of expressing his/her sexuality in order to prevent secondary infectious disease acquisition and transmission of HIV to another individual.

Once the goals have been negotiated, the intended learning outcomes (i.e. objectives) of the session are derived and can be specified. **Objectives are carefully constructed statements which indicate with precision what the client will be able to do at the end of a teaching/learning session.** Objectives are written for and directed at the client and are action verb statements, i.e. they describe what behaviour the client will be able to achieve at the end of the session. For example, a specific objective might be 'at the end of this session, the client will be able to describe high-risk sexual behaviours', or 'with the use of an anatomical model, demonstrate the correct use of a condom' (Fig. 17.4). Each action verb used in objective statements describes a specific behaviour which is observable, measurable, logical, feasible, unequivocal and relevant

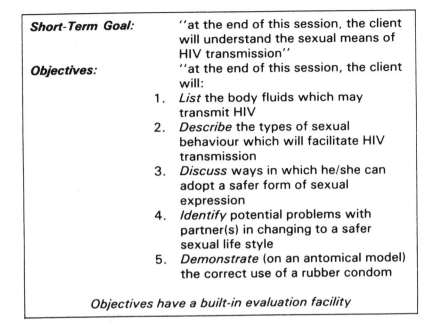

Short-Term Goal:	"at the end of this session, the client will understand the sexual means of HIV transmission"
Objectives:	"at the end of this session, the client will:
	1. *List* the body fluids which may transmit HIV
	2. *Describe* the types of sexual behaviour which will facilitate HIV transmission
	3. *Discuss* ways in which he/she can adopt a safer form of sexual expression
	4. *Identify* potential problems with partner(s) in changing to a safer sexual life style
	5. *Demonstrate* (on an antomical model) the correct use of a rubber condom

Objectives have a built-in evaluation facility

Fig. 17.4 Teaching session: safer sexual behaviour – short-term goal

(Fig. 17.5). The 'goals and objectives' at the beginning of this chapter offer another example of setting the intended learning outcomes of a planned educational initiative. Objectives are usually constructed to describe **cognitive** (i.e. thinking) and **psycho-motor skills** which will result from the teaching/learning process and, as such, have a built-in evaluation facility. Objectives can also be directed at different cognitive levels, for example knowledge, comprehension, application, analysis, synthesis and evaluation. More difficult to evaluate, but also useful, are objectives which can be directed towards **affective** (i.e. valuing, feeling and attitude formation) domains (Fig. 17.6).

Goals and specific objectives are much like a brick wall. The wall itself is the goal (or aim) and each individual brick is an objective. Initially, the short-term and long-term goals, along with the specific objectives, should be written down by the nurse in order to have a checklist to evaluate the degree of learning that has taken place after the encounter(s). Once the goals and objectives have been negotiated and specified, the nurse can select the appropriate teaching method. In patient education encounters, the most common methods used are

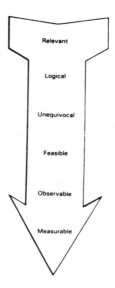

Fig. 17.5   Qualities of a specific educational objective

Cognitive	– process of thinking, of acquiring information & working with it
Affective	– incorporates values, attitudes, beliefs & feelings which create idiosyncratic reactions. Has important motivation influences
Psycho-motor	– acquisition of a motor skill perfected throughout practice

Fig. 17.6   Types and levels of learning

one-to-one discussions in which the current knowledge, attitudes and behaviour of the client are assessed, clarifying or giving additional information or facilitating the development of skills (e.g. decision-making, psycho-motor, assertion skills, etc.). **Demonstrations** are also a method commonly used in patient education encounters (e.g. the use of camouflage make-up, using a condom). In the planning stage, any teaching equipment/aids, written guidelines or literature may also be considered. A simple and brief teaching plan should be constructed, which includes the goals and objectives of the session, the step-by-step implementation of the session and a brief evaluation of what learning took place. This teaching plan should form part of the documentation of care given in the nursing care plan.

Preparing a teaching plan

This plan should first consider the teaching method or techniques which seem best suited to achieve the goals negotiated with the patient/client. The first consideration is that the method or technique chosen allows for maximum involvement of the patient. This is facilitated by using effective non-verbal communication skills, building into the plan opportunities for frequent question and answer periods and to be involved in the verbal summary of the session. If the goal is directed towards enabling the acquisition of a psycho-motor skill (e.g. preparing intravenous medication for administration through a Hickman catheter), then the teaching plan should include an opportunity for immediate supervised practice following the demonstration.

The teaching plan should include a short introduction, the main body of the teaching material, a summary and a question and answer period (Fig. 17.7).

The introduction should include the goals (both short-term and long-term) and objectives of the session and should establish the importance of the session.

The material in the main body of the session should follow a logical sequence. As the nurse will have already established during the assessment period the prior knowledge of the patient, the teaching session should be directed at working from the known to the unknown, from familiar to unfamiliar knowledge and concepts, from basic to advanced material, from questions to answers and from identified problems to solutions.

The summary should include a review of the original goals and objectives of the session and repeat the important points made during the main body of the talk.

Finally, questions and answers will help clarify information for the patient/client and allow for the first evaluation of the achievement (or non-achievement) of the short-term goal(s).

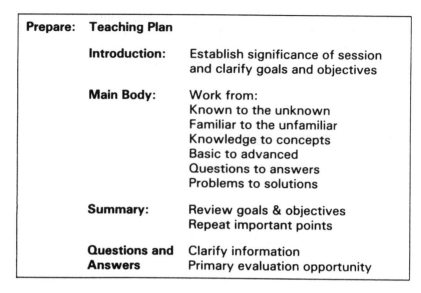

Prepare:	Teaching Plan	
	Introduction:	Establish significance of session and clarify goals and objectives
	Main Body:	Work from: Known to the unknown Familiar to the unfamiliar Knowledge to concepts Basic to advanced Questions to answers Problems to solutions
	Summary:	Review goals & objectives Repeat important points
	Questions and Answers	Clarify information Primary evaluation opportunity

Fig. 17.7   Planning an educational response – the teaching plan

Implementing patient education

Effective teaching requires effective communication skills, both verbal and non-verbal. Non-verbal communications (i.e. body language) are critical and include the following:

Proximity, i.e. how close you are to the client   Individuals with HIV infection and AIDS often feel isolated and stigmatized and effective teaching means being close to the client, without invading their personal space. Teaching sessions should not be conducted from the foot of the bed or with the nurse standing over a patient lying in bed. Either both the nurse and the patient are sitting in chairs relatively close to each other or, if the patient is in bed, the nurse is sitting near the patient's head.

Body contact, i.e. touching   Although in formal teaching practice, body contact is not generally useful, in patient education, especially with an individual who has HIV-related conditions, touching can convey many effective messages, such as 'I care and I'm here for you' and 'I'm not afraid'. Touching has to be done sensitively and is often over-done, resulting in counter-productive reactions.

Facial expressions These convey a wealth of information and a 'deadpan', non-reactive facial expression is not useful. Nurses who practise good listening skills, as described by Ewles and Simnett[6] and who are enthusiastic and responsive to the client and their material, convey a real sense of sincerity.

Eye contact This should be scanning in nature, not staring, which would make the client feel uncomfortable. Good, intermittent eye contact is needed, from speaker to listener during educational encounters. Generally, the listener (be it the nurse or the client) will look directly (straight in the eyes) at the speaker. If this doesn't happen, it is an indication that for one reason or another the listener is not paying attention to the speaker. There may be many reasons (e.g. material is uncomfortable to the listener, the language used is not being understood, the client is in pain, etc.) and this is an important clue to the speaker.

Posture This sends messages to both the health educator and client. Sitting with arms crossed and fists clenched may signal significant anxiety which precludes learning until the underlying cause of the anxiety is addressed.

Many other aspects of body language, e.g. hand and head movements, orientation (i.e. the layout of the room), physical appearance (e.g. uniform versus casual/professional clothes) and movements are all important in teaching and learning, especially in semi-formal and formal teaching environments.

Maintaining good listening skills is an essential ingredient at all stages of the teaching process. It is an active process which helps the client talk, ask questions and participate in the learning process. Effective listening assists in clarifying the client's attitudes, beliefs and values. These skills include:

- **Expressive concentration** on what the speaker is saying. This involves the non-verbal body language skills discussed previously, e.g. good eye contact, reactive facial expressions, posture and head movements (e.g. nodding in understanding), etc.
- **Inviting the client to talk**, e.g. 'How do you feel about what I've just said' or 'How can you use the information we've discussed this morning?'
- **Being attentive**, e.g. maintaining steady eye contact, making neutral noises such as 'I see . . .' or 'yes . . . ,' etc.
- **Paraphrasing** involves re-stating the essential aspects of what the client is saying, e.g. 'so, you're worried your partner will be put

off having sex if you wear a rubber condom.'

- **Reflecting feelings** verbally mirrors back to the client feelings you perceive he/she is communicating, e.g. 'you are clearly worried about how your parents will react to the news that you are gay.'
- **Reflecting meanings** adds content to feelings, e.g. 'you are frightened because you are scheduled for a bronchoscopy this afternoon.'
- **Summarizing** is useful in clarifying the material the client is giving you and should be used throughout active listening, not just at the end of the teaching session. Summarizing involves making brief statements which reflect the salient points the client has made, e.g. 'so far, it seems that what you are saying is. . . .'

In implementing the main body of the teaching session, the following principles are useful to consider:

Time   Negotiate with the patient when the session will start and ensure that you are there on time. Keep the session brief. It is far better to have several brief sessions which the client can concentrate on, rather than a long, tiring session. People who are ill or worried or who have some degree of subclinical cognitive dysfunction as a result of HIV infection, often find it difficult to concentrate for more than 15 or 20 minutes at a time.

State the most important things first   Clients will often remember the first things said and objectives should be prioritized so that critical points are discussed first.

Repeat and stress critical points   Without being tedious, it is important to repeat and re-emphasize critical points, e.g. 'the most important aspect in adopting safer sexual behaviour is to avoid penetrative sex without using a rubber condom.'

Give clear, precise and specific advice   For example, 'You will be taking foscarnet through your Hickman catheter every day, except Saturday and Sunday. It is important that you adjust your administration set so that the foscarnet takes 2 hours to run it', rather than 'take your foscarnet five days a week and run it in slowly'.

Avoid using jargon and long words and sentences   It may be appropriate to use medical terminology in order to help the client communicate easily with other health care professionals, but if medical terminology is used, it must be carefully explained to the client and, during the evaluation stage, any terminology used must be re-checked to ensure the client actually understands it.

Give written information to the client and go through the information with him/her. It is sometimes possible to have the client write down the important points covered and as this actively involves the client in the learning process, can be useful. Obviously having the client take dictation is not useful.

If the learning goals include teaching a psycho-motor skill, then the following essential principles must be included in the teaching plan:

- Demonstrate skill, using a skill analysis approach
- Ensure demonstration is clearly visible to client
- Maintain non-threatening atmosphere
- Allow immediate supervised practice
- Provide written information.

In demonstrating the skill, it is important that all the equipment (if any) used is prepared and at hand and that the demonstration is easily visible to the client. Part of the demonstration should include a skills analysis, i.e. the components of the skill are broken down into stages, starting with component 1, then component 2 and so on until the totality of the components equal the skill being taught. For example, if the client is being taught to administer his or her own aerosolized pentamidine, the skills analysis might be:

1. Attach a needle to 10 ml syringe.
2. Wipe off the rubber top of the vial of bacteriostatic water with an alcohol swab and let dry.
3. Uncap the needle-guard from the needle.
4. Insert the needle into the rubber top of the vial of water.
5. Pull back on the plunger of the syringe and draw up 6 ml of water.
6. Carefully withdraw the needle and syringe from the vial of water.
7. Put the needle guard back on the needle.
8. Wipe off the rubber top of the lyophilized pentamidine with an alcohol swab and let dry.
9. Take the needle-guard back off the needle.
10. Insert the needle into the rubber top of the pentamidine vial and inject the 6 ml of water.
11. Withdraw the needle and syringe and cover the needle again with the needle-guard.
12. Shake the vial of pentamidine and water until the pentamidine is fully dissolved.
13. Etc.

Full, simple written instructions as per the skills analysis should be left with the client.

During the learning session, the teacher needs to ensure that the atmosphere is friendly and relaxed (i.e. non-threatening) and should remain enthusiastic in order to keep the client motivated.

Following the demonstration, it is essential that an opportunity is built into the learning session for immediate supervised practice by the client so that the skills can be consolidated and reinforced. This is also part of the evaluation stage of the teaching/learning process.

If part of the learning goals is directed towards teaching the client both affective (feeling) and cognitive (thinking) skills, e.g. decision-making skills, the following points are important:

- Help the client to define the problem, e.g. 'I can't find a way to tell my wife I'm infected with HIV.'
- Clarify the client's goals, e.g. 'I don't want to infect my wife.'
- Help the client to define alternative methods of achieving the goal, e.g. 'Maybe the doctor should tell her,' or 'I won't tell her but I'll only have safer sex with her in the future.'
- Help the client to identify the advantages and disadvantages of each method, e.g. 'If I don't tell her myself, she won't trust or respect me in the future.'
- Let the client decide which is the best course of action, based on the above, and discuss with the patient his/her perception of the likely results of that decision.

Finally, in implementing planned teaching, barriers to effective communication should be identified and addressed, as discussed previously.

Evaluating the teaching session

After summarizing the main points of the session and answering the client's questions, the short-term goals and specific learning objectives are reviewed with the client and an evaluation assessment is made, i.e. the client did or did not achieve the learning objectives and the short-term goal. The long-term goals are evaluated at future teaching/learning sessions. The nurse should revisit the client the next day, if possible, to re-check the evaluation assessment and to answer any further questions the client might have. On-going assessment will identify further learning needs and the process described in this chapter is repeated.

Documentation of teaching

The teaching plan is entered into the client's notes and the teaching/learning session is documented in the Nursing Care Plan.

References

1. Henderson, V. (1964). *Basic Principles of Nursing Care.* International Council of Nurses, Geneva.
2. Riverside Health Authority (1990). *Philosophy For Nursing,* 2nd edn. Riverside Health Authority, London.
3. Ridley, N. (1989). *The Nurses, Midwives and Health Visitors (Registered Fever Nurses Amendment Rules and Training Amendment Rules) Approval Order 1989.* Statutory Instruments, United Kingdom.
4. Coutts, L.C. and Hardy, L.K. (1985). *Teaching For Health; The Nurse as Health Educator.* Churchill Livingstone, London.
5. Quinn, F.M. (1988). *The Principles and Practice of Nurse Education,* 2nd edn. Croom Helm, London.
6. Ewles, L. and Simnett, I. (1985). *Promoting Health: A Practical Guide to Health Education.* John Wiley & Sons, Chichester.

Recommended Reading

1. Coutts, L.C. and Hardy, L.K. (1985). *Teaching For Health; The Nurse as Health Educator.* Churchill Livingstone, London.
2. Ewles, L. and Simnett, I. (1985). *Promoting Health: A Practical Guide to Health Education.* John Wiley & Sons, Chichester.

18

The Management of Strategic Nursing Care

The efficient delivery of individualized patient care requires informed, perceptive nursing management. The failure to develop competent and compassionate management services results in a breakdown of direct patient care, confusion and low morale among nursing staff, distress and isolation for the patient and a negative image of the hospital. Most metropolitan hospitals now have some experience in caring for patients suffering from HIV-related disease. In the beginning of the epidemic, a general commonality in problems and issues emerged. A core of expertise has now developed which other hospitals can use to avoid the early problems associated with the admission of a patient with AIDS.

Coordination of nursing care

Nursing management should initiate the formation of an 'AIDS coordinating committee', which should have broad educational and supportive responsibilities. The committee should be composed of both experts and non-experts and be representative of the hospital community. A typical coordinating committee might have the following membership:

Experts
Infection control nurse
Microbiologist
Clinical nurse specialist
  (medical/oncology nursing)
Dietitian
Physician
Clinical psychologist
Clinical nurse specialist
  (psychiatric nursing)

Non-experts
Key Trade Union representatives
Hospital chaplain
Representative from domestic/
  housekeeping services
Representative from transport/
  portering services
Senior nurse – occupational
  health services
Unit general manager or deputy

Nurse educationalists   Senior nurse manager
Social worker/health adviser
Community nurse

The committee must have visible and aggressive support from both nursing and hospital management and from experts within the hospital. The coordinating committee should have three major areas of responsibilities .

1. The formation and adoption of universal IC precautions as well as the monitoring of their implementation.
2. Planning and implementing in-service education and training programmes for all grades of staff.
3. Advising general management on policy and long-term planning for patients with HlV-related illnesses.

Hospitals which currently have little experience in caring for patients with HlV-related illnesses should form a coordinating committee and initiate planning prior to admitting their first patient. It is inconceivable that any general hospital will not be responsible for caring for these patients in the future. Planning now will dissipate initial anxiety and confusion.

In-service education

Hospitals which have developed pro-active in-service educational programmes for their staff have been the most successful in minimizing anxiety and disruption when a patient with HIV disease is admitted. In-service education should commence with orientation/induction of new staff and be ongoing. A combination of various formats is the most useful approach, including workshops, seminars, study days and ward-based discussions and tutorials. Specialist nurse teachers and the infection control nurse are ideally placed to implement educational programmes, advised by the AIDS coordinating committee. A study day once a year on 'AIDS' is not adequate to deal with the new problems and issues posed by the admission of patients with HIV disease.

Infection control nurse

If not already in post, the recruitment of a clinical nurse specialist in infection control is absolutely essential. Comprehensive, competent and safe patient care, both in hospital and at home, cannot be ensured without the support and advice of this specialist. With the advent of HIV disease, it would seem impossible to cope without the guidance of an IC nurse.

Conditions of employment

Contracts of employment for all health care workers must clearly preclude the withdrawal of care from any patient, regardless of age, sex, sexual orientation, race, religion or presenting illness. Nursing management must make it absolutely clear that nursing personnel do not have the right to choose whom they will or will not nurse. Management must be seen to be determined in enforcing this correct obligation of employment. Staff who are reluctant to care for a patient should be counselled and given additional in-service training. If their reluctance persists, they should be dismissed. Quality assurance strategies should be designed to ensure that patients are not suffering as a result of ignorance, prejudice or unethical and judgemental attitudes projected onto them by health care workers.

Dedicated wards and clinics

Metropolitan hospitals experiencing significant admissions of patients with HIV-related disease should consider the creation of dedicated units. The advantages of these units include:

- Nursing care can be 'state of the art' and specialized care strategies can be developed to meet the complex psycho-social-medical issues seen in these patients.
- Many patients with HIV-related illness prefer being cared for in a dedicated unit.
- Motivated, concerned staff, comfortable with their own sexuality, can be recruited to these units and given additional specialist training. They will quickly gain knowledge of other available resources to enable them to formulate effective, early discharge planning.
- Units are cost-effective and have a positive impact on bed availability. Effective discharge planning, centralized care and the identification of other resource issues can most efficiently take place within these units.
- Units can attract additional funds from concerned groups in the community. There can be a positive public relations impact in their creation.
- The body of knowledge upon which the profession is based can

be increased by the expanding expertise acquired by the nursing staff in these units.

- Personnel problems are minimized and hospitals which have created these units have experienced high staff morale and a correspondingly high level of patient satisfaction.

Dedicated units must have clear admission criteria and therapeutic objectives. Their existence does not mean that patients with AIDS will not be cared for in other areas of the hospital. Many patients with HIV-related illness do not require the intensive specialist care offered by dedicated units. Hospice and terminal care facilities should also be considered as dedicated units are generally designed as active treatment units. A dedicated unit will not be effective unless it is supported by a comprehensive dedicated out-patients clinic. These clinics should be able to screen patients, initiate diagnostic procedures and maintain out-patients by providing a range of services which include intravenous rehydration, blood transfusions and intravenous chemotherapy. Clinical nurse specialists need to be recruited and trained for dedicated clinics.

Counselling services and support groups

Hospitals need to develop comprehensive counselling services for patients with HIV-related disease. Although a multi-disciplinary approach is needed for the complex problems seen in this disease, clinical psychologists have the most relevant skills and should lead the planning and implementation of these services. Health advisers, social workers and lay counsellors from concerned community groups (e.g. the Terrence Higgins Trust, London) can complement this service. If lay counsellors are used, facilities must be made available to them. Counselling is required at all stages of illness, from pre-screening counselling to bereavement support, both for in-patients and for out-patients. If a hospital is treating more than a few patients with HIV-related illnesses, a patients 'Support Group' can be established. These groups are invaluable in providing space for venting emotions and offering mutual support. They can include both in-patients and out-patients. Hospitals which have large numbers of patients with AIDS and other HIV-related conditions often provide a sophisticated range of support groups. For example, patients with Kaposi's sarcoma may form one group as they have specific problems coping with alterations in body image which patients with opportunistic infections may not have. Injecting drug users often respond only where other group members are also drug users. In addition, staff support groups are used to provide an opportunity for health care workers to explore their anxieties, frustrations and other related 'burn-out' problems. Support groups must be competently and sensitively led by a staff member especially trained for this role.

Confidentiality

Nursing management must be sensitive to the balance required between ensuring appropriate IC precautions and the need to ensure appropriate confidentiality. The implementation of universal precautions assists in maintaining confidentiality in that IC precautions are the same for all patients. Management must ensure that policies and procedures designed to ensure confidentiality are in place, understood by all staff and effectively monitored.

Public relations

Contact with the media presents both potential problems and opportunities for the hospital to assume a leadership role in health education. In dealing with the press, precise and honest information will diminish adverse publicity. It is useful if an expert and authoritative representative of the hospital staff is designated as the spokesperson for the hospital on all HIV-related issues. All hospital staff members should be required to coordinate all press communications through this individual. Maximum use should be made of written press releases when information is requested rather than verbal interviews, which are often 'reinterpreted' by the media. The overriding principle of public relations is the maintenance of patient confidentiality and dignity.

Employment of health care workers who are infected with HIV

Currently, many hospitals have experienced situations where a member of their staff has developed HIV disease or is asymptomatically seropositive for anti-HIV. This has included surgeons, dentists, nurses and ancillary staff. Excluding the rare documented incidents of gross needlestick injuries (discussed previously), these health care workers acquired HIV infection sexually. It seems obvious that, in time, all sexually active individuals may be 'at risk' for HIV infection, including health care workers. Although the occupational risk of HIV transmission is minimal (or nil if the strategies outlined in this text are diligently followed), health care workers are members of the broader community and are as much at risk sexually as any other member of the community.

As it is inconceivable that routine screening for anti-HIV could ever be implemented, most individuals who are seropositive for anti-HIV will be unknown to the employing health authority. However, occasionally this information is made known to the health authority by the employee. More commonly, health care workers who develop clinical manifestations of HIV infection consult the occupational health services and, eventually, a diagnosis of HIV disease is established.

Early in the epidemic, some hospitals and health authorities reacted inappropriately to this situation by suspending or dismissing the employee on the grounds that they posed an unacceptable IC risk to the patients of the hospital. This is quite clearly wrong and several issues need to be addressed in establishing the correct response of an employing health authority faced with this increasingly common predicament.

1. The means of transmission for HIV are well-established and well-documented. Other than injecting drug use, HIV infection is now almost exclusively a sexually transmitted disease. In a health care setting, person-to-person transmission of HIV from a health care worker to a patient, could probably only be achieved by sexual transmission. This would be an unusual, if not bizarre, event in hospital.

2. Consequently, there has only been one possible case of HIV transmission from an infected health care worker to a patient[1].

3. If a health care worker was infected with HIV, it would be essential that appropriate precautions were taken to eliminate any possibility of blood or body fluid contamination from the employee to a patient. This would include covering any cuts or abrasions on the hands with a waterproof dressing and wearing disposable gloves when engaging in direct patient care. Well-established, appropriate precautions should also be taken to prevent transmission of any infection (e.g. herpes) to a patient. However, all of the precautions required amount to no more than good clinical practice, which all health care workers have a responsibility to maintain, regardless of their serological status for anti-HIV.

4. Health care workers involved in invasive procedures, such as surgery, midwifery or dentistry, may be thought to be more of a

risk to patients if they are anti-HIV positive. Concern has been expressed that these health care workers should be reassigned to clinical duties which do not involve invasive procedures. It is essential that management create a public stance on this issue and a model policy on the employment of HIV infected health care workers can be found in Appendix 8.

A more detailed discussion of the potential risk of nosocomial transmission from an infected health care worker to a patient can be found in Chapter 13.

Patient's bill of rights

Nursing management should construct and communicate widely a philosophy of care with which both the patient and the nurse can identify. This philosophy should include a description of the patient's rights[2]. These rights should guarantee to all patients:

1. The right to quality health care in an atmosphere of human dignity without regard to age, ethnic or national origin, sex or sexual orientation, religion or presenting illness.
2. The right to receive emergency medical and surgical treatment.
3. The right to considerate, dignified and respectful care by all health care workers, regardless of the patient's physical or emotional condition.
4. The right to be informed of the name, title and function of anyone involved in their care.
5. The right to receive upon request an explanation of their current medical condition in language that they can understand.
6. The right to give or decline true informed consent and to participate in the choice of treatment. If consent for treatment is not given, the right to be informed of the likely medical consequences of their action.
7. The right to privacy to an extent consistent with providing dignified medical and nursing care.
8. The right to confidentiality.
9. The right to be informed of and to participate in their discharge planning.
10 The right to refuse to participate in research projects.
11. The right to receive, upon request, a consultation and/or care and treatment from another appropriate physician on the staff other than the one assigned to them.
12. The right, both as a patient and as a citizen, free from restraint, interference, coercion, discrimination or reprisal, to voice grievances and complaints and to recommend changes in

policies and services. This implies that patients have access upon request to senior nurse managers.

13. The right to expect visitors to be treated with courtesy and respect.

Resuscitation

In the current state of knowledge, patients with AIDS have a terminal illness. While it may be appropriate to offer ventilation and other life-support systems to patients with AIDS in the early stages, it is often not compassionate to do so in the end-stage of their illness. The patient must be involved in decisions regarding intensive care and resuscitation. It is the physician's primary responsibility to discuss this with the patient and to make the final decision. This decision must be clearly communicated to all health care workers directly involved with the care of the patient and is appropriately discussed at routine, multi-disciplinary case conferences.

Summary

The competent and compassionate management of nursing is as important as the direct nursing care delivered at the bedside. The issues discussed in this chapter must not come as a surprise to management.

Effective forward planning will facilitate the smooth running of the hospital and the delivery of quality care to all patients when patients with AIDS are admitted. Although each nurse is accountable for his or her own clinical and professional practice, nurse managers are individually accountable for providing adequate staffing levels, planning, guidance, formation of policies and procedures and for providing a philosophy of leadership, which promotes the high standards of care that all patients have a right to expect.

The 'Riverside Model'

Over 15 years of experience in caring for an escalating number of individuals, both in hospital and in the community, has been gained by the former Riverside Health Authority in London. This authority has now evolved into a variety of health care organizations, including the Hammersmith Hospitals NHS Trust and the Chelsea & Westminster Hospital NHS Trust. However, the model of care developed during the formative years of their experience with AIDS is still referred to as the 'Riverside Model'. These hospitals, and associated clinics and community nursing services, are currently caring for the majority of individuals with HIV disease in the UK. They provide comprehensive services, including dedicated in-patient and out-patient facilities. However, because of the vast number of patients being cared for, it is recognized that patients with HIV disease will be nursed in all wards and all departments of all hospitals, not just in dedicated units.

The Nursing Advisory Committee

A vast amount of nursing, educational, medical and managerial expertise in caring for patients with HIV-related illnesses has been gained and an exciting model of nursing management has emerged, committed to ensuring that all patients/clients within the authority consistently receive meaningful, non-judgemental, compassionate nursing care of the highest quality. The provision of this exemplary care is facilitated by the managerial structure of the health authority. Professional nursing advice to the authority is derived from the **Nursing Advisory Committee (NAC)**. This committee is composed of senior nurse managers and educationalists. The **AIDS Coordinating Group (Nursing)** was established to ensure that the NAC was fully informed on all the professional and managerial issues associated with HIV infection in order to advise general management appropriately.

The AIDS Coordinating Group (Nursing)

This subgroup of the NAC, composed of nursing experts in caring for patients/clients with HIV-related illnesses and senior nurse managers and educationalists, develops policies and procedures related to caring for patients with HIV infection and advises on the nursing education strategy. This strategy addresses the learning needs of both student nurses in pre-registration nursing education programmes and qualified nursing personnel (for examples of recommended educational strategies see Appendix 6). The AIDS Coordinating Group (Nursing) submits all draft policies and procedures and any further appropriate advice to the NAC for approval. Once approved by the NAC, they become part of the operational policies and procedures for nursing services within the authority.

Policies and procedures

It is essential that current infection control policies and procedures are formulated which take into account the changes in clinical practice required by the advent of HIV infection. Clearly, these policies and procedures must be based on current practice recommendations that **all** blood and body fluids from **all** patients in **all** health care settings must be regarded as potentially infectious and appropriate precautions taken. Senior nurses for infection control and other experts advise the AIDS Coordinating Group (Nursing) on infection control procedures who then drafts appropriate policies and procedures for consideration by the **Infection Control Committee**. All infection control policies are reviewed on an annual basis and current, approved procedures are distributed to all service areas within the authority.

Philosophy for Nursing

It is essential that the mission of care within the nursing services is discussed, agreed and published and, further, is widely understood by all nursing employees within the authority. The **Philosophy for Nursing** acts as the essential underpinning for all specific policy statements by the NAC and is the professional reference for all subgroups of the NAC. The Philosophy for Nursing in the Riverside Health Authority[3] (see Appendix 7) is an exciting, dynamic concept which has guided nursing services in formulating the operational policies and procedures needed to effectively manage the nursing force within the authority as they confront the complexities of caring for large numbers of patients/clients with HIV-related illness. It is critical that nursing services within all health authorities define and describe their mission of care and that it is widely understood by all nursing service/education staff.

Specific policy statements

Nursing services should develop policies for their employees on the following issues:

- Universal precautions
- Duty of care
- Confidentiality
- Consent for serological testing
- Anonymous prevalence data testing
- Employment of nurses who are infected with HIV
- Educational strategy for HIV infection.

The policy statement on **duty of care** must be discussed (and documented as discussed) with all current nursing service employees and by all prospective candidates for nursing posts within the authority at interview.

Naturally, nurse managers must ensure that all approved policies and procedures are adhered to by all nursing service employees and initiate appropriate action should there be any inconsistencies in the implementation of the operational policies and procedures of the authority. These policies should be discussed at regular service unit meetings and at all orientation/induction programmes for newly joined nursing employees. They must be available for reference, along with the current infection control procedures, in all units of service.

The creation and ongoing monitoring of these operational policies and procedures increase the security of both staff and patients/clients and ensure that the nursing care being delivered is both current and safe. Without this type of forward planning, health authorities will find that the admission of individuals with HIV-related illnesses to their hospital and community services will create chaos and detract from the smooth running of health care services. Nurse managers have a professional obligation to ensure that nursing service employees are provided with appropriate guidance and support; these policies assist with this provision.

Model operational policies and procedures, as developed by the Riverside Health Authority (i.e. the 'Riverside Model') are given in Appendix 8.

References

1. Centers for Disease Control (1990). Possible transmission of human immunodeficiency virus to a patient during an invasive dental procedure. *Morbidity and Mortality Weekly Report (MMWR)*, 27 July, **39**(29), 489–93.
2. New York City Health and Hospitals Corporation (1984). *Patient's Bill of Rights*. Office of Patient Relations, New York.
3. Dorman, M., Forrest Riley, M., Jones, J. *et al*. (1990). *Philosophy for Nursing*, 2nd edn. The Riverside Health Authority, London.

Further reading

Scott, Cherill (1994). *The Care and Treatment of People with HIV Disease and AIDS: A Nursing Perspective*. AVERT Project, The Daphne Heald Research Unit, The Royal College of Nursing, London.

19

Nursing Issues Related to Medical Management

With the recognition of HIV as the causative agent of AIDS, medical research has progressed rapidly on two fronts: towards the development of an effective treatment regime and the discovery and deployment of a biological vaccine.

Medical treatment

Current medical treatment is designed to slow viral replication and to treat and prevent episodes of opportunistic disease.

Antiviral agents

Antiviral therapy for HIV infection is based on the premise that continued viral replication is involved in both the pathogenesis and the progression of HIV disease and that suppression of HIV replication will reduce the direct and indirect effects of HIV infection.

The major drugs used today to suppress HIV replication are the dideoxynucleoside analogues, a group of drugs that inhibit the action of reverse transcriptase. The major drugs in this class are: **zidovudine** (Retrovir), **dideoxycytidine** (ddC – zalcitabine) and **dideoxyinosine** (ddI – didanosine). Other drugs in this group which are in clinical trials include **d4T** (stavudine), **3TC** and **PMEA**.

Zidovudine

Zidovudine (Retrovir), formerly known as **azidothymidine** (AZT), was discovered and introduced into the clinical care of patients with HIV-related illness by Burroughs-Wellcome in 1986. Zidovudine is chemically similar to thymidine, a substance normally found in T4-helper cells. Thymidine is one of four bases that are the 'building blocks' required to make DNA from RNA. If thymidine is replaced by zidovudine, the next 'brick' cannot be put in place because of an inappropriate chemical radical (N3) at the binding site. This inhibition of DNA synthesis is referred to as **chain termination**. Thymidine is necessary for the reverse transcriptase in HIV to convert the viral RNA into viral DNA which is then incorporated into the host cell DNA (Fig. 19.1).

By giving a thymidine analogue (i.e. 'fake' thymidine), the viral

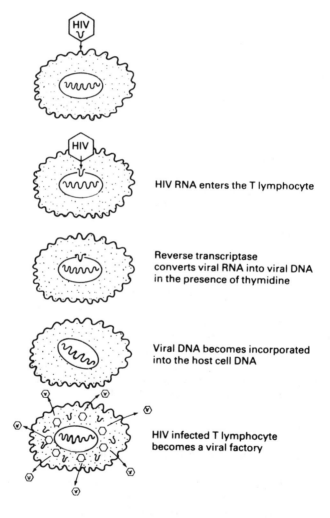

HIV RNA enters the T lymphocyte

Reverse transcriptase converts viral RNA into viral DNA in the presence of thymidine

Viral DNA becomes incorporated into the host cell DNA

HIV infected T lymphocyte becomes a viral factory

Fig. 19.1   HIV infection and replication

DNA formed (the 'transcript') is abnormal and cannot fully be integrated into the host cell DNA (Fig. 19.2). The result is that viral replication is halted.

Such an inhibition will also inhibit any other process associated with synthesis of DNA, such as natural DNA synthesis associated with red blood corpuscle production and white blood cell synthesis.

Efficacy of zidovudine therapy

The administration of zidovudine leads to clinical improvement in most patients. Patients feel well, gain weight and clearance of chronic opportunistic infections is usually seen. The immune system has a chance of recovering and the numbers of circulating T4-helper cells increase. Although zidovudine is not a cure for AIDS, it most definitely leads to a longer life of better quality. In symptomatic HIV disease, the administration of zidovudine appears to have clinical benefit lasting ± 6–9 months. Although originally thought to be of some benefit in early, asymptomatic HIV disease, zidovudine is now not thought to confer any significant benefit in symptom-free individuals in terms of survival or disease progression, irrespective of their initial CD4+ T-cell count[1]. Although there is great diversity amongst clinicians as to the optimal time to initiate zidovudine therapy, general agreement is beginning to emerge. Zidovudine is recommended for the treatment of patients with symptomatic HIV-1

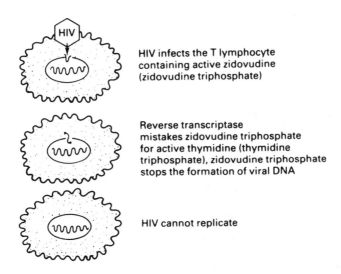

Fig. 19.2 Retrovir mode of action

disease in patients who have a CD4+ T-cell count < 500 cells/mm³, deferring therapy in patients with asymptomatic HIV infection until the CD4+ T-cell count declines to fewer than 200–300 cells/mm³[2].

Retrovir (zidovudine) comes as 100 mg and 250 mg capsules and currently is usually prescribed as 100 mg every 4 hours (600 mg total daily dose) for patients with late HIV disease. Patients with early HIV disease are generally prescribed Retrovir 100 mg every 4 hours while awake (500 mg total daily dose). Retrovir should be taken on an empty stomach[3]. Retrovir crosses the blood–brain barrier and may improve or prevent the neurological effects of HIV infection.

Zidovudine must be taken for life and is associated with significant side-effects in some individuals (Table 19.1). These side-effects include severe anaemia, which usually occurs after 4–6 weeks of therapy. Anaemia may require blood transfusions and temporary cessation of zidovudine therapy. Leucopenia and neutropenia may also be encountered and patients on zidovudine therapy should have a full blood count every 2 weeks during the early stages of treatment and then at monthly intervals. Other common side-effects include nausea, rash, headache, fever and myalgia. Patients taking zidovudine must not take paracetamol BP (acetaminophen USP) extensively, or probenecid. Methadone possibly increases plasma zidovudine concentrations. Drugs which are known to be nephrotoxic, hepatoxic or myelosuppressive (e.g. ganciclovir) should not be taken while on zidovudine therapy and patients should be cautioned about self-administration of OTC (over-the-counter) drugs. Some patients have become extremely lethargic if on zidovudine and intravenous acyclovir.

Table 19.1 Toxicity associated with nucleoside reverse transcriptase

Drug	Effect
Zidovudine	Headache, myalgia, fatigue, nausea, dyspepsia, anaemia, neutropenia, nail pigmentation, myopathy, lactic acidosis
Didanosine	Altered taste, nausea, abdominal pain, pancreatitis, hypermylasemia, hyperuricemia, peripheral neuropathy
Zalcitabine	Stomatitis, mucosal ulcers, rash, fever, pancreatitis, peripheral neuropathy
Stavudine	Headache, asthenia, confusion, hepatic toxicity, peripheral neuropathy

Monotherapy/combined therapy

It is becoming clear that reverse transcriptase inhibitors all have a limited effect in terms of clinical efficacy and patient improvements. Trials are now progressing to evaluate **combined therapy** as evidence suggests that such an approach has some benefit in relation to viral markers, but clinical efficacy has yet to be proven. **Didanosine (ddI)** and **zalcitabine (ddC)** and **stavudine** are being investigated as monotherapy for patients who cannot tolerate zidovudine, or as combination therapy, with zidovudine.

Didanosine (ddI)
Didanosine is rapidly degraded by the acidity of the stomach. Consequently, it is formulated as a chewable, buffered, dispersible tablet. A buffered powder for oral solution is also available. Both preparations are taken on an empty stomach. Since the buffering will increase, i.e. make more alkaline, the pH of the stomach, other drugs which are dependent on gastric acidity, i.e. **ketoconazole** and **dapsone**, must be taken at least 2 hours before didanosine is taken. The dose is based on body weight and two 100 mg tablets every 12 hours, or one 250 mg sachet of buffered didanosine powder every 12 hours is recommended for patients weighing $\geq$ 60 kg. Lower doses should be used for patients weighing < 60 kg[2].

Zalcitabine (ddC)
Zalcitabine is often combined with zidovudine as they show synergistic inhibitory activity against HIV *in vitro*. Zalcitabine is given orally, the recommended dose being two 0.375 mg tablets administered every 8 hours. If zidovudine is also being administered with zalcitabine, two 100 mg capsules of zidovudine are given every 8 hours[2].

Stavudine (d4T)
This is a new nucleoside reverse transcriptase inhibitor entering phase III clinical trials. Currently there are no recommendations for stavudine therapy but this drug is available for patients with HIV disease who are intolerant to zidovudine or didanosine, or who have had disease progression while receiving either of these two drugs.

Other antiretroviral drugs

There has been an explosion of scientific initiatives directed at exploiting differences between the biology of HIV and the host cells it infects. Although zidovudine is currently the only approved antiretroviral agent for HIV infection, it is likely that during the next few years, other agents will be available. If newer drugs are to be effective, the future is likely to increasingly feature the use of drugs that act at different sites of viral replication, and their use in combination, rather like the strategies used for cancer chemotherapy.

Prophylaxis of opportunistic infections

Although zidovudine therapy reduces the frequency and severity of opportunistic infections in individuals infected with HIV, patients who have CD4+ lymphocyte counts below 200 cells/mm³ (or CD4+ cells totalling less than 20 per cent of total lymphocytes) are usually advised to initiate prophylaxis against opportunistic infections commonly seen in immunocompromised individuals. Common prophylaxis regimes which the nurse should be familiar with, include the following.

Pneumocycstis carinii pneumonia

The two most common approaches are:

1. Oral **trimethoprim-sulphamethoxazole** (160 mg trimethoprim and 800 mg of sulphamethoxazole), also known as co-trimoxazole, i.e. two Septrin or Bactrim tablets, given twice daily, three times a week[4].
2. **Aerosol pentamidine** given as 300 mg once monthly. A higher dose, e.g. 600 mg, may be more effective in preventing relapses[5].

If the above two drugs are not tolerated, **dapsone,** with or without either **trimethoprim** or **pyrimethamine** may be prescribed[6]. **Pyrimethamine-sulfadoxine** (Fansidar) may also be used but seems less effective and more toxic than dapsone. Fansidar may provoke a fatal **Stevens–Johnson syndrome** and should be used with caution.

All of the above drugs are associated with common side-effects (discussed earlier in Chapter 6) which nurses should anticipate during care evaluations.

Toxoplasma gondii

Like most opportunistic infections seen in patients with symptomatic HIV disease, the cause is the activation of already present latent infection and some studies have found that 30–35 per cent of patients with AIDS have serological evidence of prior *T. gondii* infection.

T. gondii infection notoriously causes a serious, life-threatening encephalitis in late stage HIV disease, which can often be prevented by effective prophylaxis[7].

Patients infected with HIV disease should be serologically screened for *T. gondii* antibodies. If they are negative, patient education programmes should be implemented to teach the patient how to avoid acquiring *T. gondii* infection. The following precautions should be emphasized:

- Avoid eating under-cooked meats.
- Wash hands thoroughly after handling uncooked meat and avoid touching your mouth or eyes while handling uncooked meat.
- Thoroughly wash all kitchen surfaces which have come into contact with uncooked meat.
- Carefully wash all fruits and vegetables (especially lettuce) prior to cooking or eating.
- Wear household gloves when dealing with cat litter trays and when working in the garden. Wash hands thoroughly after both activities.
- If you have a cat litter tray, disinfect it frequently and empty it of cat faeces daily.

For patients who have serological evidence of past *T. gondii* infection or who have had *T. gondii* encephalitis, prophylaxis usually includes **pyrimethamine with sulphadiazine**. **Clindamycin** may be used for those patients who cannot tolerate **sulphonamides** and may be given with **pyrimethamine**. Both **dapsone** and **co-trimoxazole** (often used for PCP prophylaxis) also confer protection against infection with or re-activation of *T. gondii*.

Candida

Candida infections (usually C. *albicans* but other species may be involved) are almost universal in patients with AIDS. **Fluconazole (Diflucan)** and **clotrimazole troches** are sometimes prescribed for prophylaxis[8].

Cryptococcus neoformans

This is another fungal infection commonly seen in patients with late HIV disease. It may be prevented by the use of **fluconazole (Diflucan)**.

Cytomegalovirus infections

Either **ganciclovir** or **phosphonoformate** (Foscarnet) are used for maintenance therapy. Primary prophylaxis is not practical.

Herpes simplex infection

Acyclovir (Zovirax) is used for maintenance therapy but as acyclovir-resistant herpes simplex infections can occur, it is not usually prescribed for primary prophylaxis.

Streptococcus pneumoniae

Polyvalent pneumococcal vaccination should be offered to all HIV-infected individuals, early in the course of HIV infection.

Vaccination against HIV Infection

There is currently no biological vaccine available to protect against HIV infection, although impressive progress is being made to develop one. Several candidate vaccines have already been entered into clinical trials and it is possible that an effective vaccine may be developed during the next decade. There are two vaccine development strategies being pursued. One is to develop **preventive vaccine(s)**, which are designed to protect those who are not infected from becoming infected, should they be exposed to HIV. Another scientific tract is attempting to develop **therapeutic vaccine(s)**, which would be given following infection (**post-infection HIV vaccination**). These vaccines would restore the immune system and reduce HIV replication and the viral burden[9]. By re-priming the immune system with a therapeutic vaccine, specific neutralizing antibodies would be made and CD8+ T lymphocytes (cytotoxic 'killer' cells) could be recharged to seek out and kill those cells infected with HIV.

Screening for markers of HIV infection

Following infection with HIV, several immunological reactions can be serologically observed (Fig. 19.3).

1. Within 2–3 weeks of infection, **core antigens (p24)** can be detected in the blood. A test to detect p24 antigens is often referred to as an 'antigen test'.
2. Shortly after the appearance of p24 antigens, **IgM antibodies** appear. These antibodies can be directed against the core (gag)

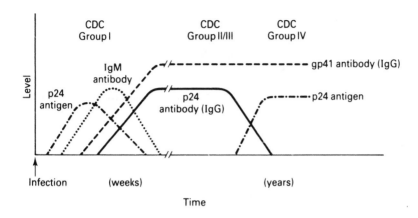

Fig. 19.3 Serological markers of HIV infection

proteins of the virus (i.e. p24, p18, p55) and the envelope (env) glycoproteins (i.e. gp120 and gp41). IgM antibodies to the virus are short-lived; IgM antibodies to p24 will be undetectable within 3–4 months. However, IgM antibodies to gp41 can be detected for a longer period. Their presence is a marker of acute (i.e. early) infection.

3. Within 3–6 months, **IgG antibodies** to the transmembrane glyco-protein (gp41) start to appear . **These antibodies are long-lasting and their detection is the basis of common serological screening tests.** IgG antibodies to other major structural gene products of HIV (i.e. gag and env proteins) are also found.

4. Shortly after the appearance of IgG antibodies to gp41, **IgG anti-bodies to p24** (i.e. **anti-p24**) start to appear. These are referred to as 'core' antibodies.

5. As the level (titre) of anti-p24 rises, the level of p24 antigen decreases to levels which are no longer detectable.

6. Shortly after this, IgM antibody titres also decrease and disap-pear.

7. Many years will now go by and IgG antibodies to both p24 and gp41 will be detectable.

8. Eventually, IgG core antibodies (i.e. anti-p24) will start to decrease and p24 antigen will re-appear. This serological event is associated with progression to clinical illness.

Types of serological tests for HIV

Any serological test used for detecting HIV infection must have a high degree of **sensitivity** (the probability that the test will be positive if the patient is infected) and **specificity** (the probability that the test will be negative if the patient is uninfected). No screening tests for any trait are ever 100 per cent sensitive and specific and, therefore, all positive test results are re-tested by another method for confirmation.

ELISA

ELISA (enzyme linked immunosorbent assay) and **EIA (enzyme immunoassay)** are the most common tests used for screening for markers of HIV infection. There are several different types of ELISA/EIA tests on the market but they all look for IgG antibodies to the transmembrane glycoprotein (gp41) and the p24 core protein. Special ELISA/EIA tests can also look for IgM antibodies to both gp41 and p24.

ELISA/EIA tests are also designed to detect p24 antigen and this test is generally referred to as the **antigen test**. Because the antigen is not detectable throughout the course of HIV infection, the antigen test is not useful as a primary tool for detecting HIV infection. Its principal use is in determining prognosis; a positive antigen test result indicates the end of the asymptomatic phase of infection and heralds the onset of AIDS[10]. It is also a useful test in resolving the infection status of infants born to HIV-infected mothers. In infants, a positive antigen test result indicates a much higher probability of infection.

ELISA/EIA tests can be designed to test for markers of both HIV-1 and HIV-2 infection. The sensitivity and specificity of ELISA/EIA tests are generally high but may vary from one laboratory to another. Therefore, a single positive ELISA/EIA result is not presumptive for infection. Diagnosis should be established by repeated, positive ELISA/EIA tests and a positive confirmatory test.

Immunofluorescent assay

The **immunofluorescent assay (IFA)** may also be used to detect HIV antibodies (especially IgM class antibodies) but is more time-consuming and requires more expertise than ELISA/EIA tests. It is used more as a research tool than a screening test.

Western blot

The **Western blot** is the most widely used **confirmatory test.** It uses gel electrophoresis to separate viral antigens, and then antibodies, so individual viral proteins can be identified. This test is accurate when properly conducted and analysed; however, it is difficult to perform and interpret. Third generation ELISA/EIA tests are becoming much more sensitive and specific and may replace Western blot as a confirmatory test.

PCR

The **PCR (polymerase chain reaction)** is a gene-amplification technique which measures HIV nucleic acid. It can detect minute amounts of HIV genetic material in infected individuals. It is not used as a general screening test but may be useful in detecting HIV infection in infants and in those rare cases where, despite indications of HIV disease, an individual consistently tests negative by ELISA/EIA.

Viral culture

Viral culture techniques can be used to isolate HIV from peripheral blood mononuclear cells (PBMCs), cell-free plasma, bone marrow cells and cerebrospinal fluid. A positive viral culture reflects a true viraemia. HIV can be cultured during primary infection or during symptomatic illness. It becomes more difficult to culture HIV during the long period of asymptomatic infection.

Rapid method tests

A new range of **rapid method tests** have now been developed which offer almost instant results and do not require laboratory equipment to interpret. These include **TESTPACK** (Abbott), **HIVCHECK** (Dupont), **GENIE** (Genetic System) and **AIDS-SUDS** (Murex). These will enable screening in a variety of sites where it is not possible to process standard HIV tests. In the UK, TESTPACK (Abbott) is the most widely used rapid method test and will detect markers of both HIV-1 and HIV-2 infection. Calypte Biomedical have also developed a kit for detecting HIV antibodies in urine. Although there is no doubt that the new rapid method tests will be useful, they present unique issues (e.g. home testing) which need to be addressed. However, they offer for the first time a realistic, inexpensive, sensitive, low-technology method for screening blood transfusions in developing countries. Tests which use urine or saliva are particularly beneficial, in that both of these media are much safer to handle than is blood.

Other monitoring tests

The long, asymptomatic period characteristic of HIV disease eventually ends with progression to symptomatic disease and AIDS. Because the span of the asymptomatic period may vary from 2 to more than 10 years, all HIV-infected individuals want an indication of their likely prognosis during the next few years.

In general, four tests are used to gauge progression of HIV infection from asymptomatic to symptomatic disease. These are **CD4+ T-cell counts, HIV p24 antigen, β_2-microglobulin** and **p24 antibody**.

A declining CD4+ T-cell count is associated with a shift into symptomatic disease, as is the re-appearance of p24 antigen, a declining (or undetectable) p24 antibody level and rising levels of β_2-microglobulin or serum neopterin.

Guidelines for counselling and testing

Counselling and testing individuals who are infected or at risk of acquiring HIV infection is an important component of a comprehensive prevention strategy.

The counselling role of the nurse

There is a very real counselling role in nursing practice and nurses, and other health care professionals, must be supported and developed in this role. In the arena of AIDS patient care, counselling involves a continuing dialogue and relationship between the client or patient and the nurse, with the aims of preventing primary infection and providing psychosocial support to those already affected. Prevention and support are complementary processes and efforts to prevent HIV infection that are not accompanied by some type of support are not likely to be effective. Excellent counselling guidelines and textbooks are available for nurses and other health care professionals (see Further reading) and the CDC's *Technical Guidance on HIV Counseling* can be found in Appendix 9.

The vast majority of people infected with HIV are unaware of their infection. The primary public health purposes of counselling and testing are to help uninfected individuals initiate and sustain behavioural changes that reduce their risk of becoming infected and to assist infected individuals in avoiding infecting others.

The benefits to the individual of being tested if their past behaviour may have exposed them to infection, include:

1. An opportunity for individual counselling and health education. Those who test negative may be reassured by their test result and increase their commitment to avoid becoming infected.
2. If their test is positive, regular monitoring of T4-helper cells (CD4+ T lymphocytes) can be initiated, and individuals so identified can take advantage of current and developing treatment strategies, designed to slow down disease progression. An example of this is the introduction of zidovudine treatment for individuals who are asymptomatically infected with HIV and have T4 counts below 500 cells/mm^3.
3. In addition, regular monitoring of health status and CD4+ T-cell counts in infected individuals will indicate when to initiate primary prophylaxis for opportunistic infections.
4. Infected individuals can also be immunized against various illnesses (e.g. pneumococcal pneumonia, influenza and hepatitis B) while their immune system is still capable of responding to vaccines.
5. For women who are infected, this information may be paramount as they make decisions in relation to having children. In addition, cervical dysplasia is more common in immunosuppressed women and HIV infection is an indication for more frequent cervical cytology (see Chapter 10).
6. For individuals undergoing medical evaluation or treatment, it may be essential to know their HIV status in order to make informed medical decisions. For example, transplant surgery should not be considered for individuals infected with HIV, as the associated immunosuppressant therapy would be contraindicated. Other drugs or treatment may also be contraindicated. In addition, regular screening for tuberculosis would be beneficial for individuals who know they are infected, as HIV infection is associated with an increased incidence of severe clinical tuberculosis (see Chapter 7).

There are also many **individual disadvantages** of being screened.

1. A negative result may falsely reassure and individuals may not follow safer sexual practices.
2. If the test results become known to anyone other than the client and those personally involved, individuals risk losing their

job and friends and may have difficulty in obtaining insurance (medical, mortgages, etc.). Unfortunately, discrimination against individuals infected with HIV is rampant, e.g. their right to travel to many foreign countries may be restricted, etc. It may be significant to some individuals (or institutions) that a particular person was tested, regardless of the result (the 'Where there's smoke, there's fire' theory).

3. A positive test result is a heavy burden to carry and some people may have psychological difficulty adjusting to this information.

The decision to be tested can only be an individual decision, based upon perceived benefits and risks.

Hospitals and other health care facilities must ensure that they have trained adequate numbers of health care professionals to implement effective pre- and post-test counselling.

It is important for nurses to remember that HIV testing has no logical place in making infection control decisions. A person can test negative and yet be infected with HIV for the following reasons:

- There is a lag between exposure and seroconversion. Although this may be only a few months, it may extend up to 6 months (or longer).
- During this time, a patient will test negative but will be infected and infectious.
- An individual may be free of HIV infection and test negative. However, he/she may become exposed the following day and then become infected and infectious.
- Some individuals (rarely) who become infected fail to demonstrate IgG antibodies detected by current screening tests (e.g. ELISA/EIA negative but PCR positive). They would test negative but be infected and infectious.
- The result may be a 'false negative', yet this patient would also be infected and infectious.
- The individual may be infected with HIV-2 and unless the screening test was designed to detect antibodies to both HIV-1 and HIV-2, it may miss HIV-2 infection.

It is because of this and because of the increasing number of individuals in the community who are becoming infected with this virus, that universal infection control precautions or body substance isolation (see Chapter 12) have become incorporated into current clinical nursing practice.

Informed consent

No individual citizen should be tested for markers of HIV infection without their true, informed consent. Informed consent implies that the reason why the test is being recommended is clearly explained to the patient in language he/she can understand. Since HIV testing is rarely an emergency, time and space should be built into the encounter so that the patient can consider the information given. Literature, clearly describing the advantages and disadvantages of being tested, should be left with the patient and an opportunity should be offered for the patient to consult with a trained counsellor. The results of the test should be equally carefully explained to the patient and, if the result is positive, appropriate post-test counselling and support arranged. The waiting period for the test result is often filled with anxiety and individuals frequently need support during this period.

Hospitals and other health care facilities must also ensure that they have created, implemented and monitored policies and procedures to ensure that informed consent is obtained prior to testing and that mechanisms exist to ensure the confidentiality of the test. If health care facilities are participating in anonymous, prevalence data testing, specific protocols and policies must be additionally established for this type of unconsented testing. Model policies for informed consent, confidentiality and anonymous prevalence data testing can be found in Appendix 8. The advocacy skills of the nurse are often critical in the area of serological testing for markers of HIV infection. In the 1990s, the 'age of AIDS', clearly we should all behave towards each other as if we were all infected. This includes our positions on sexual behaviour, infection control and making moral and ethical decisions. We should not be doing anything to our patients that we would not wish to be done to us or our loved ones.

Summary

Although impressive advances are being made in the treatment of opportunistic diseases associated with HIV infection, scientists have not yet developed drugs that will eliminate the virus from the body or restore the ability of the immune system to defend the body against repeated assaults by these pathogens. Until this has been achieved, AIDS will continue to be a fatal disease. Immense international effort is being directed towards the development of a vaccine against HIV but it remains elusive.

There seems little doubt that the escape of HIV from the animal kingdom into the human population represents an uniquely sinister

342   *Nursing Issues Related to Medical Management*

threat to the human race. The advent of AIDS may turn out to be
the most significant event of our lifetime.

References

1. Aboulker, J.P. and Swart, A.M. (1993). Preliminary analysis of the
   Concorde trial. *Lancet*, 3 April, **ii**(341), 889–90.
2. Fischl, M.A. (1994). Antiretroviral therapy strategies: B. The Miami
   perspective. In *Textbook of AIDS Medicine*, eds Broder, S., Merigan,
   T.C. Jr. and Bolognesi, D., Williams & Wilkins, Baltimore, MD,
   pp. 787–92.
3. Uandkat, J.D., Collier, A.C., Crosby, S.C. *et al.* (1990).
   Pharmacokinetics of oral zidovudine (azidothymidine) in patients
   with AIDS when administered with and without a high-fat meal.
   AIDS **4**(3), 229–32.
4. Podzamczer, D., Santín, José, J., Casanova, A. *et al.* (1993). Thrice-
   weekly cotrimoxazole is better than weekly dapsone-pyrimethamine for
   the primary prevention of *Pneumocystis carinii* pneumonia in HIV-
   infected patients. *AIDS* **7**(4), 501–6.
5. Ong, E.L. (1993). Editorial review: The role of aerosol pentamidine
   prophylaxis. *International Journal of STD & AIDS*, March/April, **4**,
   67–9.
6. Slavin, M.A., Hoy, J.F., Stewart, K. *et al.* (1992). Oral dapsone versus nebulized pentamidine for *Pneumocystis carinii* pneumonia prophylaxis: an open randomized prospective trial to assess efficacy and
   haematological toxicity. *AIDS* **6**(10), 1169–74.
7. Oksenhendler, E., Charreau, I., Tournerie, C. *et al.* (1994).
   Toxoplasma gondii infection in advanced HIV infection. *AIDS* **8**(4),
   483–7.
8. Glatt, A.E. (1993). Editorial: Therapy for oropharyngeal candidiasis
   in HIV-infected patients. *Journal of Acquired Immune Deficiency Syndromes* **6**(12), 1317–18.
9. Birx, D.L. and Redfield, R.R. (1994). Therapeutic HIV vaccines: Concept, current status, and future directions. In *Textbook of AIDS Medicine*, eds Broder, S., Merigan, T.C. Jr. and Bolognesi, D., Williams &
   Wilkins, Baltimore, MD, pp. 693–711.
10. Sloand, E.M., Pitt, E., Chiarello, R.J. *et al.* (1991). Testing: State of
    the art. *Journal of the American Medical Association* **266**, 2861–6.

Further reading

Medical management

Broder, S., Merigan, T.C. Jr. and Bolognesi, D. (1994). *Textbook of AIDS
Medicine*. Williams & Wilkins, Baltimore, MD (ISBN 0-683-01072-7.

Devita, V. Jr., Hellman, S. and Rosenberg, S.A. (1992). *AIDS: Etiology, Diagnosis, Treatment and Prevention*, 3rd edn. J.B. Lippincott, Philadelphia, PA (ISBN 0-397-51229-5).

Muma, R.D., Lyons, B.A., Borucki, M.J. *et al.* (1994). *HIV: Manual for Health Care Professionals*. Appleton & Lange, Norwalk, CT (ISBN 0-8385-0170-2).

Sande, Merle A. and Volberding, Paul A. (1992). *The Medical Management of AIDS*, 3rd edn. W.B. Saunders, Philadelphia, PA (ISBN 0-7216-6752-X).

Wormser, Gary P. (1992). *AIDS and Other Manifestations of HIV Infection*, 2nd edn. Raven Press, New York (ISBN 0-88167-881-3).

Counselling

Bor, R., Miller, R. and Goldman, E. (1992). *Theory and Practice of HIV Counselling: A Systemic Approach*. Cassell, London (ISBN 0-304-32580-5).

Burnard, P. (1992) *Counselling: A Guide to Practice in Nursing*. Butterworth-Heinemann, Oxford (ISBN 0-7506-0643-6).

Centers for Disease Control and Prevention (CDC) (1993). Technical guidance on HIV counseling. *Morbidity and Mortality Weekly Report (MMWR)*, **42**(RR-2) 11–17 (Reprinted in Appendix 9).

Dryden, W. and Feltham, C. (1992). *Brief Counselling: A Practical Guide for Beginning Practitioners*. Open University Press, London (ISBN 0-335-09972-6).

Green, J. and McCreaner, A. (1994). *Counselling in HIV Infection and AIDS*, 2nd edn. Blackwell Scientific, London.

Mulleady, G. (1992). *Counselling Drug Users about HIV and AIDS*. Blackwell Scientific, London (ISBN 0-632-02939-0).

Sherr, L. (1991). *HIV and AIDS in Mothers and Babies: A Guide to Counselling*. Blackwell Scientific, London (ISBN 0-632-02834-3).

World Health Organization (WHO) (1990). Guidelines for Counselling About HIV Infection and Disease. *WHO AIDS Series 8*, WHO, Geneva.

Appendices

Appendix 1: Revision of the CDC Surveillance Case Definition for Acquired Immunodeficiency Syndrome
(see Chapter 6)

A report by the Council of State and Territorial Epidemiologists; AIDS Program, Center for Infections Diseases, CDC. Reproduced from Centers for Disease Control (1987). *Morbidity and Mortality Weekly Report*, 14 August, 36(Suppl. 1).

Introduction

The following revised case definition for surveillance of acquired immunodeficiency syndrome (AIDS) was developed by CDC in collaboration with public health and clinical specialists. The Council of State and Territorial Epidemiologists (CSTE) has officially recommended adoption of the revised definition for national reporting of AIDS. The objectives of the revision are (a) to track more effectively the severe disabling morbidity associated with infection with human immunodeficiency virus (HIV) (including HIV-1 and HIV-2); (b) to simplify reporting of AIDS cases; (c) to increase the sensitivity and specificity of the definition through greater diagnostic application of laboratory evidence for HIV infection; and (d) to be consistent with current diagnostic practice, which in some cases includes presumptive, i.e., without confirmatory laboratory evidence, diagnosis of AIDS-indicative diseases (e.g., *Pneumocystis carinii* pneumonia, Kaposi's sarcoma).

The definition is organized into three sections that depend on the status of laboratory evidence of HIV infection (e.g., HIV antibody) (Fig. A. 1). The major proposed changes apply to patients with laboratory evidence for HIV infection: (a) inclusion of HIV encephalopathy, HIV wasting syndrome, and a broader range of specific AIDS-indicative diseases (Section II.A); (b) inclusion of AIDS patients whose indicator diseases are diagnosed presumptively (Section II.B); and (c) elimination of exclusions due to other causes of immunodeficiency (Section I.A).

Application of the definition for children differs from that for adults in two ways. First, multiple or recurrent serious bacterial infections and lymphoid interstitial pneumonia/pulmonary lymphoid hyperplasia are accepted as indicative of AIDS among children but not among adults. Second, for children < 15 months of age whose mothers are thought to have had HIV infection during the child's perinatal

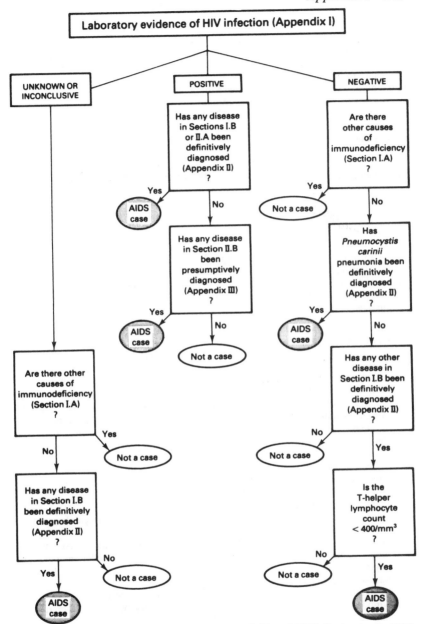

Fig. A.1 Flow diagram for revised CDC case definition of AIDS, September 1, 1987

period, the laboratory criteria for HIV infection are more stringent, since the presence of HIV antibody in the child is, by itself, insufficient evidence for HIV infection because of the persistence of passively acquired maternal antibodies < 15 months after birth. The new definition is effective immediately. State and local health departments are requested to apply the new definition henceforth to patients reported to them. The initiation of the actual reporting of cases that meet the new definition is targeted for September 1, 1987, when modified computer software and report forms should be in place to accommodate the changes. CSTE has recommended retrospective application of the revised definition to patients already reported to health departments. The new definition follows:

1987 revision of case definition for AIDS for surveillance purposes

For national reporting, a case of AIDS is defined as an illness characterized by one or more of the following 'indicator' diseases, depending on the status of laboratory evidence of HIV infection, as shown below.

1. Without laboratory evidence regarding HIV infection
If laboratory tests for HIV were not performed or gave inconclusion results (see Appendix I) and the patient had no other cause of immunodeficiency listed in Section I .A below, then any disease listed in Section I.B indicates AIDS if it was diagnosed by a definitive method (see Appendix II).

A. *Causes of immunodeficiency that disqualify diseases as indicators of AIDS in the absence of laboratory evidence for HIV infection*
1. high-dose or long-term systemic corticosteroid therapy or other immunosuppressive/cytotoxic therapy ≤ 3 months before the onset of the indicator disease
2. any of the following diseases diagnosed ≤ 3 months after diagnosis of the indicator disease: Hodgkin's disease, non-Hodgkin's lymphoma (other than primary brain lymphoma), lymphocytic leukemia, multiple myeloma, any other cancer of lymphoreticular or histiocytic tissue, or angioimmunoblastic lymphadenopathy
3. a genetic (congenital) immunodeficiency syndrome or an acquired immunodeficiency syndrome atypical of HIV infection, such as one involving hypogammaglobulinemia

B. *Indicator diseases diagnosed definitively* (see Appendix II)
1. candidiasis of the oesophaqus, trachea, bronchi, or lungs
2. cryptococcosis, extrapulmonary
3. cryptosporidiosis with diarrhea persisting > 1 month
4. cytomegalovirus disease of an organ other than liver, spleen, or lymph nodes in a patient > 1 month of age
5. herpes simplex virus infection causing a mucocutaneous ulcer that persists longer than 1 month; or bronchitis, pneumonitis, or esophagitis for any duration affecting a patient > 1 month of age
6. Kaposi's sarcoma affecting a patient < 60 years of age
7. lymphoma of the brain (primary) affecting a patient < 60 years of age
8. lymphoid interstitial pneumonia and/or pulmonary lymphoid hyperplasia (LIP/PLH complex) affecting a child < 13 years of age
9. *Mycobacterium avium* complex or *M. kansasii* disease, disseminated (at a site other than or in addition to lungs, skin, or cervical or hilar lymph nodes)

10. *Pneumocystis carinii* pneumonia
11. progressive multifocal leukoencephalopathy
12. toxoplasmosis of the brain affecting a patient > 1 month of age

II. With laboratory evidence for HIV infection

Regardless of the presence of other causes of immunodeficiency (I.A.), in the presence of laboratory evidence for HIV infection (see Appendix 1), any disease listed above (I.B.) or below (II.A or II.B) indicates a diagnosis of AIDS.

A. *Indicator diseases diagnosed definitively* (see Appendix II)
  1. bacterial infections, multiple or recurrent (any combination of at least two within a two-year period), of the following types affecting a child < 13 years of age: septicemia, pneumonia, meningitis, bone or joint infection, or abscess of an internal organ or body cavity (excluding otitis media or superficial skin or mucosal abscesses), caused by *Haemophilus, Streptococcus* (including pneumococcus), or other pyogenic bacteria
  2. coccidioidomycosis, disseminated (at a site other than or in addition to lungs or cervical or hilar lymph nodes)
  3. HIV encephalopathy (also called 'HIV dementia', 'AIDS dementia', or 'subacute encephalitis due to HIV') (see Appendix II for description)
  4. histoplasmosis, disseminated (at a site other than or in addition to lungs or cervical or hilar lymph nodes)
  5. isosporiasis with diarrhea persisting > 1 month
  6. Kaposi's sarcoma at any age
  7. lymphoma of the brain (primary) at any age
  8. other non-Hodgkin's lymphoma of B cell or unknown immunologic phenotype and the following histologic types:
     (a) small non-cleaved lymphoma (either Burkitt or non-Burkitt type) (see Appendix IV for equivalent terms and numeric codes used in the *International Classification of Diseases*, Ninth Revision, Clinical Modification)
     (b) immunoblastic sarcoma (equivalent to any of the following, although not necessarily all in combination: immunoblastic lymphoma, large-cell lymphoma, diffuse histiocytic lymphoma, diffuse undifferentiated lymphoma, or high-grade lymphoma) (see Appendix IV for equivalent terms and numeric codes used in the International Classification of Diseases, Ninth Revision, Clinical Modification)
     Note: Lymphomas are not included here if they are of T cell immunologic phenotype or their histologic type is not described or is described as 'lymphocytic', 'lymphoblastic', 'small cleaved', or 'plasmacytoid lymphocytic'
  9. any mycobacterial disease caused by mycobacteria other than *M. tuberculosis*, disseminated (at a site other than or in addition to lungs, skin, or cervical or hilar lymph nodes)
  10. disease caused by *M. tuberculosis*, extrapulmonary (involving at least one site outside the lungs, regardless of whether there is concurrent pulmonary involvement)
  11. *Salmonella* (non-typhoid) septicemia, recurrent
  12. HIV wasting syndrome (emaciation, 'slim disease') (see Appendix II for description)
B. *Indicator diseases diagnosed presumptively (by a method other than those in Appendix II)*

Note: Given the seriousness of diseases indicative of AIDS, it is generally important to diagnose them definitively, especially when therapy that would be used may have serious side-effects or when definitive diagnosis is needed for eligibility for anti-retroviral therapy. Nonetheless, in some situations, a patient's condition will not permit the performance of definitive tests. In other situations, accepted clinical practice may be to diagnose presumptively based on the presence of characteristic clinical and laboratory abnormalities. Guidelines for presumptive diagnoses are suggested in Appendix III.

1. candidiasis of the esophagus
2. cytomegalovirus retinitis with loss of vision
3. Kaposi's sarcoma
4. lymphoid interstitial pneumonia and/or pulmonary lymphoid hyperplasia (LIP/PLH complex) affecting a child < 13 years of age
5. mycobacterial disease (acid-fast bacilli with species not identified by culture), disseminated (involving at least one site other than or in addition to lungs, skin, or cervical or hilar lymph nodes)
6. *Pneumocystis carinii* pneumonia
7. toxoplasmosis of the brain affecting a patient > 1 month of age

III. With laboratory evidence against HIV infection

With laboratory test results negative for HIV infection (see Appendix I), a diagnosis of AIDS for surveillance purposes is ruled out *unless*:

A. all the other causes of immunodeficiency listed above in Section I.A are excluded; *and*

B. the patient has had either:

1. *Pneumocystis carinii* pneumonia diagnosed by a definitive method (see Appendix II); *or*
2. (a) any of the other diseases indicative of AIDS listed above in Section I.B diagnosed by a definitive method (see Appendix II), *and*
   (b) a T-helper/inducer (CD4) lymphocyte count < 400/mm^3:

Commentary

The surveillance of severe disease associated with HIV infection remains an essential, though not the only, indicator of the course of the HIV epidemic. The number of AIDS cases and the relative distribution of cases by demographic, geographic, and behavioral risk variables are the oldest indices of the epidemic, which began in 1981 and for which data are available retrospectively back to 1978. The original surveillance case definition, based on then available knowledge, provided useful epidemiologic data on severe HIV disease[1]. To ensure a reasonable predictive value for underlying immunodeficiency caused by what was then an unknown agent, the indicators of AIDS in the old case definition were restricted to particular opportunistic diseases diagnosed by reliable methods in patients without specific known causes of immunodeficiency. After HIV was discovered to be the cause of AIDS, however, and highly sensitive and specific HIV antibody tests became available, the spectrum of manifestations of HIV infection became better defined, and classification systems for HIV infection were developed[2–5]. It became apparent that some progressive, seriously disabling, and even fatal conditions (e.g. encephalopathy, wasting syndrome) affecting a substantial number of HIV infected patients were not subject to epidemiologic surveillance, as they were not included in the AIDS case definition. For reporting purposes, the revision adds to the definition most of those severe non-infectious, non-cancerous HIV-associated conditions that are categorized in CDC clinical classification systems for HIV infection among adults and children[4,5].

Another limitation of the old definition was that AIDS-indicative diseases are diagnosed presumptively (i.e. without confirmation by methods required by the old definition) in 10–15% of patients diagnosed with such diseases; thus, an appreciable proportion of AIDS cases were missed for reporting purposes[6,7]. This proportion may be increasing, which would compromise the old case definition's usefulness as a tool for monitoring trends. The revised case definition permits the reporting of these clinically diagnosed cases as long as there is laboratory evidence of HIV infection.

The effectiveness of the revision will depend on how extensively HIV antibody tests are used. Approximately one third of AIDS patients in the United States have been from New York City and San Francisco, where, since 1985, < 7% have been reported with HIV antibody test results, compared with > 60% in other areas. The impact of the revision on the reported numbers of AIDS cases will also depend on the proportion of AIDS patients in whom indicator diseases are diagnosed presumptively rather than definitively. The use of presumptive diagnostic criteria varies geographically, being more common in certain rural areas and in urban areas with many indigent AIDS patients.

To avoid confusion about what should be reported to health departments, the term 'AIDS' should refer only to conditions meeting the surveillance definition. This definition is intended only to provide consistent statistical data for public health purposes. Clinicians will not rely on this definition alone to diagnose serious disease caused by HIV infection in individual patients because there may be additional information that would lead to a more accurate diagnosis. For example, patients who are not reportable under the definition because they have either a negative HIV antibody test or, in the presence of HIV antibody, an opportunistic disease not listed in the definition as an indicator of AIDS nonetheless may be diagnosed as having serious HIV disease on consideration of other clinical or laboratory characteristics of HIV infection or a history of exposure to HIV.

Conversely, the AIDS surveillance definition may rarely misclassify other patients as having serious HIV disease if they have no HIV antibody test but have an AIDS-indicative disease with a background incidence unrelated to HIV infection, such as cryptococcal meningitis.

The diagnostic criteria accepted by the AIDS surveillance case definition should not be interpreted as the standard of good medical practice. Presumptive diagnoses are accepted in the definition because not to count them would be to ignore substantial morbidity resulting from HIV infection. Likewise, the definition accepts a reactive screening test for HIV antibody without confirmation by a supplemental test because a repeatedly reactive screening test result, in combination with an indicator disease, is highly indicative of true HIV disease. For national surveillance purposes, the tiny proportion of possibly false positive screening tests in persons with AIDS indicative diseases is of little consequence. For the individual patient, however, a correct diagnosis is critically important. The use of supplemental tests is, therefore, strongly endorsed. An increase in the diagnostic use of HIV antibody tests could improve both the quality of medical care and the function of the new case definition, as well as assist in providing counseling to prevent transmission of HIV.

Appendix I: Laboratory evidence for or against HIV infection

1. *For infection*:

When a patient has disease consistent with AIDS:

(a) a serum specimen from a patient $\geq$ 15 months of age, or from a child $<$ 15 months of age whose mother is not thought to have had HIV infection during the child's perinatal period, that is repeatedly reactive for HIV antibody by a screening test (e.g. enzyme-linked immunosorbent assay (ELISA), as long as subsequent HIV antibody tests (e.g. Western blot, immunofluorescence assay), if done, are positive; *or*

(b) a serum specimen from a child $<$ 15 months of age, whose mother is thought to have had HIV infection during the child's perinatal period, that is repeatedly reactive for HIV antibody by a screening test (e.g. ELISA), plus increased serum immunoglobulin levels and at least one of the following abnormal immunologic test results: reduced absolute lymphocyte count, depressed CD4 (T-helper) lymphocyte count, or decreased CD4/CD8 (helper:suppressor) ratio, as long as subsequent antibody tests (e.g. Western blot, immunofluorescence assay), if done, are positive; *or*

(c) a positive test for HIV serum antigen; *or*

(d) a positive HIV culture confirmed by both reverse transcriptase detection and a specific HIV antigen test or *in situ* hybridization using a nucleic acid probe; *or*

(e) a positive result on any other highly specific test for HIV (e.g. nucleic acid probe of peripheral blood lymphocytes).

2. *Against infection*:

A nonreactive screening test for serum antibody to HIV (e.g. ELISA) without a reactive or positive result on any other test for HIV infection (e.g. antibody, antigen, culture), if done.

3. *Inconclusive (neither for nor against infection)*:

(a) a repeatedly reactive screening test for serum antibody to HIV (e.g. ELISA) followed by a negative or inconclusive supplemental test (e.g. Western blot, immunofluorescence assay) without a positive HIV culture or serum antigen test, if done; *or*

(b) a serum specimen from a child $<$ 15 months of age, whose mother is thought to have had HIV infection during the child's perinatal period, that is repeatedly reactive for HIV antibody by a screening test, even if positive by a supplemental test, without additional evidence for immunodeficiency as described above (in 1 (b)) and without a positive HIV culture or serum antigen test, if done.

Appendix II: Definitive diagnostic methods for diseases indicative of AIDS

Diseases	Definitive diagnostic methods
Cryptosporidiosis	
Cytomegalovirus	
Isosporiasis	

Kaposi's sarcoma Lymphoma Lymphoid pneumonia or hyperplasia *Pneumocystis carinii pneumonia* Progressive multifocal leukoencephalopathy Toxoplasmosis	Microscopy (history or cytology).
Candidiasis	Gross inspection by endoscopy or autopsy or by microscopy (histology or cytology) on a specimen obtained directly from the tissues affected (including scrapings from the mucosal surface), not from a culture.
Coccidioidomycosis Cryptococcosis Herpes simplex virus Histoplasmosis	Microscopy (histology or cytology), culture, or detection of antigen in a specimen obtained directly from the tissues affected or a fluid from those tissues.
Tuberculosis Other mycobacteriosis Salmonellosis Other bacterial infection	Culture.
HIV encephalopathy* (dementia)	Clinical findings of disabling cognitive and/or motor dysfunction interfering with occupation or activities of daily living, or loss of behavioral developmental milestones affecting a child, progressing over weeks to months, in the absence of a concurrent illness or condition other than HIV infection that could explain the findings. Methods to rule out such concurrent illnesses and conditions must include cerebrospinal fluid examination and either brain imaging (computed tomography or magnetic resonance) or autopsy.
HIV wasting syndrome*	Findings of profound involuntary weight loss > 10% of baseline body weight plus either chronic diarrhea (at least two loose stools per day for $\geq$ 30 days) or chronic weakness and documented fever (for $\geq$ 30 days, intermittent or constant) in the absence of a concurrent illness or condition other than HIV infection that could explain the findings (e.g. cancer, tuberculosis, cryptosporidiosis, or other specific enteritis).

*For HIV encephalopathy and HIV wasting syndrome, the methods of diagnosis described here are not truly definitive, but are sufficiently rigorous for surveillance purposes.

Appendix III: Suggested guidelines for presumptive diagnosis of diseases indicative of AIDS

Diseases	Presumptive diagnostic criteria
Candidiasis of esophagus	(a) recent onset of retrosternal pain on swallowing; *and* (b) oral candidiasis diagnosed by the gross appearance of white patches or plaques on an erythematous base or by the microscopic appearance of fungal mycelial filaments in an uncultured specimen scraped from the oral mucosa.
Cytomegalovirus retinits	A characteristic appearance on serial ophthalmoscopic examinations (e.g. discrete patches of retinal whitening with distinct borders, spreading in a centrifugal manner, following blood vessels, progressing over several months, frequently associated with retinal vasculitis, hemorrhage, and necrosis). Resolution of active disease leaves retinal scarring and atrophy with retinal pigment epithelial mottling.
Mycobacteriosis	Microscopy of a specimen from stool or normally sterile body fluids or tissue from a site other than lungs, skin, or cervical or hilar lymph nodes, showing acid-fast bacilli of a species not identified by culture.
Kaposi's sarcoma	A characteristic gross appearance of an erythematous or violaceous plaque-like lesion on skin or mucous membrane. (**Note**: Presumptive diagnosis of Kaposi's sarcoma should not be made by clinicians who have seen few cases of it.)
Lymphoid interstitial pneumonia	Bilateral reticulonodular interstitial pulmonary infiltrates present on chest X-ray for ≥ 2 months with no pathogen identified and no response to antibiotic treatment.
Pneumocystis carinii pneumonia	(a) a history of dyspnea on exertion or nonproductive cough of recent onset (within the past 3 months); *and* (b) chest X-ray evidence of diffuse bilateral interstitial infiltrates or gallium scan evidence of diffuse bilateral pulmonary disease; *and* (c) arterial blood gas analysis showing an arterial pO_2 of $< 70\,mmHg$ or a low respiratory diffusing capacity ($< 80\%$ of predicted values) or an increase in the alveolar-arteriai oxygen tension gradient; *and* (d) no evidence of a bacterial pneumonia.
Toxoplasmosis of the brain	(a) recent onset of a focal neurologic abnormality consistent with intracranial disease or a reduced level of consciousness; *and* (b) brain imaging evidence of a lesion having a mass effect (on computed tomography or nuclear magnetic resonance) or the radiographic appearance of which is enhanced by injection of contrast medium; *and* (c) serum antibody to toxoplasmosis or successful response to therapy for toxoplasmosis.

Appendix IV: Equivalent terms and International Classification of Disease (ICD) codes for AIDS-indicative lymphomas

The following terms and codes describe lymphomas indicative of AIDS in patients with antibody evidence for HIV infection (Section II.A.8 of the AIDS case definition). Many of these terms are obsolete or equivalent to one another.

ICD-9-CM (1978)

Codes	Terms
200.0	**Reticulosarcoma**: lymphoma (malignant): histiocytic (diffuse) reticulum cell sarcoma: pleomorphic cell type or not otherwise specified.
200.2	**Burkitt's tumor or lymphoma**: malignant lymphoma, Burkitt's type.

ICD-O (Oncologic Histologic Types 1976)

Codes	Terms
9600/3	**Malignant lymphoma, undifferentiated cell type**: non-Burkitt's or not otherwise specified.
9601/3	**Malignant lymphoma, stem cell type**: stem cell lymphoma.
9612/3	**Malignant lymphoma, immunoblastic type**: immunoblastic sarcoma, immunoblastic lymphoma, or immunoblastic lymphosarcoma.
9632/3	**Malignant lymphoma, centroblastic type**: diffuse or not otherwise specified, or germinoblastic sarcoma: diffuse or not otherwise specified.
9633/3	**Malignant lymphoma, follicular center cell, non-cleaved**: diffuse or not otherwise specified.
9640/3	**Reticulosarcoma, not otherwise specified**: malignant lymphoma, histiocytic: diffuse or not otherwise specified reticulum cell sarcoma, not otherwise specified malignant lymphoma, reticulum cell type.
9641/3	**Reticulosarcoma, pleomorphic cell type**: malignant lymphoma, histiocytic, pleomorphic cell type reticulum cell sarcoma, pleomorphic cell type.
9750/3	**Burkitt's lymphoma or Burkitt's tumor**: malignant lymphoma, undifferentiated, Burkitt's type malignant lymphoma, lymphoblastic, Burkitt's type.

References

1. World Health Organization (1986). Acquired immunodeficiency syndrome (AIDS): WHO/CDC case definition for AIDS. *WHO Wkly Epidemiol Rec*, 61:69–72
2. Haverkos H.W., Gottlieb M.S., Killen J.Y. and Edelman R. (1985). Classification of HTLV-III/LAV-related diseases [Letter]. *J Infect Dis*; 152:1095
3. Redfield R.R., Wright D.C. and Tramont E.C. (1986). The Walter Reed staging classification of HTLV-III infection. *N Engl J Med*; 314:131–2
4. Centers for Disease Control (1986). Classification system for human T-lymphotropic virus type III/lymphadenopathy-associated virus infections. *MMWR*, 35:334–9
5. Centers for Disease Control (1987). Classification system for human immunodeficiency virus (HIV) infection in children under 13 years of age. *MMWR*, 36:225–30, 235
6. Hardy A.M., Starcher E.T., Morgan W.M., *et al.* (1987). Review of death certificates to assess completeness of AIDS case reporting. *Pub Hlth Rep*, 102(4):386–91

7. Starcher E.T., Biel J.K., Rivera-Castano R., Day J.M., Hopkins S.G., Miller J.W. (1987). The impact of presumptively diagnosed opportunistic infections and cancers on national reporting of AIDS [Abstract]. Washington, DC: III International Conference on AIDS, June 1–5

Update: 1993 Revised Classification System for HIV Infection and Expanded Surveillance Case Definition for AIDS Among Adolescents and Adults

Reproduced from Centers for Disease Control and Prevention (1992). *Morbidity and Mortality Weekly Report*, 18 December, 41 (RR-17)

Summary

CDC has revised the classification system for HIV infection to emphasize the clinical importance of the CD4+ T-lymphocyte count in the categorization of HIV-related clinical conditions. This classification system replaces the system published by CDC in 1986[1] and is primarily intended for use in public health practice. Consistent with the 1993 revised classification system, CDC has also expanded the AIDS surveillance case definition to include all HIV-infected persons who have < 200 CD4+ T-lymphocyte, or a CD4+ T-lymphocyte percentage of total lymphocytes of < 14. This expansion includes the addition of three clinical conditions – pulmonary tuberculosis, recurrent pneumonia, and invasive cervical cancer – and retains the 23 clinical conditions in the AIDS surveillance case definition published in 1987[2]; it is to be used by all states for AIDS case reporting, effective January 1, 1993.

Revised HIV classification system for adolescents and adults

The etiologic agent of acquired immunodeficiency syndrome (AIDS) is a retrovirus designated human immunodeficiency virus (HIV). The CD4+ T-lymphocyte is the primary target for HIV infection because of the affinity of the virus for the CD4 surface marker[3]. The CD4+ T-lymphocyte co-ordinates a number of important immunologic functions, and a loss of these functions results in progressive impairment of the immune response. Studies of the natural history of HIV infection have documented a wide spectrum of disease manifestations, ranging from asymptomatic infection to life-threatening conditions characterized by severe immunodeficiency, serious opportunistic infections, and cancers[4-13]. Other studies have shown a strong association between the development of life-threatening opportunistic illnesses and the absolute number (per microliter of blood) or percentage of CD4+ T-lymphocytes[14-21]. As the number of CD4+ T-lymphocytes decreases, the risk and severity of opportunistic illnesses increase.

Measures of CD4+ T-lymphocytes are used to guide clinical and therapeutic management of HIV-infected persons[22]. Antimicrobial prophylaxis and antiretroviral therapies have been shown to be most effective within certain levels of immune dysfunction[23-28]. As a result, antiretroviral therapy should be considered for all persons with CD4+ T-lymphocyte counts of < 500/μL, and prophylaxis against *Pneumocystis carinii* pneumonia, the most common serious opportunistic infection diagnosed in men and women with AIDS, is recommended for all persons with CD4+ T-lymphocyte counts of < 200/μL and for persons who have had prior episodes of

PCP. Because of these recommendations, CD4+ T-lymphocyte determinations are an integral part of medical management of HIV-infected persons in the United States.

The classification system for HIV infection among adolescents and adults has been revised to include the CD4+ T-lymphocyte count as a marker for HIV-related immunosuppression. This revision establishes mutually exclusive subgroups for which the spectrum of clinical conditions is integrated with the CD4+ T-lymphocyte count. The objectives of these changes are to simplify the classification of HIV infection, to reflect current standards of medical care for HIV-infected persons, and to categorize more accurately HIV-related morbidity.

The revised CDC classification system for HIV-infected adolescents and adults* categorizes persons on the basis of clinical conditions associated with HIV infection and CD4+ T-lymphocyte counts. The system is based on three ranges of CD4+ T-lymphocyte counts and three clinical categories and is represented by a matrix of nine mutually exclusive categories (Table 1). This system replaces the classification system published in 1986, which included only clinical disease criteria and which was developed before the widespread use of CD4+ T-cell testing[1].

CD4+ T-lymphocyte categories

The three CD4+ T-lymphocyte categories are defined as follows:

- Category 1: ≥ 500 cells/μL
- Category 2: 200–499 cells/μL
- Category 3: < 200 cells/μL

These categories correspond to CD4+ T-lymphocyte counts per microliter (μL) of blood and guide clinical and therapeutic actions in the management of HIV-infected adolescents and adults[22-28]. The revised HIV classification system also allows for the use of the percentage of CD4+ T-cells (Appendix A).**

HIV-infected persons should be classified based on existing guidelines for the medical management of HIV-infected persons[22]. Thus, the lowest accurate, but not necessarily the most recent, CD4+ T-lymphocyte count should be used for classification purposes.

Clinical Categories
The clinical categories of HIV infection are defined as follows:

Category A
Category A consists of one or more of the conditions listed below in an adolescent

---

*Criteria for HIV infection for persons ages ≥ 13 years: a) repeatedly reactive screening tests for HIV antibody (e.g., enzyme immunoassay) with specific antibody identified by the use of supplemental tests (e.g., Western blot, immuno-fluorescence assay); b) direct identification of virus in host tissues by virus isolation; c) HIV antigen detection; or d) a positive result on any other highly specific licensed test for HIV.

**Appendices not included; see original document, if necessary.

or adult (≥ 13 years) with documented HIV infection. Conditions listed in Categories B and C must not have occurred.

- Asymptomatic HIV infection
- Persistent generalized lymphadenopathy
- Acute (primary) HIV infection with accompanying illness or history of acute HIV infection[29,30]

Category B

Category B consists of symptomatic conditions in an HIV-infected adolescent or adult that are not included among conditions listed in clinical Category C and that meet at least one of the following criteria: a) the conditions are attributed to HIV infection or are indicative of a defect in cell-mediated immunity; or b) the conditions are considered by physicians to have a clinical course or to require management that is complicated by HIV infection. **Examples** of conditions in clinical Category B include, **but are not limited to:**

- Bacillary angiomatosis
- Candidiasis, oropharyngeal (thrush)
- Candidiasis, vulvo-vaginal; persistent, frequent, or poorly responsive to therapy
- Cervical dysplasia (moderate or severe)/cervical carcinoma in situ
- Constitutional symptoms, such as fever[38.5°C] or diarrhoea lasting > 1 month
- Hairy leukoplakia, oral
- Herpes zoster (shingles), involving at least two distinct episodes or more than one dermatome
- Idiopathic thrombocytopenic purpura
- Listeriosis
- Pelvic inflammatory disease, particularly if complicated by tubo-ovarian abscess
- Peripheral neuropathy

For classification purposes, Category B conditions take precedence over those in

Table 1   1993 revised classification system for HIV infection and expanded AIDS surveillance case definition for adolescents and adults*

CD4+ T-cell categories	Clinical categories		
	(A) Asymptomatic, acute (primary) HIV or PGL	(B) Symptomatic, not (A) or (C) conditions	(C) AIDS-indictor conditions
(1) > 500/μL	A1	B1	C1
(2) 200–499/μL	A2	B2	C2
(3) < 200/μL AIDS-indicator T-cell count	A3	B3	C3

*The shaded cells illustrate the expanded AIDS surveillance case definition. Persons with AIDS-indicator conditions (Category C) as well as those with CD4 lymphocyte counts < 200 cells/μL (Categories A3 or B3) will be reportable as AIDS cases in the United States and Territories, effective January 1, 1993.
PGL = persistent generalized lymphadenopathy. Clinical Category A includes acute (primary) HIV infection[29,30].

Category A. For example, someone previously treated for oral or persistent vaginal candidiasis (and who has not developed a Category C disease) but who is now asymptomatic should be classified in clinical Category B.

Category C
Category C includes the clinical conditions listed in the AIDS surveillance case definition (Appendix B). For classification purposes, once a Category C condition has occurred, the person will remain in Category C.

Expansion of the CDC surveillance case definition for AIDS

In 1991, CDC, in collaboration with the Council of State and Territorial Epidemiologists (CSTE), proposed an expansion of the AIDS surveillance case definition. This proposal was made available for public comment in November 1991 and was discussed at an open meeting on September 2, 1992. Based on information presented and reviewed during the public comment period and at the open meeting, CDC, in collaboration with CSTE, has expanded the AIDS surveillance case definition to include all HIV-infected persons with CD4+ T-lymphocyte counts of < 200 cells/μL or a CD4+ percentage of <14. In addition to retaining the 23 clinical conditions in the previous AIDS surveillance definition, the expanded definition includes **pulmonary tuberculosis (TB)**, **recurrent pneumonia**, and **invasive cervical cancer**.* This expanded definition requires laboratory confirmation of HIV infection in persons with a CD4+ T-lymphocyte count of < 200 cells/μL or with one of the added clinical conditions. This expanded definition for reporting cases to CDC becomes effective January 1, 1993.

In the revised HIV classification system, persons in subcategories A3, B3, and C3 meet the immunologic criteria of the surveillance case definition, and those persons with conditions in subcategories Cl, C2, and C3 meet the clinical criteria for surveillance purposes (Table 1).

Commentary

Revised Classification System
The revised classification system for HIV infection is based on the recommended clinical standard of monitoring CD4+ T-lymphocyte counts, since this parameter consistently correlates with HIV-related immune dysfunction and disease progression and provides information needed to guide medical management of persons infected with HIV [14-18,22-28]. The classification system also allows for use of the percentage of CD4+ T-cells instead of absolute CD4+ T-lymphocyte counts (Appendix A). Other markers of immune status – such as serum neopterin, beta-2 microglobulin, HIV p24 antigen, soluble interleukin-2 receptors, immunoglobulin A, and delayed-type hypersensitivity (DTH) skin-test reactions – may be useful in the evaluation of individual patients but are not as strongly predictive of disease progression or as specific for HIV-related immunosuppression as measures of CD4+ T-lymphocytes[14-21,31]. DTH

---

*Diagnostic criteria for AIDS-defining conditions included in the expanded surveillance case definition are presented in Appendix C and Appendix D.

skin-test reactions are often used in conjunction with the Mantoux tuberculin skin test to evaluate HIV-infected patients for TB infection and anergy[31-33].

Other systems have been proposed for classification and staging of HIV infection[1,31,34-39]. In 1990, the World Health Organization (WHO) published an interim proposal for a staging system for HIV infection and diseases that was based primarily on clinical criteria and included the use of CD4+ T-lymphocyte determinations[34]. The WHO system incorporates a performance scale and total lymphocyte counts to be used in lieu of CD4+ T-lymphocyte determinations in countries where CD4+ T-lymphocyte testing is not available.

The accuracy of CD4+ T-lymphocyte counts is important for medical care of individual patients. To assure reliability, laboratories conducting CD4+ T-lymphocyte measurements should be experienced with test procedures, have established quality assurance methods, and participate in proficiency testing programs conducted by CDC or other organizations[22,40]. CDC has published guidelines for the performance of CD4+ T-cell determinations for HIV-infected persons[41]. To assure that test results are indicative of a patient's medical condition, the health-care provider should evaluate the results with those of earlier tests and with the patient's clinical condition. In clinical practice, repeat CD4+ testing may be judged necessary in guiding therapeutic decisions for individual patients. For surveillance purposes, however, a requirement for repeat CD4+ determinations is impractical for population-based monitoring.

The revised classification system of the clinical and immunologic manifestations of HIV infection provides a framework for categorizing HIV-related morbidity and immunosuppression and will assist efforts to evaluate the overall impact of the HIV epidemic. Knowledge of the spectrum of clinical conditions and the extent of immunosuppression that may occur during the course of HIV infection is important for prompt evaluation and for provision of appropriate health services. Clinicians should be aware of the clinical conditions suggestive of HIV infection and the need for prophylactic and therapeutic interventions.

This revised HIV classification system should be used by state and territorial health departments that conduct HIV infection surveillance. Because AIDS surveillance data will continue to represent only a portion of the total morbidity caused by HIV, surveillance for HIV infection may be particularly useful in depicting the total impact of HIV on health-care and social services (42). More accurate reporting and analysis of CD4+ T-lymphocyte counts, together with HIV-related clinical conditions, should facilitate efforts to evaluate health-care and referral needs for persons with HIV infection and to project future needs for these services.

Expanded AIDS surveillance case definition

The population of HIV-infected persons with CD4+ T-lymphocyte counts of< 200 cells/μL is substantially larger than the population of persons with AIDS-defining clinical conditions[43]. The inclusion in the AIDS surveillance definition of persons with a CD4+ T-lymphocyte count of < 200 cells/μL or a CD4+ percentage < 14 will enable AIDS surveillance to reflect more accurately the number of persons with severe HIV-related immunosuppression and those at highest risk for severe HIV-related morbidity. Since the AIDS surveillance case definition was last revised in 1987, the increasing use of prophylaxis against PCP and antiretroviral therapy for persons infected with HIV has slowed the rate at which HIV-infected persons develop AIDS-defining clinical conditions[2,22-25]. For example, among homosexual/bisexual men with AIDS reported to CDC, the proportion with PCP decreased from 62% in 1988 to 46% in 1990[44]. This trend is expected to continue.

The ability of clinicians to report HIV-infected persons on the basis of CD4+ T-lymphocyte counts may also simplify the case-reporting process. A simplified AIDS surveillance case definition will be particularly important for outpatient clinics in which the availability of staff to conduct surveillance is limited and from which an increasing proportion of AIDS cases are being reported. For example, from pre-1985 to 1988, the proportion of AIDS cases reported from outpatient sites in the state of Washington increased from 6% (9/155) to 25%(55/219)[45]. A similar increase occurred in Oregon: 25% (44/1711) before 1987 to 38% (140/1051) in the first half of 1989[46].

Pulmonary tuberculosis

Throughout the world, pulmonary TB is the most common type of TB in persons with HIV infection[47]. The addition of pulmonary TB to the list of AIDS-indicator diseases is based on the strong epidemiologic link between HIV infection and the development of TB[48–50]. Persons co-infected with HIV and TB have a substantially increased risk of developing active TB compared with persons without HIV infection[48,49]. In a prospective evaluation of injecting-drug users (IDUs) with positive tuberculin skin tests, the estimated annual incidence of active TB among 49 HIV-infected IDUs was 7.9 cases/100 person-years; however, no cases of active TB occurred among 62 tuberculin-positive but HIV-sero-negative IDUs followed for as long as 30 months[48].

There is also a substantial immunologic association between HIV-infected persons and pulmonary TB when compared with HIV-infected persons with extra-pulmonary TB (a condition included in the 1987 surveillance definition). In a recent review, median CD4+ T-lymphocyte counts in HIV-infected patients with pulmonary TB ranged from 250 to 500 cells/μL[51]. In comparison, the median CD4+ lymphocyte count was 242 cells/μL in one study of persons with localized extra-pulmonary TB and ranged from 70 to 79 cells/μL in two studies of patients with disseminated or miliary TB[51–53]. In CDC's Adult and Adolescent Spectrum of HIV Disease (ASD) Project, 69% of HIV-infected persons with pulmonary TB had CD4+ T-lymphocyte counts of < 200/μL, compared with 77% of persons with extra-pulmonary TB (CDC, unpublished observations).

The addition of pulmonary TB to AIDS surveillance criteria will require continued collaboration between state and local TB and HIV/AIDS programs. Knowledge of a patient's HIV status is important for the proper medical management of TB because longer courses of therapy and prophylaxis are recommended for HIV-infected patients with TB[54]. Furthermore, HIV-infected TB patients should be a priority for epidemiologic investigation because these persons are more likely to have HIV-infected contacts than are sero-negative TB patients. TB contact follow-up among HIV-infected persons will help to ensure delivery of a full course of preventive therapy to these contacts, who are at greatly increased risk of developing active TB themselves.

Recurrent pneumonia

With the exception of conditions included in the 1987 AIDS surveillance case definition, pneumonia, with or without a bacteriologic diagnosis, is the leading cause of HIV-related morbidity and death[55,56]. In addition, several studies have shown that persons with HIV-related immunosuppression are at an increased risk of bacterial pneumonia[57–59]. For example, one study found that the yearly incidence rate of bacterial pneumonia among HIV-infected IDUs without AIDS was five times that found in non-HIV-infected IDUs[58]. Recurrent episodes of pneumonia (two or more episodes within a 1-year period) are required for AIDS case reporting because pneumonia is a relatively common diagnosis and multiple episodes of pneumonia are more strongly associated with immunosuppression than are single episodes. For example, data from the ASD Project indicate that the risk of an HIV-infected person having had one episode of pneumonia in a 12–month period is approximately five times higher among infected persons with CD4+ T-lymphocyte counts of < 200 cells/μL (320/2,411) than among those with higher CD4+ T-lymphocyte counts (90/2,792). In contrast, data from the same study indicate that the risk for multiple episodes of pneumonia in a 12–month period is approximately 20 times higher among HIV-infected persons with CD4+ T-lymphocyte counts of < 200 cells/μL (67/2,411) than among those with higher CD4+ T-cell counts (4/2,792) (CDC, unpublished observations).

Invasive cervical cancer
Several studies have found an increased prevalence of cervical dysplasia, a precursor lesion for cervical cancer, among HIV-infected women[60,61]. In a study of 310 HIV-infected women attending methadone maintenance and sexually transmitted disease clinics in New York City and Newark, New Jersey, cervical dysplasia was confirmed by biopsy and/or colposcopy in approximately 22%, a prevalence rate 10 times greater than that found among women attending family planning clinics in the United States (Wright TC, personal communication)[62]. Several studies have documented that a higher prevalence of cervical dysplasia among HIV-infected women is associated with greater immunosuppression (Wright TC, personal communication)[61,63]. In addition, HIV infection may adversely affect the clinical course and treatment of cervical dysplasia and cancer[64-69].

Invasive cervical cancer is a more appropriate AIDS-indicator disease than is either cervical dysplasia or carcinoma in situ because these latter cervical lesions are common and frequently do not progress to invasive disease[70]. Also, cervical dysplasia or carcinoma in situ among women with severe cervicovaginal infections, which are common in HIV-infected women, can be difficult to diagnose. In contrast, the diagnosis of invasive cervical cancer is generally unequivocal.

Invasive cervical cancer is preventable by the proper recognition and treatment of cervical dysplasia. Thus, the occurrence of invasive cervical cancer among all women – including those who are HIV-infected – represents missed opportunities for disease prevention. The addition of invasive cervical cancer to the list of AIDS-indicator diseases emphasizes the importance of integrating gynecologic care into medical services for HIV-infected women.

Impact on AIDS case reporting
The expanded AIDS surveillance case definition is expected to have a substantial impact on the number of reported cases. The immediate increase in case reporting will be largely attributable to the addition of severe immunosuppression to the definition; a smaller impact is expected from the addition of pulmonary TB, recurrent pneumonia, and invasive cervical cancer, since many persons with these diseases will also have CD4+ T-lymphocyte counts of < 200 cells/μL. If all of the approximately 1,000,000 persons in the United States with HIV infection were diagnosed and their immune status were known, it is estimated that 120,000–190,000 persons who do not have AIDS-indicator diseases would be found to have CD4+ T-lymphocyte counts of < 200 cells/μL[71]. However, not all of these persons are aware of their HIV infection and of those who know their HIV infection status, not all have had an

immunologic evaluation; thus, the immediate impact on the number of AIDS cases will be considerably less than 120,000–190,000. If AIDS surveillance criteria were unchanged, approximately 50,000–60,000 reported AIDS cases would be expected in 1993. Based on current levels of HIV and CD4+ testing, CDC estimates that the expanded definition could increase cases reported in 1993 by approximately 75%. Early effects of expanded surveillance will be greater than long-term effects because prevalent as well as incident cases of immunosuppression will be reported following implementation of the expanded surveillance case definition. In subsequent years, the effect on the number of reported cases is expected to be much smaller.

Uses of the HIV classification system or AIDS surveillance case definition

The revised HIV classification system and the AIDS surveillance case definition are intended for use in conducting public health surveillance. The CDC's AIDS surveillance case definition was not developed to determine whether statutory or other legal requirements for entitlement to Federal disability or other benefits are met. Consequently, this revised surveillance case definition does not alter the criteria used by the Social Security Administration in evaluating claims based on HIV infection under the Social Security disability insurance and Supplemental Security Income programs. Other organizations and agencies providing medical and social services should develop eligibility criteria appropriate to the services provided and local needs.

Confidentiality

The confidentiality of AIDS case reports – including laboratory reports of HIV test results, CD4+ T-lymphocyte test results, and medical records under review by health department staff – is of critical importance to maintaining effective HIV/AIDS surveillance. CDC and state health departments have implemented procedures and policies to maintain confidentiality and security of HIV/AIDS surveillance data[72]. CDC's efforts include a federal assurance of confidentiality, the removal of names before encrypted records are transmitted to CDC, strict guidelines for the release of aggregate data, and the inclusion of confidentiality and security safeguards as evaluation criteria for federal funding of state HIV/AIDS surveillance activities[73]. These strict criteria will continue to apply to cases reported under the expanded definition. CDC funding of surveillance co-operative agreements is dependent on the recipient's ability to ensure the physical security of case reports and on state policies or laws to protect the confidentiality of persons reported with AIDS. Failure to ensure the security and confidentiality of personal identifying information collected as part of AIDS or HIV surveillance activities will jeopardize federal surveillance funding.

CD4+ T-lymphocyte test results reported by laboratories will be an important adjunct to medical record review and provider-initiated reporting in order to increase completeness, timeliness, and efficiency of AIDS surveillance. Information from a laboratory-initiated report of a CD4+ T-lymphocyte count is insufficient for reporting a case of AIDS. Confirmation of HIV infection status and receipt of other surveillance information from the health-care provider or from medical or public health records will remain necessary.

Every effort should be made by health-care providers, laboratories, and public health agencies to protect the confidentiality of CD4+ T-lymphocyte test results, including the review of record-keeping practices in laboratories and health-care settings. Some states have considered additional means to assure the confidentiality of CD4+

T-lymphocyte test results. For example, a proposal in Oregon would allow health-care providers to send specimens to laboratories for CD4+ T-lymphocyte testing with a unique code for each person being tested. If the test result indicates a CD4+ T-lymphocyte count of 200 cells/μL, the health department would notify the health-care provider that an AIDS case report is required if the person is HIV infected, the CD4+ T-lymphocyte count is valid, and the case has not been previously reported. Informed consent for CD4+ T-lymphocyte testing should be obtained in accordance with local laws or regulations. CD4+ T-lymphocyte test results alone should not be used as a surrogate marker for HIV or AIDS. A low CD4+ T-lymphocyte count without a positive HIV test result will not be reportable, since other conditions may result in a low CD4+ T-lymphocyte count. Health-care providers must ensure that persons who have a CD4+ T-lymphocyte count of 200/μL are HIV infected before initiating treatment for HIV disease or reporting those persons as cases of AIDS.

Conclusion

The revised HIV classification system provides uniform and simple criteria for categorizing conditions among adolescents and adults with HIV infection and should facilitate efforts to evaluate current and future health-care and referral needs for persons with HIV infection. The addition of a measure of severe immunosuppression, as defined by a CD4+ T-lymphocyte count of < 200 cells/μL or a CD4+ percentage of <14, reflects the standard of immunologic monitoring for HIV-infected persons and will enable AIDS surveillance data to more accurately represent those who are recognized as being immunosuppressed, who are in greatest need of close medical follow-up, and who are at greatest risk for the full spectrum of severe HIV-related morbidity. The addition of three clinical conditions – pulmonary TB, recurrent pneumonia, and invasive cervical cancer – to AIDS surveillance criteria reflects the documented or potential importance of these diseases in the HIV epidemic. Two of these conditions (pulmonary TB and cervical cancer) are preventable if appropriate screening tests are linked with proper follow-up. The third, recurrent pneumonia, reflects the importance of pulmonary infections not included in the 1987 definition as leading causes of HIV-related morbidity and mortality. Successful implementation of expanded surveillance criteria will require the extension of existing safeguards to protect the security and confidentiality of AIDS surveillance information.

References

1. CDC. Classification system for human T-lymphotropic virus type III/ lymphadenopathy-associated virus infections. MMWR 1986; 35: 334–9.
2. CDC. Revision of the CDC surveillance case definition for acquired immuno-deficiency syndrome. MMWR 1987; 36: 1–15S.
3. McDougal JS, Kennedy MS, Sligh JM, et al. Binding of the HTLV-III/LAV to T4+ T cells by a complex of the 110K molecule and the T4 molecule. Science 1985; 231: 382–5.
4. Moss AR, Bacchetti P Natural history of HIV infection. AIDS 1989; 3: 55–61.
5. Rutherford GW, Lifson AR, Hessol NA, et al. Course of HIV-1 in a cohort of homosexual, and bisexual men: an 11 year follow-up study. Br Med J 1990; 301: 1183–8.

6. Muhoz A, Wang MC, Bass S, et al. Acquired immunodeficiency syndrome (AIDS)-free time after human immunodeficiency virus type 1 (HIV-1) seroconversion in homosexual men. Am J Epidemiol 1989; 130: 530–9.

7. Rezza G, Lazzarin A, Angarano G, et al., The natural history of HIV infection in intravenous drug users: risk of disease progression in a cohort of seroconverters. AIDS 1989; 3: 87–90.

8. Selwyn PA, Hartel D, Schoenbaum EE, et al. Rates and predictors of progression to HIV disease and AIDS in a cohort of intravenous drug users (IVDUs), 1985–1990 (abstract F.C.111). VI International Conference on AIDS, San Francisco, CA, June 22, 1990; 2: 117.

9. Medley GF, Anderson RM, Cox DR, Billard L. Incubation period of AIDS in patients infected via blood transfusion. Nature 1987; 328: 719–21.

10. Ward JW, Bush TJ, Perkins HA, et al. The natural history of transfusion-associated infection with human immunodeficiency virus. N Engl J Med 1989; 321: 947–52.

11. Goedert JJ, Kessler CM, Aledort LM, et al. A prospective study of human immunodeficiency virus type 1 infection and the development of AIDS in subjects with hemophilia. N Engl J Med 1989; 321: 1141–8.

12. Auger I, Thomas P, De Gruttola V, et al. Incubation periods for paediatric AIDS patients. Nature 1988; 336: 575–7.

13. Krasinski K, Borkowsky W, Holzman RS. Prognosis of human immunodeficiency virus in children and adolescents. Pediatr Infect Dis J 1989; 8: 216–20.

14. Goedert JJ, Biggar RJ, Melbye M, et al. Effect of T4 count and cofactors on the incidence of AIDS in homosexual men infected with human immunodeficiency virus. JAMA 1987; 257: 331–4.

15. Nicholson JKA, Spira TJ, Aloisio CH, et al. Serial determinations of HIV-1 titers in HIV-infected homosexual men: association of rising titers with CD4 T cell depletion and progression to AIDS. AIDS Res Hum Retroviruses 1989; 5: 205–15.

16. Lang W, Perkins H, Anderson RE, Royce R, Jewell N, Winkelstein W. Patterns of T lymphocyte changes with human immunodeficiency virus infection: from seroconversion to the development of AIDS. J Acquir Immune Defic Syndr 1989; 2: 63–9.

17. Lange MA, de Wolf F, Goudsmit J. Markers for progression of HIV infection. AIDS 1989; 3(suppl.1): SI53–160.

18. Taylor JM, Fahey JL, Detels R, Giorgi J. CD4 percentage, CD4 numbers, and CD4:CD8 ratio in HIV infection: which to choose and how to use. J Acquir Immune Defic Syndr 1989; 2: 114-24.

19. Masur H, Ognibene FP, Yarchoan R, et al. CD4 counts as predictors of opportunistic pneumonias in human immunodeficiency virus (HIV) infection. Ann Intern Med 1989; 111: 223–31.

20. Fahey JL, Taylor JMG, Detels R, et al. The prognostic value of cellular and serologic markers in infection with human immunodeficiency virus type 1. N Engl J Med 1990; 322: 166–72.

21. Fernandez-Cruz E, Desco M, Garcia Montes M, Longo N, Gonzalez B, Zabay JM. Immunological and serological markers predictive of progression to AIDS in a cohort of HIV-infected drug users. AIDS 1990; 4: 987–94.

22. National Institutes of Health. State-of-the-art conference on azidothymidine therapy for early HIV infection. Am J Med 1990; 89: 335–44.

23. CDC. Guidelines for prophylaxis against *Pneumocystis carinii* pneumonia for persons infected with human immunodeficiency virus. MMWR 1992; 41 (No. RR-4): 1–11.

24. Fischl MA, Richman DD, Hansen N, et al. The safety and efficacy of zidovudine (AZT) in the treatment of subjects with mildly symptomatic human immunodeficiency virus type 1 (HIV) infection: a double blind, placebo controlled trial. Ann Intern Med 1990; 112: 727–37.

25. Volberding PA, Lagakos SW, Koch MA, et al. Zidovudine in asymptomatic human immunodeficiency virus infection: a controlled trial in persons with fewer than 500 CD4-positive cells per cubic millimeter. N Engl J Med 1990; 322: 941.

26. Lagakos S, Fischl MA, Stein DS, Lim L, Volberding PA. Effects of zidovudine therapy in minority and other subpopulations with early HIV infection. JAMA 1991; 266: 2709–12.

27. Easterbrook PJ, Keruly JC, Creagh-Kirk T, et al. Racial and ethnic differences in outcome in zidovudine-treated patients with advanced HIV disease. JAMA 1991; 266: 2713–8.

28. Hamilton JD, Hartigan PM, Simberkoff MS, et al. A controlled trial of early versus late treatment with zidovudine in symptomatic human immunodeficiency virus infection. N Engl J Med 1992; 326: 437–43.

29. Ho DD, Sarngadharan MG, Resnick L, et al. Primary human T-lymphotropic virus type III infection. Ann Intern Med 1985; 103: 880–3.

30. Tindall B, Cooper DA. Primary HIV infection: host responses and intervention strategies. AIDS 1991; 5: 1–14.

31. Redfield RR, Wright DC, Tramont EC. The Walter Reed Staging Classification for HTLV-III/LAV infection. N Engl J Med 1986; 314: 131–2.

32. CDC. Guidelines for preventing the transmission of tuberculosis in health-care settings, with special focus on HIV-related issues. MMWR 1990; 39(No. RR-17): 1–29.

33. CDC. Purified protein derivative (PPD)-tuberculin anergy and HIV infection. MMWR 1991; 40 (No. RR-15): 37–43.

34. WHO. Interim proposal for a WHO staging system for HIV infection and diseases. Weekly Epidemiol Record 1990; 65: 221–4.

35. Chaisson RE, Volberding PA. Clinical manifestations of HIV infection. In: Mandell GL, Douglas RG, Bennett JE, eds. Principles and practice of infectious diseases. New York, NY. Churchill Livingstone, 1990: 1061.

36. Haverkos HW, Gottlieb MS, Killen JY, Edelman R. Classification of HTLV-III/LAV-related diseases. J Infect Dis 1985; 152: 1905.

37. Zolla-Pazner S, DesJarlais DC, Friedman SR, et al. Non-random development of immunologic abnormalities after infection with human immunodeficiency virus: implications for immunologic classification of the disease. Proc Natl Acad Sci USA 1987; 84: 5404-8.

38. Royce RA, Luckmann RS, Fusaro RE, Winkelstein W Jr. The natural history of HIV-1 infection: staging classifications of disease. AIDS 1991; 5: 355–64.

39. Justice AC, Feinstein AR, Wells CK. A new prognostic staging system for the acquired immunodeficiency syndrome. N Engl J Med 1989; 320: 1388–93.

40. Valdiserri RO, Cross GD, Gerber AR, Schwartz RE, Hearn TL. Capacity of US labs to provide TLI in support of early HIV-1 intervention. Am J Public Health 1991; 81: 491–4.

41. CDC. Guidelines for the performance of CD4+ T-cell determinations in persons with human immunodeficiency virus infections. MMWR 1992; 41 (No. RR-8): 1–12.

42. CDC. Surveillance for HIV infection-United States. MMWR 1990; 39: 853, 859–61.

43. Brookmeyer R. Reconstruction and future trends of the AIDS epidemic in the

United States. Science 1991; 253: 37–42.

44. Ciesielski CA, Fleming PL, Berkelman RL. Changing trends in AIDS-indicator diseases in the U.S.- role of therapy and prophylaxis? (abstract 254). 31st Interscience Conference on Antimicrobial Agents and Chemotherapy, Chicago, IL, 1991:141.

45. Hopkins S, Lafferty W, Honey J, Hurlich M. Trends in the outpatient diagnosis of AIDS: implications for epidemiologic analysis and surveillance (abstract T.A.P72). V International Conference on AIDS, Montreal, Canada, 1989:111.

46. Modesitt S, Espenlaub C, Klockner R, Fleming D. AIDS cases diagnosed as outpatients (abstract Th.C.736). VI International Conference on AIDS, San Francisco, CA, 1990; 1:309.

47. Raviglione MC, Narain JP, Kochi A. HIV-associated tuberculosis in developing countries: clinical features, diagnosis, and treatment. Bull WHO 1992; 70:515–26.

48. Selwyn PA, Hartel D, Lewis VA, et al. A prospective study of the risk of tuberculosis among intravenous drug users with human immunodeficiency virus infection. N Engl J Med 1989; 320:545–50.

49. Selwyn PA, Sckell BM, Alcabes P, Friedland GH, Klein RS, Schoenbaum EE. High risk of active tuberculosis in HIV-infected drug users with cutaneous anergy. JAMA 1992; 268:504–9.

50. Braun MM, Badi N, Ryder R, et al. A retrospective cohort study of the risk of tuberculosis among women of childbearing age with HIV-infection in Zaire. Am Rev Resp Dis 1991; 143:501–4.

51. De Cock KM, Soro B, Coulibaly IM, Lucas SB. Tuberculosis and HIV infection in sub-Saharan Africa. JAMA 1992; 268:1581–7.

52. Shafer RW, Chirgwin KD, Glatt AE, Dahdouh MA, Landesman SH, Suster B. HIV prevalence, immunosuppression, and drug resistance in patients with tuberculosis in an area endemic for AIDS. AIDS 1991; 5:399–405.

53. Barber TW, Craven DE, McCabe WR. Bacteremia due to *Mycobacterium tuberculosis* in patients with human immunodeficiency virus infection: a report of 9 cases and review of the literature. Medicine 1990; 69:375–83.

54. CDC. Tuberculosis and human immunodeficiency virus infection: recommendations of the Advisory Committee for the Elimination of Tuberculosis (ACET). MMWR 1989; 38: 23, 243–50.

55. Buehler JW, Devine OJ, Berkelman RL, Chevarley FM. Impact of the human immunodeficiency virus epidemic on mortality trends in young men, United States. Am J Public Health 1990; 80:1080–6.

56. Chu SY, Buehler JW, Berkelman RL. Impact of the human immunodeficiency virus epidemic on mortality in women of reproductive age, United States. JAMA 1990; 264:225–9.

57. Poisky B, Gold JW, Whimbey E, et al. Bacterial pneumonia in patients with the acquired immunodeficiency syndrome. Ann Intern Med 1986; 104:38–41.

58. Selwyn PA, Feingold AR, Hartel D, et al. Increased risk of bacterial pneumonia in HIV-infected intravenous drug users without AIDS. AIDS 1988; 2:267–72.

59. Farizo KM, Buehler JW, Chamberiand ME, et al. Spectrum of disease in persons with human immunodeficiency virus infection in the United States. JAMA 1992; 267:1798–1805.

60. Laga M, Icenogle JP, Marsella R, et al. Genital papillomavirus infection and cervical dysplasia – opportunistic complications of HIV infection. Int J Cancer 1992; 50:45–8.

61. Schafer A, Friedmann W, Mielke M, Schwartiander B, Koch MA. The increased

frequency of cervical dysplasia – neoplasia in women infected with the human immunodeficiency virus is related to the degree of immunosuppression. Am J Obstet Gynecol 1991; 164:593-9.

62. Sadeghi SB, Sadeghi A, Robboy SJ. Prevalence of dysplasia and cancer of the cervix in a nation-wide Planned Parenthood population. Cancer 1988; 61:2359-61.

63. Feingold AR, Vermund SH, Burk RD, et al. Cervical cytologic abnormalities and papillomavirus in women infected with human immunodeficiency virus. J Acquir Immune Defic Syndr 1990; 3:896-903.

64. Maiman M, Fruchter RG, Serur E, Remy JC, Feuer G, Boyce J. Human immunodeficiency virus infection and cervical neoplasia. Gynecol Oncol 1990; 38:377-82.

65. Klein RS, Adachi A, Fleming I, Ho GYF, Burk R. A prospective study of genital neoplasia and human papillomavirus (HPV) in HIV-infected women (abstract). Vol. I. Presented at the VIII International Conference on AIDS/111 STD World Congress, Amsterdam, The Netherlands, July 19–24, 1992.

66. Fruchter R, Maiman M, Serur E, Cuthill S. Cervical intraepithelial neoplasia in HIV-infected women (abstract). Vol. I. Presented at the VII International Conference on AIDS/111 STD World Congress, Amsterdam, The Netherlands, July 19–24, 1992.

67. Richart RM, Wright TC. Controversies and the management of low-grade cervical intraepithelial neoplasia. Cancer (in press).

68. Rellihan MA, Dooley DP, Burke TW, Berkland ME, Longfield RN. Rapidly progressing cervical cancer in a patient with human immunodeficiency virus infection. Gynecol Oncol 1990; 36:435-8.

69. Schwartz LB, Carcangiu ML, Bradham L, Schwartz PE. Rapidly progressive squamous carcinoma of the cervix coexisting with human immunodeficiency virus infection: clinical opinion. Gynecol Oncol 1991; 41:255-8.

70. Richart RM. Cervical intraepithelial neoplasia: a review. In: Sommers SC, ed. Pathology annual, 1973. New York: Appleton-Century-Crofts, 1973, 301-28.

71. CDC. Projections of the number of persons diagnosed with AIDS and the number of immunosuppressed HIV-infected persons – United States, 1992–1994. MMWR 1992; 41 (No. RR-18) (in press).

72. US Congress, Office of Technology Assessment. The CDC's case definition of AIDS: implications of the proposed revisions. Background Paper, OTA-BP-H-89. Washington, DC: US Government Printing Office, August 1992.

73. Torres CG, Turner ME, Harkess JR, Istre GR. Security measures for AIDS and HIV. Am J Public Health 1991; 81:208-9.

74. Kessler HA, Landay A, Pottage JC, Benson CA. Absolute number versus percentage of T-helper lymphocytes in human immunodeficiency virus infection. J Infect Dis 1990; 161:356-7.

Appendix 2: Interim Proposed World Health Organization Clinical Staging System for HIV Infection and Disease

Reproduced from WHO (1990). *Weekly Epidemiological Record*, 20 July. World Health Organization, Geneva.

The Global Programme on AIDS of the World Health Organization (WHO) has developed an interim proposed clinical staging system for HIV infection and disease. Following two technical consultations and a validation exercise, a list of clinical markers felt to have prognostic significance was assembled. The list was hierarchically organized into four prognostic categories and a performance scale was incorporated.

An internationally accepted staging system could be used to: improve clinical management of patients; establish reliable prognoses; help in designing and evaluating drug and vaccine trials; and perform studies on pathogenesis and natural history of HIV infection.

The proposed WHO Staging System is primarily based on clinical criteria. Symptoms, signs and diseases should be defined according to medical judgement. Patients, who should be confirmed HIV-antibody positive and 13 years of age or older, are clinically staged on the basis of the presence of the clinical condition, or performance score, belonging to the highest level.

A further refinement of the system would also include, in addition to the 'clinical axis', a 'laboratory axis'. The laboratory axis would subdivide each clinical category into 3 strata (A, B, C), depending on the number of CD4 lymphocytes per mm^3 (> 500, $200-500$, < 200). If CD4 counts are not available, total lymphocyte counts could be used as an alternative laboratory marker, also in 3 different strata (> 2000, $1000-2000$, < 1000). Patients would then be classified as 1A, 1B, etc. A suffix should be used to indicate if the laboratory classification is based on CD4(c) or lymphocyte[1] counts (e.g. 1Ac, 2B1). If laboratory values are not available, patients could be classified as 1X, 2X, 3X or 4X, or simply as 1, 2, 3, or 4.

Note: for staging purposes, both definitive and presumptive diagnoses are acceptable. However, if, for a particular disease, the diagnostic criteria stated in the surveillance case definition of AIDS are met, then *the case should be reported on the appropriate form*. In addition, in the UK, clinicians are asked to report deaths in HIV infected persons in whom no AIDS indicator disease was diagnosed either presumptively or definitively.

Clinical stage 1
1. Asymptomatic.
2. Persistent generalized lymphadenopathy (PGL)

Performance scale 1: asymptomatic, normal activity.

Clinical stage 2
3. Weight loss, < 10% of body weight.
4. Minor mucocutaneous manifestations (seborrheic dermatitis, prurigo, fungal nail

infections, recurrent oral ulcerations, angular cheilitis).
5. Herpes zoster, within the last 5 years.
6. Recurrent upper respiratory tract infections (i.e.. bacterial sinusitis).

And/or Performance scale 2: symptomatic, normal activity.

Clinical stage 3
7. Weight loss, > 10% of body weight.
8. Unexplained chronic diarrhoea, > 1 month.
9. Unexplained prolonged fever (intermittent or constant), > 1 month.
10. Oral candidiasis (thrush).
11. Oral hairy leukoplakia.
12. Pulmonary tuberculosis, within the past year.
13. Severe bacterial infections (i.e., pneumonia, pyomyositis).

And/or Performance scale 3: bed-ridden, < 50% of the day during the last month.

Clinical Stage 4
14. HIV wasting syndrome, as defined.
15. *Pneumocystis carinii* pneumonia.
16. Toxoplasmosis of the brain.
17. Cryptosporidiosis with diarrhoea, > 1 month.
18. Cryptococcosis, extrapulmonary.
19. Cytomegalovirus (CMV) disease of an organ other than liver, spleen or lymph nodes.
20. Herpes simplex virus (HSV) infection, mucocutaneous > 1 month, or visceral any duration.
21. Progressive multifocal leukoencephalopathy (PML).
22. Any disseminated endemic mycosis (i.e., histoplasmosis, coccidioidomycosis).
23. Candidiasis of the oesophagus, trachea, bronchi or lungs.
24. Atypical mycobacteriosis, disseminated.
25. Non-typhoid salmonella septicaemia.
26. Extrapulmonary tuberculosis.
27. Lymphoma.
28. Kaposi's sarcoma (KS).
29. HIV encephalopathy, as defined.

And/or Performance scale 4: bed-ridden, > 50% of the day during the last month.

Appendix 3: Recommendations for Prevention of HIV Transmission in Health Care Settings

A report from the US Department of Health and Human Services

Reproduced from Centers for Disease Control (1987). *Morbidity and Mortality Weekly Report*, 21 August, **36**(Suppl. 2).

Introduction

Human immunodeficiency virus (HIV), the virus that causes acquired immuno-deficiency syndrome (AIDS), is transmitted through sexual contact and exposure to infected blood or blood components and perinatally from mother to neonate. HIV has been isolated from blood, semen, vaginal secretions, saliva, tears, breast milk, cerebrospinai fluid, amniotic fluid, and urine and is likely to be isolated from other body fluids, secretions, and excretions. However, epidemiologic evidence has implicated only blood, semen, vaginal secretions, and possibly breast milk in transmission.

The increasing prevalence of HIV increases the risk that health care workers will be exposed to blood from patients infected with HIV, especially when blood and body fluid precautions are not followed for all patients. Thus, this document emphasizes the need for health care workers to consider *all* patients as potentially infected with HIV and/or other blood-borne pathogens and to adhere rigorously to infection control precautions for minimizing the risk of exposure to blood and body fluids of all patients.

The recommendations contained in this document consolidate and update CDC recommendations published earlier for preventing HIV transmission in health care settings: precautions for clinical and laboratory staffs[1] and precautions for health care workers and allied professionals[2]; recommendations for preventing HIV transmission in the workplace[3] and during invasive procedures[4]; recommendations for preventing possible transmission of HIV from tears[5]; and recommendations for providing dialysis treatment for HIV infected patients[6]. These recommendations also update portions of the 'Guideline for Isolation Precautions in Hospitals'[7] and re-emphasize some of the recommendations contained in 'Infection Control Practices for Dentistry'[8]. The recommendations contained in this document have been developed for use in health care settings and emphasize the need to treat blood and other body fluids from *all* patients as potentially infective. These same prudent precautions also should be taken in other settings in which persons may be exposed to blood or other body fluids.

Definition of health care workers

Health care workers are defined as persons, including students and trainees, whose activities involve contact with patients or with blood or other body fluids from patients in a health care setting.

Health care workers with AIDS

As of July 10, 1987, total of 1875 (5.8%) of 32 395 adults with AIDS, who had been reported to the CDC national surveillance system and for whom occupational information was available, reported being employed in a health care or clinical laboratory setting. In comparison, 6.8 million persons – representing 5.6% of the US labor force – were employed in health services. Of the health care workers with AIDS, 95% have been reported to exhibit high-risk behaviour; for the remaining 5%, the means of HIV acquisition was undetermined. Health care workers with AIDS were significantly more likely than other workers to have an undetermined risk (5% versus 3%, respectively). For both health care workers and non health care workers with AIDS, the proportion with an undetermined risk has not increased since 1982.

AIDS patients initially reported as not belonging to recognized risk groups are investigated by state and local health departments to determine whether possible risk factors exist. Of all health care workers with AIDS reported to CDC who were initially characterized as not having an identified risk and for whom follow-up information was available, 66% have been reclassified because risk factors were identified or because the patient was found not to meet the surveillance case definition for AIDS. Of the 87 health care workers currently categorized as having no identifiable risk, information is incomplete on 16 (18%) because of death or refusal to be interviewed; 38 (44%) are still being investigated. The remaining 33 (38%) health care workers were interviewed or had other follow-up information available. The occupations of these 33 were as follows: five physicians (15%), three of whom were surgeons; one dentist (3%); three nurses (9%); nine nursing assistants (27%); seven housekeeping or maintenance workers (21 %); three clinical laboratory technicians (9%); one therapist (3%); and four others who did not have contact with patients (12%). Although 15 of these 33 health care workers reported parenteral and/or other non-needlestick exposure to blood or body fluids from patients in the 10 years preceding their diagnosis of AIDS, none of these exposures involved a patient with AIDS or known HIV infection.

Risk to health care workers of acquiring HIV in health care settings

Health care workers with documented percutaneous or mucous membrane exposures to blood or body fluids of HIV infected patients have been prospectively evaluated to determine the risk of infection after such exposures. As of June 30, 1987, 883 health care workers have been tested for antibody to HIV in an ongoing surveillance project conducted by CDC[9]. Of these, 708 (80%) had percutaneous exposures to blood, and 175 (20%) had a mucous membrane or an open wound contaminated by blood or body fluid. Of 396 health care workers, each of whom had only a convalescent-phase serum sample obtained and tested ≥ 90 days post-exposure, one – for whom heterosexual transmission could not be ruled out – was seropositive for HIV antibody. For 425 additional health care workers, both acute and convalescent phase serum samples were obtained and tested; none of 74 health care workers with nonpercutaneous exposures seroconverted, and three (0.9%) of 351 with percutaneous exposures seroconverted. None of these three health care workers had other documented risk factors for infection.

Two other prospective studies to assess the risk of nosocomial acquisition of HIV infection for health care workers are ongoing in the United States. As of April 30,

1987, 332 health care workers with a total of 453 needlestick or mucous membrane exposures to the blood or other body fluids of HIV infected patients were tested for HIV antibody at the National Institutes of Health[10]. These exposed workers included 103 with needlestick injuries and 229 with mucous membrane exposures; none had seroconverted. A similar study at the University of California of 129 health care workers with documented needlestick injuries or mucous membrane exposures to blood or other body fluids from patients with HIV infection has not identified any seroconversions[11]. Results of a prospective study in the United Kingdom identified no evidence of transmission among 150 health care workers with parenteral or mucous membrane exposures to blood or other body fluids, secretions, or excretions from patients with HIV infection[12].

In addition to health care workers enrolled in prospective studies, eight persons who provided care to infected patients and denied other risk factors have been reported to have acquired HIV infection. Three of these health care workers had needlestick exposures to blood from infected patients[13–15]. Two were persons who provided nursing care to infected persons; although neither sustained a needlestick, both had extensive contact with blood or other body fluids, and neither observed recommended barrier precautions[16,17]. The other three were health care workers with non-needlestick exposures to blood from infected patients[15]. Although the exact route of transmission for these last three infections is not known, all three persons had direct contact of their skin with blood from infected patients, all had skin lesions that may have been contaminated by blood, and one also had a mucous membrane exposure.   A total of 1231 dentists and hygienists, many of whom practised in areas with many AIDS cases, participated in a study to determine the prevalence of antibody to HIV; one dentist (0.1 %) had HIV antibody. Although no exposure to a known HIV infected person could be documented, epidemiologic investigation did not identify any other risk factor for infection. The infected dentist, who also had a history of sustaining needlestick injuries and trauma to his hands, did not routinely wear gloves when providing dental care[19].

Precautions to prevent transmission of HIV

Universal precautions
Since medical history and examination cannot reliably identify all patients infected with HIV or other blood-borne pathogens, blood and body fluid precautions should be consistently used for *all* patients. This approach, previously recommended by CDC[3,4], and referred to as 'universal blood and body fluid precautions' or 'universal precautions', should be used in the care of *all* patients, especially including those in emergency care settings in which the risk of blood exposure is increased and the infection status of the patient is usually unknown[20].

1. All health care workers should routinely use appropriate barrier precautions to prevent skin and mucous membrane exposure when contact with blood or other body fluids of any patient is anticipated. Gloves should be worn for touching blood and body fluids, mucous membranes, or non-intact skin of all patients, for handling items or surfaces soiled with blood or body fluids, and for performing venepuncture and other vascular access procedures. Gloves should be changed after contact with each patient. Masks and protective eyewear or face shields should be worn during procedures that are likely to generate droplets of blood or

other body fluids to prevent exposure of mucous membranes of the mouth, nose, and eyes. Gowns or aprons should be worn during procedures that are likely to generate splashes of blood or other body fluids.

2. Hands and other skin surfaces should be washed immediately and thoroughly if contaminated with blood or other body fluids. Hands should be washed immediately after gloves are removed.

3. All health care workers should take precautions to prevent injuries caused by needles, scalpels, and other sharp instruments or devices during procedures; when cleaning used instruments; during disposal of used needles; and when handling sharp instruments after procedures. To prevent needlestick injuries, needles should not be recapped, purposely bent or broken by hand, removed from disposable syringes, or otherwise manipulated by hand. After they are used, disposable syringes and needles, scalpel blades, and other sharp items should, be placed in puncture-resistant containers for disposal; the puncture-resistant containers should be located as close as practical to the use area. Large bore reusabie needles should be placed in a puncture-resistant container for transport to the reprocessing area.

4. Although saliva has not been implicated in HIV transmission, to minimize the need for emergency mouth-to-mouth resuscitation, mouthpieces, resuscitation bags, or other ventilation devices should be available for use in areas in which the need for resuscitation is predictable.

5. Health care workers who have exudative lesions or weeping dermatitis should refrain from all direct patient care and from handling patient-care equipment until the condition resolves.

6. Pregnant health care workers are not known to be at greater risk of contracting HIV infection than health care workers who are not pregnant; however, if a health care worker develops HIV infection during pregnancy, the infant is at risk of infection resulting from perinatal transmisison. Because of this risk, pregnant health care workers should be especially familiar with and strictly adhere to precautions to minimize the risk of HIV transmission.

Implementation of universal blood and body fluid precautions for *all* patients eliminates the need for use of the isolation category of 'Blood and Body Fluid Precautions' previously recommended by CDC[7] for patients known or suspected to be infected with blood-borne pathogens. Isolation precautions (e.g. enteric, 'AFB'[7]) should be used as necessary if associated conditions, such as infectious diarrhoea or tuberculosis, are diagnosed or suspected.

Precautions for invasive procedures

In this document, an invasive procedure is defined as surgical entry into tissues, cavities, or organs or repair of major traumatic injuries (1) in an operating or delivery room, emergency department, or out-patient setting, including both physicians' and dentists' offices; (2) cardiac catheterization and angiographic procedures; (3) a vaginal or caesarean delivery or other invasive obstetric procedure during which bleeding may occur; or (4) the manipulation, cutting, or removal of any oral or perioral tissues, including tooth structure, during which bleeding occurs or the potential for bleeding exists. The universal blood and body fluid precautions listed above, combined with the precautions listed below, should be the minimum precautions for *all* such invasive procedures.

1. All health care workers who participate in invasive procedures must routinely use

appropriate barrier precautions to prevent skin and mucous membrane contact with blood and other body fluids of all patients. Gloves and surgical masks must be worn for all invasive procedures. Protective eyewear or face shields should be worn for procedures that commonly result in the generation of droplets, splashing of blood or other body fluids, or the generation of bone chips. Gowns or aprons made of materials that provide an effective barrier should be worn during invasive procedures that are likely to result in the splashing of blood or other body fluids. All health care workers who perform or assist in vaginal or caesarean deliveries should wear gloves and gowns when handling the placenta or the infant until blood and amniotic fluid have been removed from the infant's skin and should wear gloves during post-delivery care of the umbilical cord.

2. If a glove is torn or a needlestick or other injury occurs, the glove should be removed and a new glove used as promptly as patient safety permits; the needle or instrument involved in the incident should also be removed from the sterile field.

Precautions for dentistry

(General infection control precautions are more specifically addressed in previous recommendations for infection control practices for dentistry[8].

Blood, saliva, and gingival fluid from *all* dental patients should be considered infective. Special emphasis should be placed on the following precautions for preventing transmission of blood-borne pathogens in dental practice in both institutional and non-institutional settings.

1. In addition to wearing gloves for contact with oral mucous membranes of all patients, all dental workers should wear surgical masks and protective eyewear or chin-length plastic face shields during dental procedures in which splashing or spattering of blood, saliva, or gingival fluids is likely. Rubber dams, high-speed evacuation, and proper patient positioning, when appropriate, should be utilized to minimize generation of droplets and spatter.

2. Handpieces should be sterilized after use with each patient, since blood, saliva, or gingival fluid of patients may be aspirated into the handpiece or waterline. Handpieces that cannot be sterilized should at least be flushed, the outside surface cleaned and wiped with a suitable chemical germicide, and then rinsed. Handpieces should be flushed at the beginning of the day and after use with each patient. Manufacturers' recommendations should be followed for use and maintenance of waterlines and check valves and for flushing of handpieces. The same precautions should be used for ultrasonic scalers and air/water syringes.

3. Blood and saliva should be thoroughly and carefully cleaned from material that has been used in the mouth (e.g. impression materials, bite registration), especially before polishing and grinding intra-oral devices. Contaminated materials, impressions, and intra-oral devices should also be cleaned and disinfected before being handled in the dental laboratory and before they are placed in the patient's mouth. Because of the increasing variety of dental materials used intra-orally, dental workers should consult with manufacturers as to the stability of specific materials when using disinfection procedures.

4. Dental equipment and surfaces that are difficult to disinfect (e.g. light handles or X-ray-unit heads) and that may become contaminated should be wrapped with impervious backed paper, aluminum foil, or clear plastic wrap. The coverings

should be removed and discarded, and clean coverings should be put in place after use with each patient.

Precautions for autopsies or morticians' services

In addition to the universal blood and body fluid precautions listed above, the following precautions should be used by persons performing postmortem procedures:

1. All persons performing or assisting in postmortem procedures should wear gloves, masks, protective eyewear, gowns, and waterproof aprons.
2. Instruments and surfaces contaminated during postmortem procedures should be decontaminated with an appropriate chemical germicide.

Precautions for dialysis

Patients with end-stage renal disease who are undergoing maintenance dialysis and who have HIV infection can be dialyzed in hospital-based or free-standing dialysis units using conventional infection-control precautions[21]. Universal blood and body fluid precautions should be used when dialyzing *all* patients.

Strategies for disinfecting the dialysis fluid pathways of the haemodialysis machine are targeted to control bacterial contamination and generally consist of using 500–750 parts per million (ppm) of sodium hypochlorite (household bleach) for 30–40 minutes or 1.5–2.0% formaldehyde overnight. In addition, several chemical germicides formulated to disinfect dialysis machines are commercially available. None of these protocols or procedures need to be changed fordialyzing patients infected with HIV.

Patients infected with HIV can be dialyzed by either haemodialysis or peritoneal dialysis and do not need to be isolated from other patients. The type of dialysis treatment (i.e. haemodialysis or peritoneal dialysis) should be based on the needs of the patient. The dialyzer may be discarded after each use. Alternatively, centers that reuse dialyzers – i.e. a specific single-use dialyzer is issued to a specific patient, removed, cleaned, disinfected, and reused several times on the same patient only – may include HIV infected patients in the dialyzer-reuse program. An individual dialyzer must never be used on more than one patient.

Precautions for laboratories

(Additional precautions for research and industrial laboratories are addressed elsewhere[22,23].)

Blood and other body fluids from *all* patients should be considered infective. To supplement the universal blood and body fluid precautions listed above, the following precautions are recommended for health care workers in clinical laboratories.

1. All specimens of blood and body fluids should be put in a well-constructed container with a secure lid to prevent leaking during transport. Care should be taken when collecting each specimen to avoid contaminating the outside of the container and of the laboratory form accompanying the specimen.
2. All persons processing blood and body fluid specimens (e.g. removing tops from vacuum tubes) should wear gloves. Masks and protective eyewear should be worn if mucous membrane contact with blood or body fluids is anticipated. Gloves should be changed and hands washed after completion of specimen processing.
3. For routine procedures, such as histologic and pathologic studies or microbiologic culturing, a biological safety cabinet is not necessary. However, biological

safety cabinets (Class I or II) should be used whenever procedures are conducted that have a high potential for generating droplets. These include activities such as blending, sonicating, and vigorous mixing.

4. Mechanical pipetting devices should be used for manipulating all liquids in the laboratory. Mouth pipetting must not be done.

5. Use of needles and syringes should be limited to situations in which there is no alternative, and the recommendations for preventing injuries with needles outlined under universal precautions should be followed.

6. Laboratory work surfaces should be decontaminated with an appropriate chemical germicide after a spill of blood or other body fluids and when work activities are completed.

7. Contaminated materials used in laboratory tests should be decontaminated before reprocessing or be placed in bags and disposed of in accordance with institutional policies for disposal of infective waste[24].

8. Scientific equipment that has been contaminated with blood or other body fluids should be decontaminated and cleaned before being repaired in the laboratory or transported to the manufacturer.

9. All persons should wash their hands after completing laboratory activities and should remove protective clothing before leaving the laboratory.

Implementation of universal blood and body-fluid precautions for *all* patients eliminates the need for warning labels on specimens since blood and other body fluids from all patients should be considered infective.

Environmental considerations for HIV transmission

No environmentally mediated mode of HIV transmission has been documented. Nevertheless, the precautions described below should be taken routinely in the care of *all* patients.

Sterilization and disinfection

Standard sterilization and disinfection procedures for patient care equipment currently recommended for use[25,25] in a variety of health care settings – including hospitals, medical and dental clinics and offices, haemodialysis centers, emergency care facilities, and long-term nursing care facilities – are adequate to sterilize or disinfect instruments, devices, or other items contaminated with blood or other body fluids from persons infected with blood-borne pathogens including HIV[21,23].

Instruments or devices that enter sterile tissue or the vascular system of any patient or through which blood flows should be sterilized before reuse. Devices or items that contact intact mucous membranes should be sterilized or receive high-level disinfection, a procedure that kills vegetative organisms and viruses but not necessarily large numbers of bacterial spores. Chemical germicides that are registered with the US Environmental Protection Agency (EPA) as 'sterilants' may be used either for sterilization or for high-level disinfection depending on contact time.

Contact lenses used in trial fittings should be disinfected after each fitting by using a hydrogen peroxide contact lens disinfecting system or, if compatible, with heat (78°C–80°C [172.4°F–176.0°F]) for 10 minutes.

Medical devices or instruments that require sterilization or disinfection should be thoroughly cleaned before being exposed to the germicide, and the manufacturer's instructions for the use of the germicide should be followed. Further, it is important that the manufacturer's specifications for compatibility of the medical device with chemical germicides be closely followed. Information on specific label claims of commercial germicides can be obtained by writing to the Disinfectants Branch, Office of Pesticides, Environmental Protection Agency, 401 M Street, SW, Washington, D.C. 20460.

Studies have shown that HIV is inactivated rapidly after being exposed to commonly used chemical germicides at concentrations that are much lower than used in practice[27-30]. Embalming fluids are similar to the types of chemical germicides that have been tested and found to completely inactivate HIV. In addition to commercially available chemical germicides, a solution of sodium hypochlorite (household bleach) prepared daily is an inexpensive and effective germicide. Concentrations ranging from approximately 500 ppm (1:100 dilution of household bleach) sodium hypochlorite to 5000 ppm (1:10 dilution of household bleach) are effective depending on the amount of organic material (e.g. blood, mucus) present on the surface to be cleaned and disinfected. Commercially available chemical germicides may be more compatible with certain medical devices that might be corroded by repeated exposure to sodium hypochlorite, especially to the 1:10 dilution.

Survival of HIV in the environment
The most extensive study on the survival of HIV after drying involved greatly concentrated HIV samples, i.e. 10 million tissue-culture infectious doses per milliliter[31]. This concentration is at least 100 000 times greater than that typically found in the blood or serum of patients with HIV infection. HIV was detectable by tissue culture techniques 1–3 days after drying, but the rate of inactivation was rapid. Studies performed at CDC have also shown that drying HIV causes a rapid (within several hours) 1–2 log (90–99%) reduction in HIV concentration. In tissue culture fluid, cell-free HIV could be detected up to 15 days at room temperature, up to 11 days at 37°C (98.6°F), and up to one day if the HIV was cell associated.

When considered in the context of environmental conditions in health care facilities, these results do not require any changes in currently recommended sterilization, disinfection, or housekeeping strategies. When medical devices are contaminated with blood or other body fluids, existing recommendations include the cleaning of these instruments, followed by disinfection or sterilization, depending on the type of medical device. These protocols assume 'worst-case' conditions of extreme virologic and microbiologic contamination, and whether viruses have been inactivated after drying plays no role in formulating these strategies. Consequently, no changes in published procedures for cleaning, disinfecting, or sterilizing need to be made.

Housekeeping
Environmental surfaces such as walls, floors, and other surfaces are not associated with transmission of infections to patients or health care workers. Therefore, extraordinary attempts to disinfect or sterilize these environmental surfaces are not necessary. However, cleaning and removal of soil should be done routinely.

Cleaning schedules and methods vary according to the area of the hospital or institution, type of surface to be cleaned, and the amount and type of soil present. Horizontal surfaces (e.g. bedside tables and hard-surfaced flooring) in patient care areas are usually cleaned on a regular basis, when soiling or spills occur, and when patient is discharged. Cleaning of walls, blinds, and curtains is recommended only if they are visibly soiled. Disinfectant fogging is an unsatisfactory method of decontaminating air and surfaces and is not recommended.

Disinfectant-detergent formulations registered by EPA can be used for cleaning environmental surfaces, but the actual physical removal of microorganisms by scrubbing is probably at least as important as any antimicrobial effect of the cleaning agent used. Therefore, cost, safety, and acceptability by house-keepers can be the main criteria for selecting any such registered agent. The manufacturers' instructions for appropriate use should be followed.

Cleaning and decontaminating spills of blood or other body fluids

Chemical germicides that are approved for use as 'hospital disinfectants' and are tuberculocidal when used at recommended dilutions can be used to decontaminate spills of blood and other body fluids. Strategies for decontaminating spills of blood and other body fluids in a patient care setting are different than for spills of cultures or other materials in clinical, public health, or research laboratories. In patient care areas, visible material should first be removed and then the area should be decontaminated. With large spills of cultured or concentrated infectious agents in the laboratory, the contaminated area should be flooded with a liquid germicide before cleaning, then decontaminated with fresh germicidal chemical. In both settings, gloves should be worn during the cleaning and decontaminating procedures.

Laundry

Although soiled linen has been identified as a source of large numbers of certain pathogenic microorganisms, the risk of actual disease transmission is negligible. Rather than rigid procedures and specifications, hygienic and common-sense storage and processing of clean and soiled linen are recommended[26]. Soiled linen should be handled as little as possible and with minimum agitation to prevent gross microbial contamination of the air and of persons handling the linen. All soiled linen should be bagged at the location where it was used; it should not be sorted or rinsed in patient care areas. Linen soiled with blood or body fluids should be placed and transported in bags that prevent leakage. If hot water is used, linen should be washed with detergent in water at least 71°C (160°F) for 25 minutes. If low-temperature (< 70°C (158°F)) laundry cycles are used, chemicals suitable for low-temperature washing at proper use concentration should be used.

Infective waste

There is no epidemiologic evidence to suggest that most hospital waste is any more infective than residential waste. Moreover, there is no epidemiologic evidence that hospital waste has caused disease in the community as a result of improper disposal. Therefore, identifying wastes for which special precautions are indicated is largely a matter of judgement about the relative risk of disease transmission. The most practi-cal approach to the management of infective waste is to identify those wastes with the potential for causing infection during handling and disposal and for which some spe-cial precautions appear prudent. Hospital wastes for which special precautions appear prudent include microbiology laboratory waste, pathology waste, and blood speci-mens or blood products. While any item that has had contact with blood, exudates, or secretions may be potentially infective, it is not usually considered practical or necessary to treat all such waste as infective[23,26]. Infective waste, in general, should either be incinerated or should be autoclaved before disposal in a sanitary landfill. Bulk blood, suctioned fluids, excretions, and secretions may be carefully poured down a drain connected to a sanitary sewer. Sanitary sewers may also be used to dispose of other infectious wastes capable of being ground and flushed into the sewer.

Implementation of recommended precautions

Employers of heatth care workers should ensure that policies exist for:

1. Initial orientation and continuing education and training of all health care workers – including students and trainees – on the epidemiology, modes of transmission, and prevention of HIV and other blood-borne infections and the need for routine use of universal blood and body-fluid precautions for *all* patients.
2. Provision of equipment and supplies necessary to minimize the risk of infection with HIV and other blood-borne pathogens.
3. Monitoring adherence to recommended protective measures. When monitoring reveals a failure to follow recommended precautions, counseling, education, and/or retraining should be provided, and, if necessary, appropriate disciplinary action should be considered.

Professional associations and labor organizations, through continuing education efforts, should emphasize the need for health care workers to follow recommended precautions.

Serologice testing for HIV infection

Backgound
A person is identified as infected with HIV when a sequence of tests, starting with repeated enzyme immunoassays (EIA) and including a Westem blot or similar, more specific assay, are repeatedly reactive. Persons infected with HIV usually develop antibody against the virus within 6–12 weeks after infection.

The sensitivity of the currently licensed EIA tests is at least 99% when they are performed under optimal laboratory conditions on serum specimens from persons infected for ≥ 12 weeks. Optimal laboratory conditions include the use of reliable reagents, provision of continuing education of personnel, quality control of procedures, and participation in performance evaluation programs. Given this performance, the probability of a false negative test is remote except during the first several weeks after infection, before detectable antibody is present. The proportion of infected persons with a false negative test attributed to absence of antibody in the early stages of infection is dependent on both the incidence and prevalence of HIV infection in a population (Table 1).

The specificity of the currently licensed EIA tests is approximately 99% when repeatedly reactive tests are considered. Repeat testing of initially reactive specimens by EIA is required to reduce the likelihood of laboratory error. To increase further the specificity of serologic tests, laboratories must use a supplemental test, most often the Westem blot, to validate repeatedly reactive EIA results. Under optimal laboratory conditions, the sensitivity of the Western blot test is comparable to or greater than that of a repeatedly reactive EIA, and the Western blot is highly specific when strict criteria are used to interpret the test results. The testing sequence of a repeatedly reactive EIA and a positive Western blot test is highly predictive of HIV infection, even in a population with a low prevalence of infection (Table 2). If the Western blot test result is indeterminant, the testing sequence is considered equivocal for HIV infection. When this occurs, the Western blot test should be repeated on the same serum sample, and, if still indeterminant, the testing sequence should be repeated on a sample collected 3–6 months later. Use of other supplemental tests may aid in interpreting of results on samples that are persistently indeterminant by Western blot.

Testing of patients

Previous CDC recommendations have emphasized the value of HIV serologic testing of patients for: (1) management of parenteral or mucous membrane exposures of health care workers, (2) patient diagnosis and management, and (3) counselling and serologic testing to prevent and control HIV transmission in the community. In addition, more recent recommendations have stated that hospitals, in conjunction with state and local health departments, should periodically determine the prevalence of HIV infection among patients from age groups at highest risk of infection[32].

Adherence to universal blood and body fluid precautions recommended for the care of all patients will minimize the risk of transmission of HIV and other blood-borne pathogens from patients to health care workers. The utility of routine HIV serologic testing of patients as an adjunct to universal precautions is unknown. Results of such testing may not be available in emergency or outpatient settings. In addition, some recently infected patients will not have detectable antibody to HIV (Table 1).

Personnel in some hospitals have advocated serologic testing of patients in settings in which exposure of health care workers to large amounts of patients' blood may be

Table 1 Estimated annual number of patients infected with HIV not detected by HIV-antibody testing in a hypothetical hospital with 10 000 admissions/year. The estimates are based on the following assumptions: (1) the sensitivity of the screening test is 99% (i.e. 99% of HIV infected persons with antibody will be detected); (2) persons infected with HIV will not develop detectable antibody (seroconvert) until 6 weeks (1.5 months) after infection; (3) new infections occur at an equal rate throughout the year; (4) calculations of the number of HIV infected persons in the patient population are based on the mid-year prevalence, which is the beginning prevalence plus half the annual incidence of infections

Beginning prevalence of HIV infection	Annual incidence of HIV infection	Approximate number of HIV infected patients	Approximate number of HIV infected patients not detected
5.0%	1.0%	550	17–18
5.0%	0.5%	525	11–12
1.0%	0.2%	110	3–4
1.0%	0.1%	105	2–3
0.1%	0.02%	11	0–1
0.1%	0.01%	11	0–1

anticipated. Specific patients for whom serologic testing has been advocated include those undergoing major operative procedures and those undergoing treatment in critical care units, especially if they have conditions involving uncontrolled bleeding. Decisions regarding the need to establish testing programmes for patients should be made by physicians or individual institutions. In addition, when deemed appropriate, testing of individual patients may be performed on agreement between the patient and the physician providing care.

In addition to the universal precautions recommended for all patients, certain additional precautions for the care of HIV infected patients undergoing major surgical operations have been proposed by personnel in some hospitals. For example, surgical procedures on an HIV infected patient might be altered so that hand-to-hand passing of sharp instruments would be eliminated; stapling instruments rather than hand-suturing equipment might be used to perform tissue approximation; electro-cautery devices rather than scalpels might be used as cutting instruments; and, even though uncomfortable, gowns that totally prevent seepage of blood onto the skin of members of the operative team might be worn. While such modifications might further minimize the risk of HIV infection for members of the operative team, some of these techniques could result in prolongation of operative time and could potentially have an adverse effect on the patient.

Testing programmes, if developed, should include the following principles:

- Obtaining consent for testing.
- Informing patients of test results, and providing counselling for seropositive patients by properly trained persons.
- Assuring that confidentiality safeguards are in place to limit knowledge of test results to those directly involved in the care of infected patients or as required by law.
- Assuring that identification of infected patients will not result in denial of needed care or provision of suboptimal care.
- Evaluating prospectively (1) the efficacy of the program in reducing the incidence of parenteral, mucous membrane, or significant cutaneous exposures of health care workers to the blood or other body fluids of HIV infected patients and (2) the effect of modified procedures on patients.

Table 2 Predictive value of positive HIV antibody tests in hypothetical populations with different prevalences of infection

	Prevalence of infection	Predictive value of positive test[1]
Repeatedly reactive enzyme immunoassay (EIA)[2]	0.2%	28.41%
	2.0%	80.16%
	20.0%	98.02%
Repeatedly reactive EIA followed by positive Western blot (WB)[3]	0.2%	99.75%
	2.0%	99.97%
	20.0%	99.99%

[1] Proportion of persons with positive test results who are actually infected with HIV.
[2] Assumes EIA sensitivity of 99.0% and specificity of 99.5%.
[3] Assumes WB sensitivity of 99.0% and specificity of 99.9%.

Testing of health care workers

Although transmission of HIV from infected health care workers to patients has not been reported, transmission during invasive procedures remains a possibility. Transmission of hepatitis B virus (HBV) – a blood-borne agent with a considerably greater potential for nosocomial spread – from health care workers to patients has been documented. Such transmission has occurred in situations (e.g. oral and gynaecologic surgery) in which health care workers, when tested, had very high concentrations of HBV in their blood (at least 100 million infectious virus particles per millilitre, a concentration much higher than occurs with HIV infection), and the health care workers sustained a puncture wound while performing invasive procedures or had exudative or weeping lesions or microlacerations that allowed virus to contaminate instruments or open wounds of patients[33,34].

The hepatitis B experience indicates that only those health care workers who perform certain types of invasive procedures have transmitted HBV to patients. Adherence to recommendations in this document will minimize the risk of transmission of HIV and other blood-borne pathogens from health care workers to patients during invasive procedures. Since transmission of HIV from infected health care workers performing invasive procedures to their patients has not been reported and would be expected to occur only very rarely, if at ail, the utility of routine testing of such health care workers to prevent transmission of HIV cannot be assessed. If consideration is given to developing a serologic testing programme for health care workers who perform invasive procedures, the frequency of testing, as well as the issues of consent, confidentially, and consequences of test results – as previously outlined for testing programmes for patients – must be addressed.

Management of infected health care workers

Health care workers with impaired immune systems resulting from HIV infection or other causes are at increased risk of acquiring or experiencing serious complications of infectious disease. Of particular concern is the risk of severe infection following exposure to patients with infectious diseases that are easily transmitted if appropriate precautions are not taken (e.g. measles, varicella). Any health care worker with an impaired immune system should be counselled about the potential risk associated with taking care of patients with any transmissible infection and should continue to follow existing recommendations for infection control to minimize risk of exposure to other infectious agents[7,35]. Recommendations of the Immunization Practices Advisory Committee (ACIP) and institutional policies concerning requirements for vaccinating health care workers with live virus vaccines (e.g. measles, rubella) should also be considered.

The question of whether workers infected with HIV – especially those who perform invasive procedures – can adequately and safely be allowed to perform patient care duties or whether their work assignments should be changed must be determined on an individual basis. These decisions should be made by the health care worker's personal physician(s) in conjunction with the medical directors and personnel health service staff of the employing institution or hospital.

Management of exposures

If a health care worker has a parenteral (e.g. needlestick or cut) or mucous membrane (e.g. splash to the eye or mouth) exposure to blood or other body fluids or has a cutaneous exposure involving large amounts of blood or prolonged contact with blood – especially when the exposed skin is chapped, abraded, or afflicted with dermatitis – the source patient should be informed of the incident and tested for serologic evidence of HIV infection after consent is obtained. Policies should be developed for testing source patients in situations in which consent cannot be obtained (e.g. an unconscious patient).

If the source patient has AIDS, is positive for HIV antibody, or refuses the test, the health care worker should be counselled regarding the risk of infection and evaluated clinically and serologically for evidence of HIV infection as soon as possible after the exposure. The health care worker should be advised to report and seek medical evaluation for any acute febrile illness that occurs within 12 weeks after the exposure. Such an illness – particularly one characterized by fever, rash, or lymphadenopathy – may be indicative of recent HIV infection. Seronegative health care workers should be retested 6 weeks post-exposure and on a periodic basis thereafter (e.g.1 2 weeks and 6 months after exposure) to determine whether transmission has occured. During this follow-up period – especially the first 6–12 weeks after exposure, when most infected persons are expected to seroconvert – exposed health care workers should follow US Public Health Service (PHS) recommendations for preventing transmission of HIV [36, 37],

No further follow-up of a health care worker exposed to infection as described above is necessary if the source patient is seronegative unless the source patient is at high risk of HIV infection. in the latter case, a subsequent specimen (e.g. 12 weeks following exposure) may be obtained from the health care worker for antibody testing. If the source patient cannot be identified, decisions regarding appropriate follow-up should be individualized. Serologic testing should be available to all health care workers who are concerned that they may have been infected with HIV.

If a patient has a parenteral or mucous membrane exposure to blood or other body fluid of a health care worker, the patient should be informed of the incident, and the same procedure outlined above for management of exposures should be followed for both the source health care worker and the exposed patient.

References

1. CDC (1982). Acquired immunodeficiency syndrome (AIDS): Precautions for clinical and laboratory staffs. *MMWR*, 31:577–80
2. CDC (1983). Acquired immunodeficiency syndrome (AIDS): Precautions for health-care workers and allied professionals. *MMWR*, 32:450–1
3. CDC (1985). Recommendations for preventing transmission of infection with human T-lymphotropic virus type III/lymphadenopathy-associated virus in the workplace. *MMWR*, 34:681–6, 691–5
4. CDC (1986). Recommendations for preventing transmission of infection with human T-lymphotropic virus type III/lymphadenopathy-associated virus during invasive procedures. *MMWR*, 35:221–3
5. CDC (1985). Recommendations for preventing possible transmission of human T-lymphotropic virus type III/lymphadenopathy-associated virus from tears.

MMWR, 34:533–4

6. CDC (1986). Recommendations for providing dialysis treatment to patients infected with human T-lymphotropic virus type III/lymphadenopathy-associated virus infection. *MMWR*, 35:376–8, 383

7. Garner, J.S. and Simmons, B.P. (1983). Guideline for isolation precautions in hospitals. *Infect Control*, (suppl):245–325

8. CDC (1986). Recommended infection control practices for dentistry. *MMWR*, 35:237–42

9. McCray, E. (1986). The Cooperative Needlestick Surveillance Group. Occupational risk of the acquired immunodeficiency syndrome among health care workers. *N Engl J Med*. 314:1127–32

10. Henderson, D.K., Saah, A.J., Zak, B J., et al. (1986). Risk of nosocomial infection with human T-cell lymphotropic virus type III/lymphadenopathy-associated virus in a large cohort of intensively exposed health care workers. *Ann Intern Med*. 104:644–7

11. Gerberding, J.L., Bryant-LeBlanc, C.E., Nelson, K., et al. (1987). Risk of transmitting the human immunodeficiency virus, cytomegalovirus, and hepatitis B virus to health care workers exposed to patients with AIDS and AIDS-related conditions. *J Infect Dis*, 156:1–8

12. McEvoy, M., Porter, K., Mortimer, P., Simmons, N. and Shanson, D. (1987). Prospective study of clinical, laboratory, and ancillary staff with accidental exposures to blood or other body fluids from patients infected with HIV. *Br Med J*. 294:1595–7

13. Anonymous. (1984). Needlestick transmission of HTLV–III from a patient infected in Africa. *Lancet* 2:1376–7

14. Oksenhendler, E., Harzic, M., Le Roux, J.M., Rabian, C., Clauvel, J.P. (1986). HIV infection with seroconversion after a superficial needlestick injury to the finger. *N Engl J Med*. 315:582

15. Neisson-Vernant, C., Arfi, S., Mathez, D., Leibowitch, J. and Monplaisir, N. (1986). Needlestick HIV seroconversion in a nurse. *Lancet*, 2:814

16. Grint P. and McEvoy, M. (1985). Two associated cases of the acquired immune deficiency syndrome (AIDS). *PHLS Commun Dis Rep*, 42:4

17. CDC (1986). Apparent transmission of human T-lymphotropic virus type III/lymphadenopathy-associated virus from a child to a mother providing health care. *MMWR*, 35:76–9

18. CDC (1987). Update: Human immunodeficiency virus infections in health care workers exposed to blood of infected patients. *MMWR*, 36:285–9

19. Kline, R.S., Phelan, J., Friedland, G.H., et al. (1985). Low occupational risk for HIV infection for dental professionals (Abstract). In *Abstracts from the III International Conference on AIDS*, 1–5 June. Washington, DC, 155

20. Baker, J.L., Kelen, G.D., Sivertson, K.T. and Quinn, T.C. (1987). Unsuspected human immunodeficiency virus in critically ill emergency patients. *JAMA*, 257:2609–11

21. Favero, M.S. (1985). Dialysis-associated diseases and their control. In *Hospital infections* Bennet, J.V. and Brachman, P.S. (eds), pp 267–84. Little, Brown and Company, Boston.

22. Richardson, J.H., and Barkley, W.E. (eds). (1984). Biosafety in microbiological and biomedical laboratories, US Department of Health and Human Services, Public Health Service, Washington, DC. HHS publication no. (CDC) 84–8395

23. CDC. (1986). Human T-lymphotropic virus type III/lymphadenopathy-associated

virus: Agent summary statement. *MMWR*, 35:540–2, 547–9

24. Environmental Protection Agency, (1986). EPA guide for infectious waste management. Environmental Protection Agency, Washington, DC, US. May (Publication no. EPA/530–SW–86–014)

25. Favero, M.S. (1985). Sterilization, disinfection, and antisepsis in the hospital. In *Manual of clinical microbiology*, 4th ed. American Society for Microbiology, Washington, DC. 1 29–37

26. Garner, J.S. and Favero, M.S. (1985). Guideline for handwashing and hospital environmental control, Public Health Service, Centers for Disease Control, Atlanta: HHS publication no. 99–1117

27. Spire, B., Montagnier, L., Barré-Sinoussi, F. and Chermann, J.C. (1984). Inactivation of lymphadenopathy associated virus by chemical disinfectants. *Lancet*, 2:899–901

28. Martin, L.S., McDougal, J.S. and Loskoski, S.L. (1985). Disinfection and inactivation of the human T-lymphotropic virus type III/lymphadenopathy-associated virus. *J Infect Dis*, 152:400–3

29. McDougal, J 2 S., Martin, L.S., Cort, S. P., et al. (1985) . Thermal inactivation of the immunodeficiency syndrome virus-III/lymphadenopathy-associated virus, with special reference to antithemophilic factor. *J Clin Invest*, 76:875–7

30. Spire, B., Barré-Sinoussi, F., Dormont, D., Montagnier, L. and Chermann, J.C. (1985). Inactivation of lymphadenopathy-associated virus by heat, gamma rays, and ultraviolet light. *Lancet*, 1:188–9

31. Resnik, L., Veren, K., Salahuddin, S.Z., Tondreau, S. and Markham, P.D. (1986). Stability and inactivation of HTLV-III/LAV under clinical and laboratory environments. *JAMA*, 255:1887–91

32. CDC. (1987). Public Health Service (PHS) guidelines for counseling and antibody testing to prevent HIV infection and AIDS. *MMWR*, 3:509–15

33. Kane, M.A. and Lettau, L.A. (1985). Transmission of HBV from dental personnel to patients. *J Am Dent Assoc*, 110:634–6

34. Lettau, L, A., Smith, J.D., Williams, D., *et al.* (1986). Transmission of hepatitis B with resultant restriction of surgical practice. *JAMA*, 255:934–7

35. Williams, W.W. (1983). Guideline for infection control in hospital personnel. *Infect Control*, 4 (suppl):326–49

36. CDC (1983). Prevention of acquired immune deficiency syndrome (AIDS): Report of interagency recommendations. *MMWR*, 32:101–3

37. CDC (1985). Provisional Public Health Service inter-agency recommendations for screening donated blood and plasma for antibody to the virus causing acquired immunodeficiency syndrome. *MMWR*, 34:1–5

Update: Universal Precautions for Prevention of Transmission of Human Immunodeficiency Virus, Hepatitis B Virus, and Other Bloodborne Pathogens in Health-care Settings

Reproduced from Centers for Disease Control (1988). *Morbidity and Mortality Weekly Report*, June, **37**(24)

Introduction

The purpose of this report is to clarify and supplement the CDC publication entitled 'Recommendations for Prevention of HIV Transmission in Health-Care Settings'[1].

In 1983, CDC published a document entitled 'Guideline for Isolation Precautions in Hospitals[2] that contained a section entitled 'Blood and Body Fluid Precautions.' The recommendations in this section called for blood and body fluid precautions when a patient was known or suspected to be infected with bloodborne pathogens. In August 1987, CDC published a document entitled 'Recommendations for Prevention of HIV Transmission in Health-Care Settings[1]. In contrast to the 1983 document, the 1987 document recommended that blood and body fluid precautions be consistently used for all patients regardless of their bloodborne infection status. This extension of blood and body fluid precautions to all patients is referred to as 'Universal Blood and Body Fluid Precautions' or 'Universal Precautions.' Under universal precautions, blood and certain body fluids of all patients are considered potentially infectious for human immunodeficiency virus (HIV), hepatitis B virus (HBV), and other bloodborne pathogens.

Universal precautions are intended to prevent parenteral, mucous membrane, and nonintact skin exposures of health-care workers to bloodborne pathogens. In addition, immunization with HBV vaccine is recommended as an important adjunct to universal precautions for health-care workers who have exposures to blood[3,4].

Since the recommendations for universal precautions were published in August 1987, CDC and the Food and Drug Administration (IFDA) have received requests for clarification of the following issues: 1) body fluids to which universal precautions apply, 2) use of protective barriers, 3) use of gloves for phlebotomy, 4) selection of gloves for use while observing universal precautions, and 5) need for making changes in waste management programs as a result of adopting universal precautions.

Body fluids to which universal precautions apply

Universal precautions apply to blood and to other body fluids containing visible blood. Occupational transmission of HIV and HBV to health-care workers by blood is documented[4,5]. **Blood is the single most important source of HIV, HBV, and other bloodborne pathogens in the occupational setting. Infection control efforts for HIV,**

HBV, and other bloodborne pathogens must focus on preventing exposures to blood as well as on delivery of HBV immunization.

Universal precautions also apply to semen and vaginal secretions. Although both of these fluids have been implicated in the sexual transmission of HIV and HBV, they have not been implicated in occupational transmission from patient to health-care worker. This observation is not unexpected, since exposure to semen in the usual health-care setting is limited, and the routine practice of wearing gloves for performing vaginal examinations protects health-care workers from exposure of potentially infectious vaginal secretions.

Universal precautions also apply to tissues and to the following fluids: cerebrospinal fluid (CSF), synovial fluid, pleural fluid, peritoneal fluid, pericardial fluid, and amniotic fluid. The risk of transmission of HIV and HBV from these fluids is unknown: epidemiologic studies in the health-care and community setting are currently inadequate to assess the potential risk to health-care workers from occupational exposures to them. However, HIV has been isolated from CSF, synovial, and amniotic fluid[6–8], and HBsAg has been detected in synovial fluid, amniotic fluid, and peritoneal fluid[9–11]. One case of HIV transmission was reported after a percutaneous exposure to bloody pleural fluid obtained by needle aspiration[12]. Whereas aseptic procedures used to obtain these fluids for diagnostic or therapeutic purposes protect health-care workers from skin exposures, they cannot prevent penetrating injuries due to contaminated needles or other sharp instruments.

Body fluids to which universal precautions do not apply

Universal precautions do not apply to feces, nasal secretions, sputum, sweat, tears, urine, and vomitus unless they contain visible blood. The risk of transmission of HIV and HBV from these fluids and materials is extremely low or nonexistent. HIV has been isolated and HBsAg has been demonstrated in some of these fluids; however, epidemiologic studies in the health-care and community setting have not implicated these fluids or materials in the transmission of HIV and HBV infections[13,14]. Some of the above fluids and excretions represent a potential source for nosocomial and community-acquired infections with other pathogens, and recommendations for preventing the transmission of nonbloodborne pathogens have been published[2].

Precautions for other body fluids in special settings

Human breast milk has been implicated in perinatal transmission of HIV, and HBsAg has been found in the milk of mothers infected with HBV[10,13]. However, occupational exposure to human breast milk has not been implicated in the transmission of HIV and HBV infection to health-care workers. Moreover, the health-care worker will not have the same type of intensive exposure to breast milk as the nursing neonate. Whereas universal precautions do not apply to human breast milk, gloves may be worn by health-care workers in situations where exposures to breast milk might be frequent, for example, in breast milk banking.

Saliva of some persons infected with HBV has been shown to contain HBV-DNA at concentrations 1/1,000 to 1 /10,000 of that found in the infected person's serum[15]. HBsAg-positive saliva has been shown to be infectious when injected into experimental animals and in human bite exposures[16–18]. However, HBsAg-positive saliva has not been shown to be infectious when applied to oral mucous membranes in experimental primate studies[18] or through contamination of musical instruments or cardiopulmonary resuscitation dummies used by HBV carriers[19,20]. Epidemiologic studies of nonsexual household contacts of HIV-infected patients, including several small series in which HIV transmission failed to occur after bites or after percutaneous inoculation or contamination of cuts and open wounds with saliva from HIV-infected patients, suggest that the potential for salivary transmission of HIV is remote[5,13,14,21,22]. One case report from Germany has suggested the possibility of transmission of HIV in a household setting from an infected child to a sibling through a human bite[23]. The bite did not break the skin or result in bleeding. Since the date of seroconversion to HIV was not known for either child in this case, evidence for the role of saliva in the transmission of virus is unclear[23]. Another case report suggested the possibility of transmission of HIV from husband to wife by contact with saliva during kissing[24]. However, follow-up studies did not confirm HIV infection in the wife[21].

Universal precautions do not apply to saliva. General infection control practices already in existence – including the use of gloves for digital examination of mucous membranes and endotracheal suctioning, and handwashing after exposure to saliva – should further minimize the minute risk, if any, for salivary transmission of HIV and HBV[1,25] Gloves need not be worn when feeding patients and when wiping saliva from skin.

Special precautions, however, are recommended for dentistry[1]. Occupationally acquired infection with HBV in dental workers has been documented[4], and two possible cases of occupationally acquired HIV infection involving dentists have been reported[5,26]. During dental procedures, contamination of saliva with blood is predictable, trauma to health-care workers' hands is common, and blood spattering may occur. Infection control precautions for dentistry minimize this potential for nonintact skin and mucous membrane contact of dental health-care workers to blood-contaminated saliva of patients. In addition, the use of gloves for oral examinations and treatment in the dental setting may also protect the patient's oral mucous membranes from exposures to blood, which may occur from breaks in the skin of dental workers' hands.

Use of protective barriers

Protective barriers reduce the risk of exposure of the health-care worker's skin or mucous membranes to potentially infective materials. For universal precautions, protective barriers reduce the risk of exposure to blood, body fluids containing visible blood, and other fluids to which universal precautions apply. Examples of protective barriers include gloves, gowns, masks, and protective eyewear. Gloves should reduce the incidence of contamination of hands, but they cannot prevent penetrating injuries due to needles or other sharp instruments. Masks and protective eyewear or face shields should reduce the incidence of contamination of mucous membranes of the mouth, nose, and eyes.

Universal precautions are intended to supplement rather than replace recommendations for routine infection control, such as handwashing and using gloves to prevent gross microbial contamination of hands[27]. Because specifying the types of barriers needed for every possible clinical situation is impractical, some judgment must be exercised.

The risk of nosocomial transmission of HIV, HBV, and other bloodborne pathogens can be minimized if health-care workers use the following general guidelines:

1. Take care to prevent injuries when using needles, scalpels, and other sharp instruments or devices; when handling sharp instruments after procedures; when cleaning used instruments; and when disposing of used needles. Do not recap used needles by hand; do not remove used needles from disposable syringes by hand; and do not bend, break, or otherwise manipulate used needles by hand. Place used disposable syringes and needles, scalpel blades, and other sharp items in puncture-resistant containers for disposal. Locate the puncture-resistant containers as close to the use area as is practical.
2. Use protective barriers to prevent exposure to blood, body fluids containing visible blood, and other fluids to which universal precautions apply. The type of protective barrier(s) should be appropriate for the procedure being performed and the type of exposure anticipated.
3. Immediately and thoroughly wash hands and other skin surfaces that are contaminated with blood, body fluids containing visible blood, or other body fluids to which universal precautions apply.

Glove use for phlebotomy

Gloves should reduce the incidence of blood contamination of hands during phlebotomy (drawing blood samples), but they cannot prevent penetrating injuries caused by needles or other sharp instruments. The likelihood of hand contamination with blood containing HIV, HBV, or other bloodborne pathogens during phlebotomy depends on several factors: 1) the skill and technique of the health-care worker, 2) the frequency with which the health-care worker performs the procedure (other factors being equal, the cumulative risk of blood exposure is higher for a health-care worker who performs more procedures), 3) whether the procedure occurs in a routine or emergency situation (where blood contact may be more likely), and 4) the prevalence of infection with bloodborne pathogens in the patient population. The likelihood of infection after skin exposure to blood containing HIV or HBV will depend on the concentration of virus (viral concentration is much higher for hepatitis B than for HIV), the duration of contact, the presence of skin lesions on the hands of the health-care worker, and – for HBV – the immune status of the health-care worker. Although not accurately quantified, the risk of HIV infection following intact skin contact with infective blood is certainly much less than the 0.5% risk following percutaneous needlestick exposures[5]. In universal precautions, *all* blood is assumed to be potentially infective for bloodborne pathogens, but in certain settings (e.g., volunteer blood-donation centers) the prevalence of infection with some bloodborne pathogens (e.g., HIV, HBV) is known to be very low. Some institutions have relaxed recommendations for using gloves for phlebotomy procedures by skilled phlebotomists in settings where the prevalence of bloodborne pathogens is known to be very low.

Institutions that judge that routine gloving for *all* phlebotomies is not necessary should periodically reevaluate their policy. Gloves should always be available to health-care workers who wish to use them for phlebotomy. In addition, the following general guidelines apply:

1. Use gloves for performing phlebotomy when the health-care worker has cuts, scratches or other breaks in his/her skin.

2. Use gloves in situations where the health care worker judges that hand contamination with blood may occur, for example, when performing phlebotomy on an uncooperative patient.
3. Use gloves for performing finger and/or heel sticks on infants and children.
4. Use gloves when persons are receiving training in phlebotomy.

Selection of gloves

The Center for Devices and Radiological Health, FDA, has responsibility for regulating the medical glove industry. Medical gloves include those marketed as sterile surgical or nonsterile examination gloves made of vinyl or latex. General purpose utility ('rubber') gloves are also used in the health-care setting, but they are not regulated by FDA since they are not promoted for medical use. There are no reported differences in barrier effectiveness between intact latex and intact vinyl used to manufacture gloves. Thus, the type of gloves selected should be appropriate for the task being performed.
The following general guidelines are recommended:

1. Use sterile gloves for procedures involving contact with normally sterile areas of the body.
2. Use examination gloves for procedures involving contact with mucous membranes, unless otherwise indicated, and for other patient care or diagnostic procedures that do not require the use of sterile gloves.
3. Change gloves between patient contacts.
4. Do not wash or disinfect surgical or examination gloves for reuse. Washing with surfactants may cause 'wicking,' i.e., the enhanced penetration of liquids through undetected holes in the glove. Disinfecting agents may cause deterioration.
5. Use general-purpose utility gloves (e.g., rubber household gloves) for housekeeping chores involving potential blood contact and for instrument cleaning and decontamination procedures. Utility gloves may be decontaminated and reused but should be discarded if they are peeling, cracked, or discolored, or if they have punctures, tears, or other evidence of deterioration.

Waste management

Universal precautions are not intended to change waste management programs previously recommended by CDC for health-care settings[1]. Policies for defining, collecting, storing, decontaminating, and disposing of infective waste are generally determined by institutions in accordance with state and local regulations. Information regarding waste management regulations in health-care settings may be obtained from state or local health departments or agencies responsible for waste management.
Reported by: Center for Devices and Radiological Health, Food and Drug Administration. Hospital Infections Program, AIDS Program, and Hepatitis B, Div of Viral Diseases, Center for Infectious Diseases, National Institute for Occupational Safety and Health, CDC.
Editorial Note: Implementation of universal precautions does not eliminate the need for other category- or disease-specific isolation precautions, such as enteric precautions for infectious diarrhea or isolation for pulmonary tuberculosis[1,2]. In addition to universal precautions, detailed precautions have been developed for the following procedures and/or settings in which prolonged or intensive exposures to blood occur:

invasive procedures, dentistry, autopsies or morticians' services, dialysis, and the clinical laboratory. These detailed precautions are found in the August 21, 1987, 'Recommendations for Prevention of HIV Transmission in Health-Care Settings'[1]. In addition, specific precautions have been developed for research laboratories[28].

References

1. Centers for Disease Control. Recommendations for prevention of HIV transmission in health-care settings. MMWR 1987;36 (suppl no. 2S).
2. Garner JS, Simmons BP. Guideline for isolation precautions in hospitals. Infect Control 1983:4:245–325.
3. Immunization Practices Advisory Committee. Recommendations for protection against viral hepatitis. MMWR 1985;34:313–24,329–35.
4. Department of Labor, Department of Health and Human Services. Joint advisory notice: protection against occupational exposure to hepatitis B virus (HBV) and human immunodeficiency virus (HIV). Washington, DC:US Department of Labor, US Departrnent of Health and Human Services, 1987.
5. Centers for Disease Control. Update: Acquired immunodeficiency syndrome and human immunodeficiency virus infection among health-care workers. MMWR 1988:37:229–34,239.
6. Hollander H. Levy JA. Neurologic abnormalities and recovery of human immunodeficiency virus from cerebrospinal fluid. Ann Intern Med 1987; 106:692–5.
7. Wirthrington RH, Cornes P, Harris JRW, et al. Isolation of human immunodeficiency virus from synovial fluid of a patient with reactive arthritis. Br Med J 1987;294:484.
8. Mundy DC, Schinazi RF, Gerber AR, Nahmias AJ, Randall HW. Human immunodeficiency virus isolated from amniotic fluid. Lancet 1987; 2:459–60.
9. Onion DK, Crumpacker CS, Gilliland BC. Arthritis of hepatitis associated with Australia antigen. Ann Intem Med 1971; 75:29–33.
10. Lee AKY, Ip HMH, Wong VCW. Mechanisms of maternal-fetal transmission of hepatitis B virus. J infect Dis 1978; 138:668–71.
11. Bond WW, Petersen NJ, Gravelle CR, Favero MS. Hepatitis B virus in peritoneal dialysis fluid: A potential hazard. Dialysis and Transplantation 1982;11:592–600.
12. Oskenhendler E, Harzic M, Le Roux J-M, Rabian C, Clauvel JP. HIV infection with seroconversion after a superficial needlestick injury to the finger (Letter). N Engl J Med 1986; 315:582.
13. Lifson AR: Do alternate modes for transmission of human immunodeficiency virus exist? A review. JAMA 1988;259:1353–6.
14. Friedland GH, Saltzman BR, Rogers MF, et al. Lack of transmission of HTLV-III/LAV infection to household contacts of patients with AIDS or AIDS-related complex with oral candidiasis. N Engl J Med 1986;314:344–9.
15. Jenison SA, Lemon SM, Baker LN, Newbold JE. Quantitative analysis of hepatitis B virus DNA in saliva and semen of chronically infected homosexual men. J Infect Dis 1987;156:299–306.
16. Cancio-Bello TP, de Medina M, Shorey J. Valledor MD, Schiff E,R. An institutional outbreak of hepatitis B related to a human biting carrier. J Infect Dis 1982;146:652–6.
17. MacQuarrie MB, Forghani B. Wolochow DA. Hepatitis B transmitted by a human

bite. JAMA 1 974;230:723–4.

18. Scott RM, Snitbhan R, Bancroft WH, Alter HJ, Tingpalapong M. Experimental transmission of hepatitis B virus by semen and saliva. J Insect Dis 1980; 142:67–71.

19. Glaser JB, Nadler JP. Hepatitis B virus in a cardiopulmonary resuscitation training course: Risk of transmission from a surface antigen-positive participant. Arch Intern Med 1985;145:1653–5.

20. Osterholm MT, Bravo ER, Crosson JT, et al. Lack of transmission of viral hepatitis type B after oral exposure to HBsAg-positive saliva. Br Med J 1979;2:1263–4.

21. Curran JW, Jaffe HW, Hardy AM, et al. Epidemiology of HIV infection and AIDS in the United States. Science 1988;239:610–6.

22. Jason JM, McDougal JS, Dixon G. et al. HTLV-III/LAV antibody and immune status of household contacts and sexual partners of persons with hemophilia. JAMA 1986;255:212–5.

23. Wahn V, Kramer HH, Voit T, Büster HT, Scrampical B, Scheid A. Horizontal transmission of HIV infection between two siblings (Letter). Lancet 1986;2:694.

24. Salahuddin SZ, Groopman JE, Markham PD, et al. HTLV-III in symptom-free seronegative persons. Lancet 1984;2:1418–20.

25. Simmons BP, Wong ES. Guideline for prevention of nosocomial pneumonia. Atlanta: US Department of Health and Human Services, Public Health Service, Centers for Disease Control, 1982.

26. Klein RS, Phelan JA, Freeman K, et al. Low occupational risk of human immunodeficiency virus infection among dental professionals. N Engl J Med 1988;318:86–90.

27. Garner JS, Favero MS. Guideline for handwashing and hospital environmental control, 1985. Atlanta: US Department of Health and Human Services, Public Health Service, Centers for Disease Control, 1985; HHS publication no. 99–117.

28. Centers for Disease Control. Agent summary statement for human immunodeficiency virus and report on laboratory-acquired infection with human immunodeficiency virus. MMWR 1988; 37 (suppl. no. S4:1S–22S).

Appendix 4: Guidelines for Preventing the Transmission of Tuberculosis in Health-Care Settings, with Special Focus on HIV-related Issues*

Samuel W. Dooley, Jr., Kenneth G. Castro, Mary D. Hutton, Robert J. Mullan, Jacquelyn A. Polder and Dixie E. Snider

Reproduced from Centers for Disease Control (1990). *Morbidity and Mortality Weekly Report*, 7 December, **39**(RR-17).

Summary

The transmission of tuberculosis is a recognized risk in health-care settings. Several recent outbreaks of tuberculosis in health-care settings, including outbreaks involving multidrug-resistant strains of Mycobacterium tuberculosis, have heightened concern about nosocomial transmission. In addition, increases in tuberculosis cases in many areas are related to the high risk of tuberculosis among persons infected with the human immunodeficiency virus (HIV). Transmission of tuberculosis to persons with HIV infection is of particular concern because they are at high risk of developing active tuberculosis if infected. Health-care workers should be particularly alert to the need for preventing tuberculosis transmission in settings in which persons with HIV infection receive care, especially settings in which cough-inducing procedures (e.g., sputum induction and aerosolized pentamidine (AP) treatments) are being performed.

Transmission is most likely to occur from patients with unrecognized pulmonary or laryngeal tuberculosis who are not on effective antituberculosis therapy and have not been placed in tuberculosis (acid-fast bacilli (AFB)) isolation. Health-care facilities, in which persons at high risk for tuberculosis work or receive care, should periodically review their tuberculosis policies and procedures, and determine the actions necessary to minimize the risk of tuberculosis transmission in their particular settings.

The prevention of tuberculosis transmission in health-care settings requires that all of the following basic approaches be used: a) prevention of the generation of infectious airborne particles (droplet nuclei) by early identification and treatment of persons with tuberculous infection and active tuberculosis, b) prevention of the spread of infectious droplet nuclei into the general air circulation by applying source-control methods, c) reduction of the number of infectious droplet nuclei in air contaminated with them, and d) surveillance of health-care-facility personnel for tuberculosis and tuberculous infection. Experience has shown that when inadequate attention is given to any of these approaches, the probability of

---

*This document was prepared in consultation with experts in tuberculosis, acquired immunodeficiency syndrome, infection-control and hospital epidemiology, microbiology, ventilation and industrial hygiene, respiratory therapy, nursing, and emergency medical services.

tuberculosis transmission is increased. Specific actions to reduce the risk of tuberculosis transmission should include a) screening patients for active tuberculosis and tuberculous infection, b) providing rapid diagnostic services, c) prescribing appropriate curative and preventive therapy, d) maintaining physical measures to reduce microbial contamination of the air, e) providing isolation rooms for persons with, or suspected of having, infectious tuberculosis, f) screening health-care-facility personnel for tuberculous infection and tuberculosis, and g) promptly investigating and controlling outbreaks.

Although completely eliminating the risk of tuberculosis transmission in all health-care settings may be impossible, adhering to these guidelines should minimize the risk to persons in these settings.

I. Introduction

A. Purpose of document

The purpose of this document is to review the mode and risk of tuberculosis transmission in health-care settings and to make recommendations for reducing the risk of transmission to persons in health-care settings – including workers, patients, volunteers, and visitors. The document may also serve as a useful resource for educating health-care workers about tuberculosis. Several outbreaks of tuberculosis in health-care settings, including outbreaks involving multidrug-resistant strains of *M. tuberculosis,* have been reported to CDC during the past 2 years[1] (CDC, unpublished data). In addition, CDC has recently received numerous requests for information about reducing tuberculosis transmission in health-care settings. Much of the increased concern is due to the occurrence of tuberculosis among persons infected with HIV[2], who are at increased risk of contracting tuberculosis both from reactivation of a latent tuberculous infection[3] and from a new infection[4]. Therefore, in this document, emphasis is given to the transmission of tuberculosis among persons with HIV infection, although the majority of patients with tuberculosis in most areas of the country do not have HIV infection.

These recommendations consolidate and update previously published CDC recommendations[5–10]. The recommendations are applicable to all settings in which health care is provided. In this document, the term 'tuberculosis,' in the absence of modifiers, refers to a clinically apparent active disease process caused by *M. tuberculosis* (or, rarely, *M. bovis* or *M. africanum*). The terms 'health-care-facility personnel' and 'health-care-facility workers' refer to all persons working in a health-care setting – including physicians, nurses, aides, and persons not directly involved in patient care (e.g., dietary, housekeeping, maintenance, clerical, and janitorial staff, and volunteers).

B. Epidemiology, transmission, and pathogenesis of tuberculosis

Tuberculosis is not evenly distributed throughout all segments of the population of the United States. Groups known to have a high incidence of tuberculosis include blacks, Asians and Pacific Islanders, American Indians and Alaskan Natives, Hispanics, current or past prison inmates, alcoholics, intravenous (IV) drug users, the elderly, foreign-born persons from areas of the world with a high prevalence of tuberculosis (e.g., Asia, Africa, the Caribbean, and Latin America), and persons living in the same household as members of these groups[5].

M. tuberculosis is carried in airborne particles, known as droplet nuclei, that can be generated when persons with pulmonary or laryngeal tuberculosis sneeze, cough, speak, or sing[11]. The particles are so small (1–5 microns) that normal air currents keep them airborne and can spread them throughout a room or building[12]. Infection occurs when a susceptible person inhales droplet nuclei containing *M. tuberculosis,* and bacilli become established in the alveoli of the lungs and spread throughout the body. Two to ten weeks after initial human infection with *M. tuberculosis,* the immune response usually limits further multiplication and spread of the tuberculosis bacilli. For a small proportion of newly infected persons (usually <1%), initial infection rapidly progresses to clinical illness. However, for another group (approximately 5%–10%), illness develops after an interval of months, years, or decades, when the bacteria begin to replicate and produce disease[11]. The risk of progression to active disease is markedly increased for persons with HIV infection[3].

The probability that a susceptible person will become infected depends upon the concentration of infectious droplet nuclei in the air. Patient factors that enhance transmission are discussed more fully in section II.B.3. Environmental factors that enhance transmission include a) contact between susceptible persons and an infectious patient in relatively small, enclosed spaces, b) inadequate ventilation that results in insufficient dilution or removal of infectious droplet nuclei, and c) recirculation of air containing infectious droplet nuclei.

Tuberculosis transmission is a recognized risk in health-care settings[13–21]. The magnitude of the risk varies considerably by type of health-care setting, patient population served, job category, and the area of the facility in which a person works. The risk may be higher in areas where patients with tuberculosis are provided care before diagnosis (e.g., clinic waiting areas and emergency rooms) or where diagnostic or treatment procedures that stimulate patient coughing are performed. Nosocomial transmission of tuberculosis has been associated with close contact with infectious patients, as well as procedures such as bronchoscopy[16], endotracheal intubation and auctioning with mechanical ventilation[17,18], open abscess irrigation[19], and autopsy[20,21]. Sputum induction and aerosol treatments that induce cough may also increase the potential for tuberculosis transmission[22]. Health-care workers should be particularly alert to the need for preventing tuberculosis transmission in health-care settings in which persons with HIV infection receive care, especially if cough-inducing procedures such as sputum induction and AP treatments are being performed.

II. General principles of tuberculosis control in health-care settings

A. Approaches to tuberculosis control
An effective tuberculosis-control program requires the early identification, isolation, and treatment of persons with active tuberculosis. Health-care facilities in which persons at high risk for tuberculosis work or receive care should periodically review their tuberculosis policies and procedures, and determine the actions necessary to minimize the risk of tuberculosis transmission in their particular settings. The prevention of tuberculosis transmission in health-care settings requires that all of the following basic approaches be used: a) preventing the generation of infectious droplet nuclei, b) preventing the spread of infectious droplet nuclei into the general air circulation, c) reducing the number of infectious droplet nuclei in air contaminated with them, d) following guidelines for cleaning, disinfecting, and sterilizing contaminated items, and e) conducting surveillance for tuberculosis transmission to health-care-facility personnel. Experience has shown that when inadequate attention is given to any of these

measures, the probability of tuberculosis transmission is increased.

Specific actions to reduce the risk of tuberculosis transmission should include the following:

- Screening patients for active tuberculosis and tuberculous infection.
- Providing rapid diagnostic services.
- Prescribing appropriate curative and preventive therapy.
- Maintaining physical measures to reduce microbial contamination of the air.
- Providing isolation rooms for persons with, or suspected of having, infectious tuberculosis.
- Screening health-care-facility personnel for tuberculous infection and tuberculosis.
- Promptly investigating and controlling outbreaks.

B. Preventing generation of infectious droplet nuclei

1. Early identification and treatment of persons with tuberculous infection

Early identification of persons with tuberculous infection and application of preventive therapy are effective in preventing the development of tuberculosis[5]. Persons at increased risk of tuberculosis (see section I.B.), or for whom the consequences of tuberculosis may be especially severe, should be screened for tuberculous infection to identify those for whom preventive treatment is indicated. The tuberculin skin test is the only method currently available that demonstrates infection with *M. tuberculosis* in the absence of active tuberculosis[11].

2. Early identification and treatment of persons with active tuberculosis

An effective means of preventing tuberculosis transmission is preventing the generation of infectious droplet nuclei by persons with infectious tuberculosis. This can be accomplished by early identification, isolation, and treatment of persons with active tuberculosis. Tuberculosis may be more difficult to diagnose among persons with HIV infection; the diagnosis may be overlooked because of an atypical clinical or radiographic presentation and/or the simultaneous occurrence of other pulmonary infections (e.g. *Pneumocystis carinii* pneumonia (PCP)). Among persons with HIV infection, the difficulty in making a diagnosis may be further compounded by impaired responses to tuberculin skin tests[23,24], low sensitivity of sputum smears for detecting AFB[25], or overgrowth of cultures with *Mycobacterium avium* complex (MAC) among patients with both MAC and *M. tuberculosis* infections [26].

A diagnosis of tuberculosis should be considered for any patient with persistent cough or other symptoms compatible with tuberculosis, such as weight loss, anorexia, or fever. Diagnostic measures for identifying tuberculosis should be instituted among such patients. These measures include history, physical examination, tuberculin skin test, chest radiograph, and microscopic examination and culture of sputum or other appropriate specimens[11,27]. Other diagnostic methods, such as bronchoscopy or biopsy, may be indicated in some cases[28,29]. The probability of tuberculosis is increased by finding a positive reaction to a tuberculin skin test or a history of a positive skin test, a history of previous tuberculosis, membership in a group at high risk for tuberculosis (see section I.B.), or a history of exposure to tuberculosis. Active tuberculosis is strongly suggested if the diagnostic evaluation reveals AFB in sputum, a chest radiograph is suggestive of tuberculosis, or the person has symptoms highly suggestive of tuberculosis (e.g., productive cough, night sweats, anorexia, and weight loss). Tuberculosis may occur simultaneously with other pulmonary infections, such as PCP.

a. Tuberculin skin test. The Mantoux technique (intradermal injection of 0.1 ml of purified protein derivative (PPD) containing 5 tuberculin units (TU)) should be used as a diagnostic aid to detect tuberculous infection, Although tuberculin skin tests are < 100% sensitive and specific for detection of infection with *M. tuberculosis*, no better diagnostic method has been devised. Tuberculin skin tests should be interpreted according to current guidelines[5,11]. For persons with HIV infection, a reaction of ≥ 5 mm is considered positive.

A negative skin test does not rule out tuberculosis disease or infection. Because of the possibility of a false-negative result, *the tuberculin skin test should never be used to exclude the possibility of active tuberculosis among persons for whom the diagnosis is being considered, even if reactions to other skin-test antigens are positive.* Persons with HIV infection are more likely to have false-negative skin tests than are persons without HIV infection[23,24,30]. The likelihood of a false-negative skin test increases as the stage of HIV infection advances (CDC/Florida Department of Health and Rehabilitative Services/New York City Department of Health, unpublished data). For this reason, a history of a positive tuberculin reaction is meaningful, even if the current skin-test result is negative.

b. Chest radiograph. The radiographic presentation of pulmonary tuberculosis among patients with HIV infection may be unusual[31]. Typical apical cavitary disease is less common among persons with HIV infection. They may have infiltrates in any lung zone, often associated with mediastinal and/or hilar adenopathy, or they may have a normal chest radiograph.

c. Bacteriology. Smear and culture examination of three to five sputum specimens collected on different days is the main diagnostic procedure for pulmonary tuberculosis[11]. Sputum smears that fail to demonstrate AFB do not exclude the diagnosis of tuberculosis. Studies indicate that 50%–80% of patients with pulmonary tuberculosis have positive sputum smears. Sputum smears from patients with HIV infection and pulmonary tuberculosis may be less likely to reveal AFB than those from immunocompetent patients, a finding believed to be consistent with the lower frequency of cavitary pulmonary disease observed among HIV-infected persons[23,25].

A positive sputum culture, with organisms identified as *M. tuberculosis*, provides a definitive diagnosis of tuberculosis. Conventional laboratory methods may require 4–8 weeks for species identification; however, the use of radiometric culture techniques and genetic probes facilitates more rapid detection and identification of mycobacteria[32,33]. Mixed mycobacterial infection (either simultaneous or sequential) may occur and may obscure the recognition of *M. tuberculosis* clinically and in the laboratory[26]. The use of genetic probes for both MAC and *M. tuberculosis* may be useful for identifying mixed mycobacterial infections in clinical specimens.

3. Determining infectiousness of tuberculosis patients

The infectiousness of a person with tuberculosis correlates with the number of organisms that are expelled into the air, which, in turn, correlates with the following factors: a) anatomic site of disease, b) presence of cough or other forceful expirational maneuvers, c) presence of AFB in the sputum smear, d) willingness or ability of the patient to cover his or her mouth when coughing, e) presence of cavitation on chest radiograph, f) length of time the patient has been on adequate chemotherapy, g) duration of symptoms, and h) administration of procedures that can enhance coughing (e.g., sputum induction).

The most infectious persons are those with pulmonary or laryngeal tuberculosis. Those with extrapulmonary tuberculosis are usually not infectious, with the following exceptions: a) nonpulmonary disease located in the respiratory tract or oral cavity, or b) extrapulmonary disease that includes an open abscess or lesion in which the concentration of organisms is high, especially if drainage from the abscess or lesion is extensive[19]. Although the data are limited, findings suggest that tuberculosis patients with acquired immunodeficiency syndrome (AIDS), if smear positive, have infectiousness similar to that of tuberculosis patients without AIDS (CDC/New York City Department of Health, unpublished data).

Infectiousness is greatest among patients who have a productive cough, pulmonary cavitation on chest radiograph, and AFB on sputum smear[6]. Infection is more likely to result from exposure to a person who has unsuspected pulmonary tuberculosis and who is not receiving antituberculosis therapy or from a person with diagnosed tuberculosis who is not receiving adequate therapy, because of patient noncompliance or the presence of drug-resistant organisms. Administering effective antituberculosis medications has been shown to be strongly associated with a decrease in infectiousness among persons with tuberculosis[34]. Effective chemotherapy reduces coughing, the amount of sputum, and the number of organisms in the sputum. However, the length of time a patient must be on effective medication before becoming non-infectious varies[35]; some patients are never infectious, whereas those with unrecognized or inadequately treated drug-resistant disease may remain infectious for weeks or months. Thus, decisions about terminating isolation precautions should be made on a case-by-case basis.

In general, persons suspected of having active tuberculosis and persons with confirmed tuberculosis should be considered infectious if cough is present, if cough-inducing procedures are performed, or if sputum smears are known to contain AFB, and if these patients are not on chemotherapy, have just started chemotherapy, or have a poor clinical or bacteriologic response to chemotherapy. A person with tuberculosis who has been on adequate chemotherapy for at least 2–3 weeks and has had a definite clinical and bacteriologic response to therapy (reduction in cough, resolution of fever, and progressively decreasing quantity of bacilli on smear) is probably no longer infectious. Most tuberculosis experts agree that noninfectiousness in pulmonary tuberculosis can be established by finding sputum free of bacilli by smear examination on three consecutive days for a patient on effective chemotherapy. Even after isolation precautions have been discontinued, caution should be exercised when a patient with tuberculosis is placed in a room with another patient, especially if the other patient is immunocompromised.

C. Preventing spread of infectious droplet nuclei via source-control methods

In high-risk settings, certain techniques can be applied to prevent or to reduce the spread of infectious droplet nuclei into the general air circulation. The application of these techniques, which are called source-control methods because they entrap infectious droplet nuclei as they are emitted by the patient, or 'source'[36], is especially important during performance of medical procedures likely to generate aerosols containing infectious particles.

1. Local exhaust ventilation

Local exhaust ventilation is a source-control technique that removes airborne contaminants at or near their sources[37]. The use of booths for sputum induction or administration of aerosolized medications (e.g., AP) is an example of local exhaust ventilation for preventing the spread of infectious droplet nuclei generated by these procedures into the general air circulation. Booths used for source control should be equipped with exhaust fans that remove nearly 100% of airborne particles during the time interval between the departure of one patient and the arrival of the next. The time required for removing a given percentage of airborne particles from an enclosed space depends upon the number of air exchanges per hour (Table 1), which is determined by the capacity of the exhaust fan in cubic feet per minute (cfm), the number of cubic feet of air in the room or booth, and the rate at which air is entering the room

Table 1 Air changes per hour and time in minutes required for removal efficiencies of 90%, 99% or 99.9% of airborne contaminants*

Air changes per hour	Minutes required for a removal efficiency of		
	90%	99%	99.9%
1	138	276	414
2	69	138	207
3	46	92	138
4	35	69	104
5	28	55	83
6	23	46	69
7	20	39	59
8	17	35	52
9	15	31	46
10	14	28	41
11	13	25	38
12	12	23	35
13	11	21	32
14	10	20	30
15	9	18	28
16	9	17	26
17	8	16	24
18	8	15	23
19	7	15	22
20	7	14	21
25	6	11	17
30	5	9	14
35	4	8	12
40	3	7	10
45	3	6	9
50	3	6	8

*Table prepared according to the formula $t_2 = (\ln (C_2/C_1)/-(Q/V)\cdot 60$, which is an adaptation of formula for rate of purging airborne contaminants, with $t_1 = 0$ and assuming perfect mixing of the air in the space[69]. $C_2/C_1 = 1 - $ (removal efficiency/100).

or booth at the intake source.

The exhaust fan should maintain negative pressure in the booth with respect to adjacent areas, so that air flows into the booth. Maintaining negative pressure in the booth minimizes the possibility that infectious droplet nuclei in the booth will move into adjacent rooms or hallways. Ideally, the air from these booths should be exhausted directly to the outside of the building (away from air-intake vents, people, and animals, in accordance with federal, state, and local regulations concerning environmental discharges). If direct exhaust to the outside is impossible, the air from the booth could be exhausted through a properly designed, installed, and maintained high efficiency particulate air (HEPA) filter; however, the efficacy of this method has not been demonstrated in clinical settings (see section II.D.2.a.).

2. Other source-control methods

A simple but important source-control technique is for infectious patients to cover all coughs and sneezes with a tissue, thus containing most liquid drops and droplets before evaporation can occur[38]. A patient's use of a properly fitted surgical mask or disposable, valveless particulate respirator (PR) (see section II.D.2.c.) also may reduce the spread of infectious particles. However, since the device would need to be worn constantly for the protection of others, it would be practical in only very limited circumstances (e.g., when a patient is being transported within a medical facility or between facilities).

D. Reducing microbial contamination of air

Once infectious droplet nuclei have been released into room air, they should be eliminated or reduced in number by ventilation, which may be supplemented by additional measures (e.g., trapping organisms by high-efficiency filtration or killing organisms with germicidal ultraviolet (UV) irradiation (100–290 nanometers)). Health-care-facility workers may also reduce the risk of inhaling contaminated air by using PRs.

Although for the past 2–3 decades ventilation and, to a lesser extent, UV lamps and face masks have been used in health-care settings to prevent tuberculosis transmission, few published data exist on which to evaluate their effectiveness and liabilities or to draw conclusions about the role each method should play. From a theoretical standpoint, none of the four methods (ventilation, UV irradiation, high efficiency filtration, and face masks) appears to be ideal. None of the methods used alone or in combination can completely eliminate the risk of tuberculosis transmission; however, when used with the other infection-control measures outlined in this document, they can substantially reduce the risk.

1. General ventilation

Ventilation standards for indoor air quality have been published by the American Society of Heating, Refrigerating, and Air Conditioning Engineers, Inc. (ASHRAE)[39]. Specific recommendations for health-care facilities have been published by ASHRAE[40] and by the Federal Health Resources and Services Administration[41]. Meeting these standards should reduce the probability of tuberculosis transmission in clinical settings; however, some highly infectious patients may transmit infection even if these ventilation standards are met.

a. Dilution and removal of airborne contaminants. Appropriate ventilation maintains air quality by two processes – dilution and removal of airborne contaminants[42]. Dilution reduces the concentration of contaminants in a room by introducing air that does not contain those contaminants into the room. Air is then removed from the room by exhaust, direct to the outside, or, by recirculation into the general ventilation system of the building. Continuously recirculating air in a room or in a building may result in the accumulation or concentration of infectious droplet nuclei. Air that is likely to be contaminated with infectious droplet nuclei should be exhausted to the outside, away from intake vents, people, and animals, in accordance with federal, state, and local regulations for environmental discharges.

b. Air mixing. Proper ventilation requires that within-room mixing of air (ventilation efficiency) must be adequate[42]. Air mixing is enhanced by locating air-supply outlets at ceiling level and exhaust inlets near the floor, thus providing downward movement of clean air through the breathing zone to the floor area for exhaust.

c. Direction of air flow. For control of tuberculosis transmission, the direction of air flow is as important as dilution. The direction of air flow is determined by the differences in air pressure between adjacent areas, with air flowing from higher pressure areas to lower pressure areas.

In an area occupied by a patient with infectious tuberculosis, air should flow into the potentially contaminated area (the patient's room) from adjacent areas. The patient's room is said to be under lower or negative pressure.

Proper air flow and pressure differentials between areas of a health-care facility are difficult to control because of open doors, movement of patients and staff, temperature, and the effect of vertical openings (e.g., stairwells and elevator shafts)[40]. Air-pressure differentials can best be maintained in completely closed rooms. An open door between two areas may reduce any existing pressure differential and could reduce or eliminate the desired effect. Therefore, doors should remain closed, and the close fit of all doors and other closures of openings between pressurized areas should be maintained. For critical areas in which the direction of air flow must be maintained while allowing for patient or staff movement between adjacent areas, an appropriately pressurized anteroom may be indicated.

Examples of factors that can change the direction of air flow include the following: a) dust in exhaust fans, filters, or ducts, b) malfunctioning fans, c) adjustments made to the ventilation system elsewhere in the building, or d) automatic shut down of outside air introduction during cold weather. In areas where the direction of air flow is important, trained personnel should monitor air flow frequently to ensure that appropriate conditions are maintained.

Each area to which an infectious tuberculosis patient might be admitted should be evaluated for its potential for the spread of tuberculosis bacilli. Modifications to the ventilation system, if needed, should be made by a qualified ventilation engineer. Individual evaluations should address factors such as the risk of tuberculosis among the patient population served, special procedures that may be performed, and ability to make the necessary changes.

Too much ventilation in an area can create problems. In addition to incurring additional expense in return for marginal benefits, occupants bothered by the drafts may elect to shut down the system entirely. Furthermore, if the concentration of infectious droplet nuclei in an area is high, the levels of ventilation that are practical to achieve may be inadequate to completely remove the contaminants[43].

2. *Potential supplemental approaches*

a. *HEPA filtration*

For general-use areas (e.g., emergency rooms and waiting areas) of health-care facilities, recirculating the air is an alternative to using large percentages of outside air for general ventilation. If air is recirculated, care must be taken to ensure that infection is not transmitted in the process. Although they can be expensive, HEPA filters, which remove at least 99.97% of particles >0.3 microns in diameter, have been shown to be effective in clearing the air of *Aspergillus* spores, which are in the size range of 1.5–6 microns[44–46]. The ability of HEPA filters to remove tuberculosis bacilli from the air has not been studied, but tuberculosis-containing droplet nuclei are approximately 1–5 microns in diameter, about the same size as *Aspergillus* spores; therefore, HEPA filters theoretically should remove infectious droplet nuclei. HEPA filters may be used in general-use areas, but should not be used to recirculate air from a tuberculosis isolation room back into the general circulation.

Applications in preventing nosocomial *Aspergillus* infection have included using HEPA filters in centralized air-handling units and using whole-wall HEPA filtration units with laminar air flow in patient rooms. In addition, portable HEPA filtration units, which filter the air in a room rather than filtering incoming air, have been effective in reducing nosocomial *Aspergillus* infections[45,46]. Such units have been used as an interim solution for retrofitting old areas of hospitals. Although these units should not be substituted for other accepted tuberculosis isolation procedures, they may be useful in general-use areas (e.g., waiting rooms and emergency rooms) where an increased risk of exposure to tuberculosis may exist, and where other methods of air control may be inadequate.

When HEPA filters are to be installed at a facility, qualified personnel must assess and design the air-handling system to assure adequate supply and exhaust capacity. Proper installation, testing, and meticulous maintenance are critical if a HEPA filter system is used[40]. Improper design, installation, or maintenance could permit infectious particles to circumvent filtration and escape into the ventilation[42]. The filters should be installed to prevent leakage between filter segments and between the filter bed and its frame. A regular maintenance program is required to monitor HEPA filters for possible leakage and for filter loading. A manometer should be installed in the filter system to provide an accurate means of objectively determining the need for filter replacement. Installation should allow for maintenance without contaminating the delivery system or the area served.

HEPA-filtered, recirculated air should not be used if the contaminants contain carcinogenic agents. Qualified personnel should maintain, decontaminate, and dispose of HEPA filters.

b. Germicidal UV irradiation

The use of germicidal UV lamps (wavelengths 100–290 nm) to prevent tuberculosis transmission in occupied spaces is controversial. UV lamps installed in the exhaust air ducts from the rooms of patients with infectious tuberculosis were shown to prevent infection of guinea pigs, which are highly susceptible to tuberculosis[34].

On the basis of this finding, other studies[47–50], and the experience of tuberculosis clinicians and mycobacteriologists during the past 2–3 decades, CDC has continued to recommend UV lamps (with appropriate safeguards to prevent short-term overexposure) as a supplement to ventilation in settings where the risk of tuberculosis transmission is high[6,8,11,51–54]. Their efficacy in clinical settings has not been demonstrated under controlled conditions, but there is a theoretical and experiential basis for believing they are effective[43,55,56]. Thus, individual health-care facilities may need to consider, on a case-by-case basis, using these lamps in settings with a high risk of tuberculosis transmission (see section I.B.). UV lamps are less effective in areas with a relative humidity of > 70%[57]. The potential for serious adverse effects of short- and long-term exposure to germicidal UV has been identified as a major concern[58] (NIOSH, unpublished report (Health Hazard Evaluation Report, HETA 90-122-L2073)).

The two most common types of UV installation are wall- or ceiling-mounted room fixtures for disinfecting the air within a room and irradiation units for disinfecting air in supply ducts. Wall- or ceiling-mounted fixtures act by disinfecting upper room air, and their effectiveness depends in part upon the mixing of air in the room. Organisms must be carried by air currents from the lower portion of the room to within the range of the UV radiation from the fixtures. These fixtures are most likely to be effective in locations where ceilings are high, but some protection may be afforded in areas with ceilings as low as 8 feet. To be maximally effective, lamps should be left on day and night[59].

Installing UV lamps in ventilation ducts may be beneficial in facilities that recirculate the air. UV exposure of air in ducts can be direct and more intense than that provided by room fixtures and may be effective in disinfecting exhaust air. Duct installations provide no protection against tuberculosis transmission to any person who is in the room with an infectious patient. As with HEPA filters, UV installations in ducts may be used in general-use areas but should not be used to recirculate air from a tuberculosis isolation room back into the general circulation.

The main concern about UV lamps is safety. Short-term overexposure to UV irradiation can cause keratoconjunctivitis and erythema of the skin[60]. However, with proper installation and maintenance, the risk of short-term overexposure is low. Long-term exposure to UV irradiation is associated with increased risk of basal cell carcinoma of the skin and with cataracts[58]. To prevent overexposure of health-care-facility personnel and patients, UV lamp configurations should meet applicable safety guidelines[60].

When UV lamps are used in air-supply ducts, a warning sign should be placed on doors that permit access to the duct lamps. The sign should indicate that looking at the lamps is a safety hazard. In addition, warning lights outside doors permitting access to duct lamps should indicate whether the lamps are on or off. The duct system should be engineered to prevent UV emissions from the duct radiating into potentially occupied spaces.

Consultation from a qualified expert should be obtained before and after UV lamps are installed. After installation, the safety and effectiveness of UV irradiation must be checked with a UV meter and fixtures adjusted as necessary. Bulbs should be periodically checked for dust, cleaned as needed, and replaced at the end of the rated life of the bulb. Maintenance personnel should be cautioned that fixtures should be turned off before inspection or servicing. A timing device that turns on a red light at the end of the rated life of the lamp is available to alert maintenance personnel that the lamp needs to be replaced.

c. Disposable PRs for filtration of inhaled air.

1.) For persons exposed to tuberculosis patients. Appropriate masks, when worn by health-care providers or other persons who must share air space with a patient who has infectious tuberculosis, may provide additional protection against tuberculosis transmission. Standard surgical masks may not be effective in preventing inhalation of droplet nuclei[61], because some are not designed to provide a tight face seal and to filter out particulates in the droplet nucleus size range (1–5 microns). A better alternative is the disposable PR. PRs were originally developed for industrial use to protect workers. Although the appearance and comfort of PRs may be similar to that of cup-shaped surgical masks, they provide a better facial fit and better filtration capability.

However, the efficacy of PRs in protecting susceptible persons from infection with tuberculosis has not been demonstrated.

PRs may be most beneficial in the following situations: a) when appropriate ventilation is not available and the patient's signs and symptoms suggest a high potential for infectiousness, b) when the patient is potentially infectious and is undergoing a procedure that is likely to produce bursts of aerosolized, infectious particles or to result in copious coughing or sputum production, regardless of whether appropriate ventilation is in place, and c) when the patient is potentially infectious, has a productive cough, and is unable or unwilling to cover coughs.

Comfort influences the acceptability of PRs. Generally, the more efficient the PRs, the greater is the work of breathing through them and the greater the perceived discomfort. A proper fit is vital to protect against inhaling droplet nuclei. When gaps are present, air will preferentially flow through the gaps, allowing the PR to function more like a funnel than a filter, thus providing virtually no protection[61].

2.) For tuberculosis patients. Masks or PRs worn by patients with suspected or confirmed tuberculosis may be useful in selected circumstances (see section II.C.2.). PRs used by patients should be valveless. Some PRs have valves to release expired air, and these would not be appropriate for patients to use.

E. Decontamination: cleaning, disinfecting, and sterilizing

Guidelines for cleaning, disinfecting, and sterilizing equipment have been published[10,62,63]. The rationale for cleaning, disinfecting, or sterilizing patient-care equipment can be understood more readily if medical devices, equipment, and surgical materials are divided into three general categories (critical items, semi-critical items, and non-critical items) based on the potential risk of infection involved in their use.

Critical items are instruments such as needles, surgical instruments, cardiac catheters, or implants that are introduced directly into the bloodstream or into other normally sterile areas of the body. These items should be sterile at the time of use.

Semi-critical items are items such as noninvasive, flexible and rigid fiberoptic endoscopes or bronchoscopes, endotracheal tubes, or anesthesia-breathing circuits that may come in contact with mucous membranes but do not ordinarily penetrate body surfaces. Although sterilization is preferred for these instruments, a high-level disinfection procedure that destroys vegetative microorganisms, most fungal spores, tubercle bacilli, and small, nonlipid viruses may be used. Meticulous physical cleaning before sterilization or high-level disinfection is essential.

Non-critical items are those that either do not ordinarily touch the patient or touch only intact skin. Such items include crutches, bedboards, blood pressure cuffs, and various other medical accessories. These items do not transmit tuberculous infection. Consequently, washing with a detergent is usually sufficient.

Facility policies should identify whether cleaning, disinfecting, or sterilizing an item is indicated to decrease the risk of infection. Procedures for each item depend on its intended use. Generally, critical items should be sterilized, semi-critical items should be sterilized or cleaned with high-level disinfectants, and non-critical items need only be cleaned with detergents or low-level disinfectants. Decisions about decontamination processes should be based on the intended use of the item and not on the diagnosis of the patient for whom the item was used. Selection of chemical disinfectants depends on the intended use, the level of disinfection required, and the structure and material of the item to be disinfected.

Although microorganisms are normally found on walls, floors, and other surfaces, these environmental surfaces are rarely associated with transmission of infections to patients or health-care-facility personnel. This is particularly true with organisms such as tubercle bacilli, which generally require inhalation by the host for infection to occur. Therefore, extraordinary attempts to disinfect or sterilize environmental surfaces are rarely indicated. However, routine cleaning (which can be achieved with a hospital-grade, Environmental Protection Agency-approved germicide/disinfectant) is recommended[63]. The same routine, daily cleaning procedures used in other hospital or facility rooms should be used to clean rooms of patients who are on AFB isolation precautions.

F. Conducting surveillance for tuberculosis transmission to health-care-facility personnel

A tuberculosis screening and prevention program for health-care-facility personnel should be established for protecting both health-care-facility personnel and patients. Personnel with tuberculous infection without evidence of current (active) disease should be identified, because preventive treatment with isoniazid may be indicated[5]. In addition, the screening program will enable public health personnel to evaluate the effectiveness of current infection-control practices. Recommendations for screening and surveillance are detailed in section III.A.7.

III. Recommendations

The following recommendations are divided into two categories: a) general recommendations applicable to all health-care settings, including special precautions for cough-inducing procedures, and b) recommendations for selected, specific health-care settings. Facilities should adapt these recommendations as appropriate for individual circumstances.

A. Recommendations applicable to all health-care settings

1. Early identification and preventive treatment of persons who have tuberculous infection and are at high risk for active tuberculosis

- Persons belonging to groups at risk for tuberculosis (see section I.B.) should be screened with a Mantoux tuberculin skin test. Those with positive skin tests should be evaluated for preventive therapy according to current guidelines[5].
- All persons with HIV infection or with risk factors for HIV infection should be given a Mantoux tuberculin skin test. Those with positive skin tests or histories of positive skin tests, for whom diagnostic evaluation for active tuberculosis is negative, should be evaluated for preventive therapy according to current guidelines[5].

2. Early identification and treatment of persons with active tuberculosis

- Vigorous efforts should be made to identify patients with active tuberculosis in a timely manner and to place them on appropriate therapy (see section II.B.2.). Pulmonary tuberculosis should always be included in the differential diagnosis of persons with pulmonary signs or symptoms, and appropriate diagnostic measures should be instituted.

- For patients with pulmonary signs or symptoms that are initially ascribed to other etiologies, evaluation for co-existing tuberculosis should be repeated if the patient does not respond to appropriate therapy for the presumed etiology of the pulmonary abnormalities (see section II.B.2.).
- In health-care facilities, isolation precautions should be applied to patients who are suspected or confirmed to have active tuberculosis and who may be infectious (see sections II.B.3 and III.B.I.a.).
- Procedure-specific precautions should be applied for cough-inducing or aerosol-generating procedures (see section III.A.5.).
- Patients with suspected or confirmed tuberculosis should be reported to the appropriate health department so that standard procedures for identifying and evaluating tuberculosis contacts can be initiated.

3. Ventilation

- Staff of inpatient facilities should either include an engineer or other professional with expertise in ventilation or industrial hygiene, or the facility should have this expertise available from a consultant. These persons should work closely with the infection-control committee in the control of airborne infections.
- Ventilation for health-care facilities should be developed and maintained in consultation with experts in ventilation engineering who also have hospital ventilation experience. Facility design should meet local and state requirements. Specific recommendations for health-care facilities have been published by ASHRAE and HRSA[40,41] (see section II.D.).
- The direction of air flow in health-care facilities should be set up and maintained so that air flows from clean areas to less clean areas. In areas of a facility in which tuberculosis transmission is a potential problem, direction of air flow should be monitored frequently. Periodic checks with smoke tubes or smoke sticks provide a sensitive indication of air flow direction (see section II.D.I.c.).
- Facilities serving populations with a high prevalence of tuberculosis may need to enhance ventilation or use supplemental approaches in areas of the facility where patients with tuberculosis are likely to be found (e.g., waiting areas, emergency rooms, radiology suites, or treatment rooms) or where skin tests of personnel demonstrate an increased risk of tuberculosis transmission (see section II.D.2.).

4. Potential supplemental environmental approaches

a. High-efficiency filtration

- If air from potentially contaminated general-use areas (e.g., emergency rooms or clinic waiting areas) cannot be exhausted directly to the outside, HEPA filters with test efficiencies of $\geq$ 99.97% may be useful for removing infectious organisms from air before recirculation in a room or before return to common supply ducts. If HEPA filters are used, they must be designed, installed, maintained and disposed of, in accordance with all applicable regulations and manufacturers' recommendations (see section II.D.2.a.). HEPA filters should not be used to recirculate air from a tuberculosis isolation room back into the general circulation.

b. *Germicidal UV irradiation*

- For settings in which the risk of tuberculosis transmission is high (see section I.B.), UV lamps have been used to supplement ventilation (see section II.D.2.b.). The decision to use UV lamps should be made on a case-by-case basis. If UV lamps are used, applicable safety guidelines should be followed (see section II.D.2.b.). UV lamps are not recommended for use in small rooms or booths where nebulizing devices will be used. UV units installed in ducts should not be used to recirculate air from a tuberculosis isolation room back into the general circulation.

c. *Disposable PRs for filtration of inhaled air*

- PRs (see section II.D.2.c) should be provided by health-care facilities and worn by persons in the same room with a patient whose signs and symptoms suggest a high potential for infectiousness and by those performing procedures that are likely to produce bursts of droplet nuclei, such as bronchoscopy, endotracheal auctioning, and administration of AP.
- Wearers should be adequately trained in the use and disposal of PRs and should carefully follow manufacturers' instructions. Ideally, a respirator program consistent with the guidelines found in Department of Health and Human Services (DHHS), National Institute for Occupational Safety and Health (NIOSH), Publication No. 87–116, *Guide to Industrial Respiratory Protection*[64] and the requirements of the Occupational Safety and Health Administration (OSHA), General Industry Occupational Safety and Health Standards[29]. Code of Federal Regulations (Part 1910.134) should be implemented. Such a program includes training, fit testing, care and maintenance, and medical monitoring.

5. *Procedure-specific precautions*

a. *Diagnostic sputum induction*

- Sputum induction performed on patients who may have tuberculosis should be carried out in an individual room or booth with negative pressure relative to adjacent rooms and hallways, ideally with room or booth air exhausted directly to the outside and away from all windows and air intake ducts (see section II.C.1.). Patients should remain in the booth or treatment room (or go outside, weather permitting) and not return to common waiting areas until coughing has subsided. Time should be allowed between patients so that any droplet nuclei that have been introduced into the air can be removed. This time will vary according to the efficiency of the ventilation or filtration used (Table 1). Health-care-facility personnel collecting induced sputum should wear PRs if it is necessary for them to be in the room with the patient during the procedure (see section II.D.2.c.).

b. *Administration of AP*

- All patients should be screened for active tuberculosis before AP therapy is initiated. Screening should include medical history, tuberculin skin test, and a baseline chest radiograph (see section II.B.2).

- Before each subsequent AP treatment, patients should be evaluated for symptoms highly suggestive of tuberculosis, such as the development of a productive cough or cough and fever. If such symptoms are elicited, a diagnostic evaluation should be initiated.
- If active tuberculosis is found or suspected, the patient should be placed on antituberculosis chemotherapy. AP treatments should be administered to patients who may have active tuberculosis *only* in a room or booth as described for sputum induction.
- Ideally, AP treatments for all patients should be administered in an individual room or booth as described for sputum induction (see sections II.C.1 and III.A.5.a). Adequate time should be allowed between patients for removal of residual pentamidine and any infectious organisms from the air when treatment rooms or booths are to be reused (Table 1).
- Workers administering AP should wear PRs whenever they must be in the room or booth during administration of AP to patients who have, or are at high risk of having, tuberculosis (see section II.D.2.c.).
- After they have received AP, patients should not return to common waiting areas until coughing subsides.

c. *Bronchoscopy*

- Bronchoscopy should be performed in rooms that have adequate ventilation, good distribution of air flow, and air exhausted directly to the outside – in accordance with federal, state, and local regulations for environmental discharges – or recirculated through HEPA filters. Ideally, bronchoscopy should be performed in rooms with negative pressure relative to adjacent areas. If bronchoscopy must be performed in positive-pressure rooms (such as operating rooms), the risk of infectious tuberculosis should be ruled out beforehand.
- Additional protection may be afforded by local exhaust ventilation employed near the patient's head to exhaust most organisms near their source (see section II.C.1.) or by the use of UV lamps in treatment areas where bronchoscopies are performed (see section II.D.2.b.).
- Persons who must be in the room with the patient during bronchoscopy should wear PRs (see section II.D.2.c.).

d. *Endotracheal intubation/suctioning*

- Rooms occupied by intubated patients who may have active tuberculosis should be provided with ventilation as described for patient isolation rooms (see section III.B.l.a.). Persons performing endotracheal suctioning on patients who have suspected or confirmed active tuberculosis should wear PRs.

e. *Other procedures*

- Other aerosol treatments, cough-inducing procedures, or aerosol generating procedures should be administered as described for AP administration (see section II.C.1.).

6. Decontamination: cleaning, disinfecting, and sterilizing

- Decisions about decontamination processes should be based on the intended use of the item and not on the diagnosis of the patient for whom the item was used (see section II.E.).

- Generally, critical items should be sterilized, semi-critical items should be sterilized or cleaned with high-level disinfectants, and non-critical items need only be cleaned with detergents or low-level disinfectants. Meticulous physical cleaning before sterilization or a high level of disinfection is essential (see section II.E.).

- The same routine, daily cleaning procedures used in other hospital or facility rooms should be used to clean rooms of patients who are on AFB isolation precautions (see section II.E.).

7. Conducting surveillance for tuberculosis transmission

a. Surveillance and reporting

- Health-care facilities providing care to patients at risk for tuberculosis should maintain active surveillance for tuberculosis among patients and health-care-facility personnel and for skin-test conversions among health-care-facility personnel. When tuberculosis is suspected or diagnosed, public health authorities should be notified so that appropriate contact investigation can be performed. Data on the occurrence of tuberculosis and skin-test conversions among patients and health-care-facility personnel should be collected and analyzed to estimate the risk of tuberculosis transmission in the facility and to evaluate the effectiveness of infection-control and screening practices.

- At the time of employment, all health-care-facility personnel, including those with a history of Bacillus of Calmette and Guerin (BCG) vaccination, should receive a Mantoux tuberculin skin test unless a previously positive reaction can be documented or completion of adequate preventive therapy or adequate therapy for active disease can be documented.

- Initial and follow-up tuberculin skin tests should be administered and interpreted according to current guidelines[5,11].

- Health-care-facility personnel with a documented history of a positive tuberculin test, or adequate treatment for disease or preventive therapy for infection, should be exempt from further screening unless they develop symptoms suggestive of tuberculosis.

- Periodic retesting of PPD-negative health-care workers should be conducted to identify persons whose skin tests convert to positive[11]. In general, the frequency of repeat testing should be based on the risk of developing new infection. Health-care-facility workers who may be frequently exposed to patients with tuberculosis or who are involved with potentially high-risk procedures (e.g., bronchoscopy, sputum induction, or aerosol treatments given to patients who may have tuberculosis) should be retested at least every 6 months. Health-care-facility personnel in other areas should be retested annually. Data on skin-test conversions should be periodically reviewed so that the risk of acquiring new infection may be estimated for each area of the facility. On the basis of this analysis, the frequency of retesting may be altered accordingly.

b. Evaluation of health-care-facility personnel after unprotected exposure to tuberculosis

- In addition to periodic screening, health-care-facility personnel and patients should be evaluated if they have been exposed to a potentially infectious tuberculosis patient for whom the infection-control procedures outlined in this document have not been taken. Unless a negative skin test has been documented within the preceding 3 months, each exposed health-care-facility worker (except those already known to be positive reactors) should receive a Mantoux tuberculin skin test as soon as possible after exposure and should be managed in the same way as other contacts[5]. If the initial skin test is negative, the test should be repeated 12 weeks after the exposure ended. Exposed persons with skin-test reactions ≥ 5 mm or with symptoms suggestive of tuberculosis should receive chest radiographs. Persons with previously known positive skin-test reactions, who have been exposed to an infectious patient, do not require a repeat skin test or a chest radiograph unless they have symptoms suggestive of tuberculosis.

c. Evaluation and management of health-care-facility personnel with positive skin tests or symptoms that may be due to tuberculosis

- Health-care-facility personnel with positive tuberculin skin tests or with skin test conversions on repeat testing or after exposure should be clinically evaluated for active tuberculosis[11]. Persons with symptoms suggestive of tuberculosis should be evaluated regardless of skin test results. If tuberculosis is diagnosed, appropriate therapy should be instituted according to published guidelines[65]. Personnel diagnosed with active tuberculosis should be offered counseling and HIV-antibody testing[27].

- Health-care-facility personnel who have positive tuberculin skin tests or skin test conversions but do not have clinical tuberculosis should be evaluated for preventive therapy according to published guidelines[5,65]. Personnel with positive skin tests should be evaluated for risk of HIV infection. If HIV infection is considered a possibility, counseling and HIV-antibody testing should be strongly encouraged[27].

- All persons with a history of tuberculosis or positive tuberculin tests are at risk for contracting tuberculosis in the future. These persons should be reminded periodically that they should promptly report any pulmonary symptoms. If symptoms of tuberculosis should develop, the person should be evaluated immediately.

d. Routine and follow-up chest radiographs

- Routine chest films are not required for asymptomatic, tuberculin negative health-care-facility personnel. After the initial chest radiograph is taken, personnel with positive skin-test reactions do not need repeat chest radiographs unless symptoms develop that may be due to tuberculosis[66].

e. Work restrictions

- Health-care-facility personnel with current pulmonary or laryngeal tuberculosis pose a risk to patients and other personnel while they are infectious; therefore, stringent work restrictions for these persons are necessary. They should be excluded from work until adequate treatment is instituted, cough is resolved, and sputum is free of bacilli on three consecutive smears. Health-care-facility personnel with current tuberculosis at sites other than the lung or larynx usually do not need to be excluded from work if concurrent pulmonary tuberculosis has been ruled out. Personnel who discontinue treatment before the recommended course of therapy has been completed should not be allowed to work until treatment is resumed, an adequate response to therapy is documented, and they have negative sputum smears on three consecutive days.

- Health-care-facility personnel who are otherwise healthy and receiving preventive treatment for tuberculous infection should be allowed to continue usual work activities.

- Health-care facility personnel who cannot take or do not accept or complete a full course of preventive therapy should have their work situations evaluated to determine whether reassignment is indicated. Work restrictions may not be necessary for otherwise healthy persons who do not accept or complete preventive therapy. These persons should be counseled about the risk of contracting disease and should be instructed to seek evaluation promptly if symptoms develop that may be due to tuberculosis, especially if they have contact with high-risk patients (i.e., patients at high risk for severe consequences if they become infected).

f. Consultation

- Consultation on tuberculosis surveillance, screening, and other methods to reduce tuberculosis transmission should be available from state health department tuberculosis-control programs. Facilities are encouraged to use the services of health departments in planning and implementing their surveillance and screening programs.

B. Precautions for Specific Settings

1. Hospitals and other inpatient facilities

a. Tuberculosis (AFB) isolation precautions

- In hospitals and other inpatient facilities, any patient suspected or known to have infectious tuberculosis should be placed in AFB isolation in a private room.

- ASHRAE[40] and HRSA[41] have published recommendations for ventilation in AFB isolation rooms. These recommendations specify that rooms should have at least six total air changes per hour, including at least two outside air changes per hour, with sufficient within-room air distribution to dilute or remove tuberculosis bacilli from locations where health-care-facility personnel or visitors are likely to be exposed.

- The direction of air flow should be set up and maintained so that air flows into the room from the hallway (negative pressure) to minimize possible spread of tuberculosis bacilli into the general health-care setting.

- The direction of air flow should be monitored while the room is being used for AFB isolation. The use of flutter strips provides a means of constantly observing the direction of air flow. Smoke tubes or smoke sticks are also a quick, simple means of determining the direction of air flow.

- Air from the room should be exhausted directly to the outside of the building and away from intake vents, people, and animals, in accordance with federal, state, and local regulations concerning environmental discharges. Germicidal UV lamps may be considered as a supplement to ventilation to further decrease the number of infectious droplet nuclei in the air (see sections II.D.2.b. and III.A.4.b.).

- Isolation-room doors must be kept closed to maintain control over the direction of air flow.

- Optionally, a separate anteroom may serve as an airlock to minimize the potential for droplet nuclei to spread from the patient's area to adjacent areas. To work effectively, the anteroom must have directional airflow.

- Persons who enter a room in which AFB isolation precautions are in place should wear PRs (see section II.D.2.c.).

- The patient should remain in the isolation room with the door closed and should be instructed to cover nose and mouth with a tissue during coughing and sneezing. If the patient must leave the room (e.g., for a medical procedure that cannot be done at the bedside) while potentially infectious, s/he should wear a properly fitted surgical mask or valveless PR (see section II.C.2.).

- AFB isolation precautions may be discontinued and the patient placed in a private room when s/he is improving clinically, cough has substantially decreased, and the number of organisms on sequential sputum smears is decreasing. Usually, this occurs within 2–3 weeks after tuberculosis medications are begun. Failure to take medications as prescribed and the presence of drug-resistant disease are the two most common reasons for a patient's remaining infectious. When a patient is likely to be infected with drug-resistant organisms, AFB precautions should be applied until the patient is improving and the sputum smear is negative for AFB. Placing a tuberculosis patient in a room with other patients is not advisable, especially immunosuppressed patients, until the sputum smear is free of bacilli on three consecutive days (see section II.B.3.).

b. *Transport, radiology,* and *treatment rooms*

- When a patient who may have infectious tuberculosis must be transported outside the AFB isolation room, s/he should wear a properly fitted surgical mask or valveless PR (see section II.C.2.).

- Ideally, an area in the treatment or radiology department should be specially ventilated for AFB isolation patients. If this is not possible, the patient should be returned to the isolation room as soon as is practical.

- Health-care-facility workers performing procedures on patients with potentially infectious tuberculosis should wear a PR, especially if the procedure itself induces cough (see section II.D.2.c.).

- Treatment rooms in which patients who have undiagnosed pulmonary disease, and who are at high risk for active tuberculosis, are evaluated, should meet the ventilation standards for AFB isolation rooms. ASHRAE recommends that treatment rooms have at least six air changes per hour[40].

- Treatment rooms in which cough-inducing procedures are performed should meet the specifications outlined under procedure-specific precautions.

c. *Intensive-care units (ICUs)*

- ASHRAE recommends that ventilation in ICUs should provide at least six total air changes per hour, including at least two outside air changes per hour[40]. If air is recirculated in the ICU, it should be passed through properly designed, installed, and maintained HEPA filters before being recirculated.
- Installation of UV lamps might be considered in ICUs in which there is a high risk of tuberculosis transmission (see section I.B.).
- Any ICU patient who may have infectious tuberculosis should be placed in a private room in which ventilation meets the recommendations for AFB isolation.
- Endotracheal suctioning of patients who may have infectious tuberculosis should be carried out as described under procedure-specific precautions (see section III.A.5.d.)
- ICU patients with undiagnosed pulmonary symptoms who may have infectious tuberculosis should have respiratory secretions submitted for AFB smear and culture (see section II.B.2.).

d. *Emergency rooms*

- Ventilation in emergency rooms, including waiting areas, should be designed and maintained to reduce the risk of tuberculosis transmission,[39–41]. ASHRAE recommends that emergency room waiting areas have at least 10 air changes per hour[40].
- In facilities serving populations with a high incidence of tuberculosis (see section I.B.), germicidal UV lamps and/or HEPA filters in the emergency room may provide additional benefit when used to supplement ventilation (see section II.D.2.).

e. *Laboratories*

- Laboratories should adhere to previously published recommendations concerning control of tuberculosis transmission[67].

f. *Autopsy rooms*

- ASHRAE recommends that autopsy rooms have ventilation that provides at least 12 total air changes per hour[40]. In addition, these rooms should have good distribution of air flow in the room, negative pressure with respect to adjacent areas, and room air exhausted directly to the outside of the building. PRs should be worn by personnel performing procedures that may aerosolize infectious particles (e.g., sawing, irrigating).

g. *Hospices*

- All tuberculosis-control recommendations for inpatient facilities apply to hospices.

h. *Nursing homes*

- Published recommendations for prevention and control of tuberculosis in nursing homes should be followed[68].

i. *Correctional facilities*

- Published recommendations for prevention and control of tuberculosis in correctional facilities should be followed[54]. Prison medical facilities should follow the recommendations outlined in this document.

2. Ambulatory-care facilities

- Health-care employers in outpatient settings should be aware of the risk of tuberculosis among their patient population. They should be especially aware of the increased risk among persons who have both HIV infection and tuberculous infection, and they should develop infection-control policies accordingly.
- Persons who have HIV infection or who are otherwise at risk for contracting tuberculosis should receive a tuberculin skin test, and the results should be noted in the patient's medical record. Tuberculosis diagnostic procedures should be initiated if signs and symptoms of tuberculosis develop (see section II.B.2.).
- Ambulatory patients who have pulmonary symptoms of uncertain etiology should be instructed to cover their mouths and noses when coughing or sneezing; they should spend a minimum of time in common waiting areas (see section II.C.2.).
- Personnel who are the first point of contact in facilities serving patients at risk for tuberculosis should be trained to recognize, and bring to the attention of the appropriate person, any patients with symptoms suggestive of tuberculosis (see section II.B.2.), such as a productive cough > 3 weeks' duration, especially when accompanied by other tuberculosis symptoms, such as weight loss, fever, fatigue, and anorexia.
- Ventilation in clinics serving patients who are at high risk for tuberculosis (see section 1.B.) should be designed and maintained to reduce the risk of tuberculosis transmission[39–41] (see section II.D.). This is particularly important if immunosuppressed patients are treated in the same or a nearby area. In some settings, (see section I.B.), enhanced ventilation or air-disinfection techniques, e.g., HEPA filters or germicidal UV lamps (see sections 11.D.2.a. and 11.D.2.b.) may be appropriate for common areas such as waiting rooms. Air from clinics serving patients at high risk for tuberculosis should not be recirculated unless it is first passed through an effective high-efficiency filtration system.
- In outpatient settings where cough-inducing procedures are carried out, procedure-specific AFB precautions should be implemented (see sections II.C. and III.A.5.).

3. Emergency medical services

- When emergency-medical-response personnel or others must transport patients with confirmed or suspected, active tuberculosis, a mask or valveless PR should be fitted on the patient. If this is not possible, the worker should wear a PR (see sections II.C.2. and II.D.2.c.). If feasible, the rear windows of the vehicle should be kept open and the heating and air conditioning system set on a nonrecirculating cycle.
- Emergency-response personnel should be routinely screened for tuberculosis at regular intervals. They should also be included in the follow-up of contacts of a patient with infectious tuberculosis (see section III.A.7.).

4. Home-health services

- For persons visiting the home of patients with suspected or confirmed infectious tuberculosis, precautions may be necessary to prevent exposure to air

containing droplet nuclei until infectiousness has been eliminated by chemotherapy. These precautions include instructing patients to cover coughs and
sneezes. The worker should wear a PR when entering the home or the patient's
room.

- Respiratory precautions in the home may be discontinued when the patient is
improving clinically, cough has decreased, and the number of organisms in
the sputum smear is decreasing. Usually this occurs within 2–3 weeks after
tuberculosis medications are begun. Failure to take medications as prescribed
and the presence of drug-resistant disease are the two most common reasons
for a patient's failure to improve clinically. Home health-care personnel can
assist in preventing tuberculosis transmission by educating the patient about
the importance of taking medications as prescribed (unless adverse effects are
seen).
- If immunocompromised persons or young children live in the home with a
patient who has infectious, pulmonary or laryngeal tuberculosis, temporary
relocation should be considered until the patient has negative sputum smears.
- If cough-inducing procedures (such as AP) are performed in the home of a
patient who may have infectious tuberculosis, they should be administered
in a well-ventilated area away from other household members. Persons who
perform these procedures should wear PRs while performing them.
- Home health-care workers should be included in an employer-sponsored tuberculosis screening and prevention program (see section III.A.7.).
- Early identification and treatment of persons with tuberculosis is important.
Home health-care personnel and patients who are at risk for contracting active
tuberculosis should be reminded periodically of the importance of having pulmonary symptoms evaluated.
- Close contacts of any patient with active, infectious tuberculosis should be
evaluated for tuberculous infection and managed according to CDC and American Thoracic Society guidelines[5,65].

IV. Research Needs

Additional research is needed regarding the airborne transmission of tuberculosis, including the following: a) better quantitating of the risk of tuberculosis
transmission in a variety of health-care settings, b) assessing the acceptability,
efficacy, adverse impact, and cost-effectiveness of currently available methods
for preventing transmission, and c) developing better methods for preventing
transmission. These needs also extend to other infections transmitted by the
airborne route. Currently, large numbers of immunosuppressed persons, including
patients infected with HIV, are being brought together in health-care settings in
which procedures are used that induce the generation of droplet nuclei. Research
is needed to fill many of the gaps in current knowledge and to lead to new and
better guidelines for protecting patients and personnel in these settings.

V. Glossary of Abbreviations

AFB. Acid-fast bacilli-organisms that retain certain stains, even after being washed
with acid alcohol. Most are mycobacteria. When seen on a stained smear of sputum

or other clinical specimen, a diagnosis of tuberculosis should be considered.

AIDS. Acquired immunodeficiency syndrome – an advanced stage of disease caused by infection with the human immunodeficiency virus (HIV). A patient with AIDS is especially susceptible to other infections.

AP. Aerosolized pentamidine – drug treatment given to patients with HIV infection to treat or to prevent *Pneumocystis carinii* pneumonia. The drug is put into solution, the solution is aerosolized, and the patient inhales the aerosol.

ASHRAE. American Society of Heating, Refrigerating, and Air Conditioning Engineers, Inc.

HEPA. High-efficiency particulate air filter.

HIV. Human immunodeficiency virus – the virus that causes AIDS.

HRSA. Health Resources and Services Administration.

PCP. *Pneumocystis carinii* pneumonia – this organism does not cause disease among persons with a normal immune system.

PR. A disposable, particulate respirator (respiratory protective device (face mask) that is designed to filter out particles 1–5 microns in diameter.

Tuberculous infection. A condition in which tuberculosis organisms *(M. tuberculosis, M. bovis, or M. africanum)* are present in the body, but no active disease is evident.

Tuberculosis transmission. Spread of tuberculosis organisms from one person to another, usually through the air.

UV. Ultraviolet.

References

1. CDC. Nosocomial transmission of multidrug-resistant tuberculosis to health care workers and HIV-infected patients in an urban hospital – Florida. MMWR 1990; 39:718–22.
2. Pitchenik AR, Fertel D, Bloch AB. Mycobacterial disease: epidemiology, diagnosis, treatment, and prevention. Clin Chest Med 1988; 9:425–41.
3. Selwyn PA, Hartel D, Lewis VA, et al. A prospective study of the risk of tuberculosis among intravenous drug users with human immunodeficiency virus infection. N Eng J Med 1989; 320:545–50.
4. Di Perri G, Cruciani M, Danzi MC, et al. Nosocomial epidemic of active tuberculosis among HIV-Infected patients. Lancet 1989; 23/30:1502–04.
5. CDC. Screening for tuberculosis and tuberculous infection in high-risk populations, and The use of preventive therapy for tuberculous infection in the United States: recommendations of the Advisory Committee for Elimination of Tuberculosis. MMWR 1990; 39(no. RR-8).
6. American Thoracic Society, CDC. Control of tuberculosis. Am Rev Respir Dis 1983; 128: 336–42.
7. American Thoracic Society, Ad Hoc Committee of the Scientific Assembly on

Tuberculosis. Screening for pulmonary tuberculosis in institutions. Am Rev Respir Dis 1977; 1 15:901–6.
8. CDC. Guidelines for prevention of TB transmission in hospitals. Atlanta, Georgia: US Department of Health and Human Services, Public Health Service, 1982; DHHS publication no.(CDC)82–8371.
9. Williams WW. Guideline for infection control in hospital personnel. Infect Control 1983; 4(suppl):326–49.
10. Garner JS, Simmons BP. Guideline for isolation precautions in hospitals. Infect Control 1983; 4(suppl):245–325.
11. American Thoracic Society, CDC. Diagnostic standards and classification of tuberculosis. Am Rev Respir Dis 1990; 142:725–35.
12. Wells WF. Aerodynamics of droplet nuclei. In: Airborne contagion and air hygiene. Cambridge: Harvard University Press, 1955:14–9.
13. Barrett-Connor E. The epidemiology of tuberculosis in physicians. JAMA 1979; 241:33–8.
14. Brennen C, Muder RR, Muraca PW. Occult endemic tuberculosis in a chronic care facility. Infect Control Hosp Epidemiol 1988; 9:548–52.
15. Goldman KP. Tuberculosis in hospital doctors. Tubercle 1988; 69:237–40.
16. Catanzaro A. Nosocomial tuberculosis. Am Rev Respir Dis 1982; 125:559–62.
17. Ehrenkranz NJ, Kicklighter JL. Tuberculosis outbreak in a general hospital: evidence of airborne spread of infection. Ann Intern Med 1972; 77:377–82.
18. Haley CE, McDonald RC, Rossi L, et al. Tuberculosis epidemic among hospital personnel. Infect Control Hosp Epidemiol 1989; 10:204-10.
19. Hutton MD, Stead WW, Cauthen GM, et al. Nosocomial transmission of tuberculosis associated with a draining tuberculous abscess. J Infect Dis 1990; 161:286–95.
20. Kantor HS, Poblete R, Pusateri SL. Nosocomial transmission of tuberculosis from unsuspected disease. Am J Med 1988; 84:833–8.
21. Lundgren R, Norrman E, Asberg I. Tuberculous infection transmitted at autopsy. Tubercle 1987; 68:147–50.
22. CDC. Mycobacterium tuberculosis transmission in a health clinic – Florida, 1988. MMWR 1989;38:256–64.
23. Pitchenik AE, Cole C, Russell BW, et al. Tuberculosis, atypical mycobacterlosis, and the acquired immunodeficiency syndrome among Haitian and non-Haitian patients in South Florida. Ann Intern Med 1984; 101:641–5.
24. Maayan S, Wormser GP, Hewlett D, et al. Acquired immunodeficiency syndrome (AIDS) in an economically disadvantaged population. Arch Intern Med 1985; 145:1607–12.
25. Klein NC, Duncanson FP, Lenox TH III, et al. Use of mycobacterial smears in the diagnosis of pulmonary tuberculosis in AIDS/ARC patients. Chest 1989; 95:1190–2.
26. Burnens AP, Vurma-Rapp U. Mixed mycobacterial cultures – occurrence in the clinical laboratory. Zbl Bakt 1989; 271:85–90.
27. CDC. Tuberculosis and human immunodeficiency virus infection: recommendations of the Advisory Committee for the Elimination of Tuberculosis (ACET). MMWR 1989; 38:236–8, 243–50.
28. Willcox, PA, Benator SR, Potgieter PD. Use of flexible fiberoptic bronchoscope in diagnosis of sputum-negative pulmonary tuberculosis. Thorax 1982; 37:598–601.
29. Willcox PA, Potgieter PD, Bateman ED, Benator SR. Rapid diagnosis of sputum-negative miliary tuberculosis using the flexible fiberoptic bronchoscope. Thorax 1986; 41:681–4.

30. Canessa PA, Fasano L, Lavecchia MA, Torraca A, Schiattone ML. Tuberculin skin test in asymptomatic HIV seropositive carriers [Letter]. Chest 1989; 96:1215–6.
31. Pitchenik AE, Rubinson HA. The radiographic appearance of tuberculosis in patients with the acquired imm‧ne deficiency syndrome (AIDS) and pre-AIDS. Am Rev Respir Dis 1985; 131:393–6.
32. Kiehn TE, Cammarata R. Laboratory diagnosis of mycobacterial infection in patients with acquired immunodeficiency syndrome. J Clin Microbiol 1986; 24:708–11.
33. Crawford JT, Eisenach KD, Bates JH. Diagnosis of tuberculosis: present and future. Semin Resp Infect 1989; 4:171–81.
34. Riley RL, Mills CC, O'Grady F, Sultan LU, Wittstadt F, Shivpuri DN. Infectiousness of air from a tuberculosis ward. Amer Rev Respir Dis 1962; 85:511–25.
35. Noble RC. Infectiousness of pulmonary tuberculosis after starting chemotherapy: review of the available data on an unresolved question. Am J Infect Control 1981; 9:6–10.
36. Woods JE. Cost avoidance and productivity in owning and operating buildings [state of the art review]. Occup Med 1989; 4:753–70.
37. American Conference of Governmental Industrial Hygienists. Industrial ventilation: a manual of recommended practice. Lansing, Michigan: ACGIH, 1988.
38. Riley RL. Airborne infection. Am J Med 1974; 57:466–75.
39. American Society of Heating, Refrigerating, and Air Conditioning Engineers. Ventilation for acceptable indoor air quality. Atlanta, Georgia: ASHRAE, Inc., 1989 Standard 62-1989.
40. American Society of Heating, Refrigerating, and Air Conditioning Engineers. 1987 ASHRAE handbook: heating, ventilating, and air-conditioning systems and applications. Atlanta, Georgia: American Society of Heating, Refrigerating, and Air Conditioning Engineers, Inc., 1987:23.1–23.12.
41. Health Resources and Services Administration. Guidelines for construction and equipment of hospital and medical facilities. Rockville, Maryland.: US Department of Health & Human Services, Public Health Service, 1984;PHS publication no.(HRSA)84-14500.
42. Woods JE, Rask DR. Heating, ventilation, air-conditioning systems: the engineering approach to methods of control. In: Kundsin RB, ed. Architectural design and indoor microbial pollution. New York: Oxford University Press, 1988:123–53.
43. Riley RL, Nardell EA. Clearing the air: the theory and application of UV air disinfection. Am Rev Respir Dis 1989; 139:1286–94.
44. Sherertz RJ, Belani A, Kramer BS, et al. Impact of air filtration on nosocomial *Aspergillus* infections. Am J Med 1987; 83:709–18.
45. Rhame FS, Streifel AJ, Kersey JH, McGlave PB. Extrinsic risk factors for pneumonia in the patient at high risk of infection. Am J Med 1984; 76:42–52.
46. Opal SM, Asp AA, Cannady PB, Morse PL, Burton LJ, Hammer PG. Efficacy of infection control measures during a nosocomial outbreak of disseminated *Aspergillus* associated with hospital construction. J Infect Dis 1986; 153:63–47.
47. Collins FM. Relative susceptibility of acid-fast and non-acid-fast bacteria to ultraviolet light. Appl Microbiol 1971; 21:411–13.
48. David HL, Jones WD Jr, Newman CM. Ultraviolet light inactivation and photoreactivation in the mycobacteria. Infect Immun 1971; 4:318–19.
49. David HL. Response of mycobacteria to ultraviolet light radiation. Am Rev Respir Dis 1973; 108:1175–85.
50. Riley RL, Knight M, Middlebrook G. Ultraviolet susceptibility of BCG and virulent

tubercle bacilli. Am Rev Respir Dis 1976; 113:413–18.
51. National Tuberculosis and Respiratory Disease Association. Guidelines for the general hospital in the admission and care of tuberculous patients. Am Rev Respir Dis 1969; 99:631–3.
52. CDC. Notes on air hygiene: summary of conference on air disinfection. Arch Environ Health 1971; 22:473–4.
53. Schieffelbein CW Jr, Snider DE Jr. Tuberculosis control among homeless populations. Arch Intern Med 1988; 148:1843–6.
54. CDC. Prevention and control of tuberculosis in correctional institutions: recommendations of the Advisory Committee for the Elimination of Tuberculosis, MMWR 1989; 38:313–20,325.
55. Stead WW. Clearing the air: the theory and application of ultraviolet air disinfection [Letter]. Am Rev Respir Dis 1989; 140:1832.
56. Macher JM. Ultraviolet radiation and ventilation to help control tuberculosis transmission: guidelines prepared for California Indoor Air Quality Program. Berkeley, CA: Air and Industrial Hygiene Laboratory, 1989.
57. Riley RL, Kaufman JE. Effect of relative humidity on the inactivation of airborne *Serratia marcescens* by ultraviolet radiation. Appl Microbiol 1972; 23:1113–20.
58. The biological effects of ultraviolet radiation (with emphasis on the skin). In: Urbach F, ed. Proceedings of the Ist International Conference Sponsored Jointly by the Skin and Cancer Hospital, Temple University Health Sciences Center and the International Society of Biometeorology. Oxford, England: Pergamon Press, 1969.
59. Riley RL. Ultraviolet air disinfection for control of respiratory contagion. In: Kundsin RB, ed. Architectural design and indoor microbial pollution. New York: Oxford University Press, 1988:175–97.
60. National Institute for Occupational Safety and Health. Criteria for a recommended standard . . . occupational exposure to ultraviolet radiation. Washington, DC: National Institute for Occupational Safety and Health, 1972; publication no. (HSM) 73–110009.
61. Pippin DJ, Verderame RA, Weber KK. Efficacy of face masks in preventing inhalation of airborne contaminants. J Oral Maxillofac Surg 1987; 45:319–23.
62. Rutala WA. APIC guidelines for selection and use of disinfectants. Am J Infect Control 1990; 18:99–117.
63. Garner JS, Favero MS. Guideline for handwashing and hospital environmental control. Atlanta, Georgia: US Department of Health and Human Services, Public Health Service, CDC, 1985.
64. NIOSH. Guide to industrial respiratory protection. Cincinnati, Ohio: US Department of Health and Human Services, Public Health Service, Centers for Disease Control, National Institute for Occupational Safety and Health. 1987; DHHS (NIOSH) publication no. 87-116.
65. American Thoracic Society, CDC. Treatment of tuberculosis and tuberculosis infection in adults and children, 1986. Am Rev Respir Dis 1986; 134:355–63.
66. Barrett-Connor E. The periodic chest roentgenogram for the control of tuberculosis in health care personnel. Am Rev Respir Dis 1980; 122:153–5.
67. Strong BE, Kubica GP. Isolation and identification of *Mycobacterium tuberculosis.* Atlanta, Georgia: US Department of Health and Human Services, Public Health Service, CDC, 1981; HHS publication no.(CDC)81-8390.
68. CDC. Prevention and control of tuberculosis in facilities providing long-term care to the elderly. MMWR 1990; 39(No. RR-10).

69. Mutchler JE. Principles of ventilation. In: National Institute for Occupational Safety and Health. The industrial environment – its evaluation and control. Washington, DC: National Institute for Occupational Safety and Health, 1973.

Appendix 5: Social History Form (see Chapter 16)

```
                        SOCIAL HISTORY

Name _____  Age _____
Hospital identification number _____  Ward _____
Date of admission/nursing assessment _____
Address _____

_____

_____ (Telephone number) _____
Next of kin and address _____

_____

_____ (Telephone number) _____
General practitioner and address _____

_____

_____ (Telephone number) _____
Admitting consultant _____

Next of kin informed of admission:    YES/NO
Comment _____

_____

GP informed of admission:    YES/NO
Comment _____

_____

Reason for admission _____

_____
```

Accommodation

Own   Rented   Private   Council   Sheltered

House   Flat   Room   Which floor? _____

Stairs _____

Toilet (which floor?) _____

Heating _____ Central heating

Cooking facilities _____

Coin Metres for   Heating   YES/NO   Electricity   YES/NO

Accommodation shared with _____

_____

Pets _____ _____

Pets being looked after by _____

Keys to accommodation with _____

Is accommodation now secure?   YES/NO

If no, what action being taken? _____

Employer and address _____

_____

_____ (Telephone number) _____

Does employer need to be informed of admission?   YES/NO

If yes, who is informing employer? _____

Date employer notified _____

Name/position of individual notified _____

_____

COMMUNITY SERVICES

Service	On admission			On discharge	
	Known	Frequency	Informed of admission	Needed	Arrangement
District Nurse					
Health Visitor					
Home Help					
Community Physiotherapist					
Community Occupational Therapist					
Social Worker					
Meals on Wheels					
Volunteer					
Other (Specify)					
Comments:					

SOCIAL HISTORY/DISCHARGE PLANS

Medications	
Medication being taken on admission	Medication to be taken home on discharge

Medications (patient education)

Date/Time/Name and position of individual instructing patient on discharge medications

Date _____ Time _____ Health professional _____

Assessment of patient education:

Does patient understand how to self-administer medications?   YES/NO

Is patient aware of common side-effects of medication and how to detect signs/symptoms of side-effects and reactions?   YES/NO

Has patient been given *written* instructions on how to self-administer medications, their side-effects and how and when to obtain new supply?   YES/NO

If patient on zidovudine (Retrovir – AZT), has he/she been issued with a timed medication device and instructed on how to use it?   YES/NO

Have all medications/instructions been listed on discharge summary to community nursing services?   YES/NO

Transportation: Indicate below arrangements made for patient's transportation home

Ordered by _____ Date _____

If patient lives alone, who will accompany patient home and see him/her safely in their home?

Requisites for health: State discharge status for the following self-care requisites

The need for adequate respiration:

The need for adequate hydration:

The need for adequate nutrition:

The need for urinary and faecal elimination:

The need to control body temperature:

The need for movement and mobilization:

The need for a safe environment:

The need for personal cleansing and dressing:

The need for expression and communication:

The need for working and playing:

The need for adequate rest and sleep:

The need to maintain psychological equilibrium:

The need to worship according to his/her own faith:

The need to express sexuality:

Has patient education on safer sex been implemented?   YES/NO

Needs associated with dying:

DISCHARGE PLANNING MEETINGS

Notes of Discharge Planning Meetings. Enter summary of Discharge Planning arrangements agreed (date and sign each entry)

Original social history assessment completed by:

_____ Date _____

(Nurse to *print* name)

Signature _____

Final Social History/Discharge Plans completed by:

_____ Date _____

(Nurse responsible for safe discharge of
patient – to *print* name)

Signature _____

NB   A copy of this form is to be sent to Community Nursing Service on
       day of discharge and original filed in patient's case notes.

Appendix 6: Model AIDS Educational Strategy for Pre-registration Nursing Programmes

Pre-registration courses

Aims
Students will be facilitated to explore and develop their knowledge, skills and attitudes related to the care of patients with HIV-related illnesses to enable them to provide a high standard of individualized nursing care in a safe, caring and compassionate environment.

Learning outcomes
The student should be able to:

1. Utilize a knowledge of the nature and transmission of HIV and HIV-related illnesses when assessing and planning nursing care.
2. Effectively demonstrate a knowledge of the prevention and control of infection when planning and implementing individualized patient care.
3. Show an awareness of the differing lifestyles which may influence the needs of individuals.
4. Explore and recognize their fears, feelings, acceptance and prejudices towards the lifestyles and needs of individuals affected by HIV-related illnesses and develop appropriate coping techniques.
5. Demonstrate empathy, understanding and sensitivity in identifying and meeting the special needs of individuals infected with HIV, their family and friends.
6. Participate in identifying and meeting individuals' health education needs and relate these to patient education and primary prevention.
7. Use the above knowledge, skills and attitudes to provide safe, sensitive individualized nursing care.

A wide variety of teaching styles and methods will be used during the course according to the experience and preference of the teacher and the resources available. The use of workshops, discussion groups, seminars, tutorials, videos and clinical supervision and practice will be included.

Stage of preparation	Content
Common Foundation Programme	identification of human needs.
	Sociology and health to include effects of education, lifestyle and occupation on individual health status.
	The use of an appropriate model of care (nursing construct) to meet the health care deficits of individuals infected with HIV.
	Introduction to interviewing and counselling skills.

Classification, transmission and destruction of pathogens and its application to the individual's response to infection.

The prevention and control of cross infection to include the principles of Universal Precautions.

Care of the patient with local and/or systemic infections.

Introduction to the care of the terminally ill patient.

Ethical and professional issues in nursing to include the district philosophy in nursing policy, patients' rights, consent, confidentiality, freedom of choice, standards of care and professional responsibility and accountability.

Care of the patient with HIV and HIV-related illnesses.

Students will be working in practice settings where there may be patients with AIDS or HIV-related illnesses. Their knowledge, skills and attitudes related to the care of these patients will be explored and appropriate guidance and supervision given by nursing staff.

Students are encouraged to share and discuss their practice experiences. This provides opportunities for problem solving, reassurance and information related to nursing practices and policies.

Branch
Programmes

Care of patients with AIDS and HIV-related illnesses is presented in greater detail to include both hospital and community care and related health education. Included may be visits to special clinics and specialist speakers from outside support agencies.

As the students progress through the branch their know ledge, skills and attitudes are further developed with the inclusion of:
- counselling, communication and interviewing skills
- the process of grief and the special needs of terminally ill individuals and their family and friends
- the principles of teaching, learning and evaluation
- the application of nursing research and health education to nursing practice and patient education
- ethico-legal aspects of patient care and their effect on the professional responsibility and accountability of the registered nurse.

Community nursing services.

Intended learning outcomes.
All qualified nurses, nursing auxiliaries and health care assistants will undertake training to extend their knowledge and skills in reference to caring for patients/clients with HIV related illnesses in the community. Staff will also have the opportunity to explore

their attitude towards people with HIV infection.
For all groups of staff to gain an understanding of:

1. The nature and cause of HIV infection.
2. The clinical consequences of infection.
3. The means of HIV transmission.
4. The aspects of confidentiality particular to HIV infection.
5. The systems available for obtaining further information and making referrals.
6. All district policies and procedures relating to HIV infection.
7. Clarification of management/professional clinical issues.
8. The attitudes which are necessary for staff to give confident, compassionate and competent care to people with HIV infection; and the factors which prevent individual members of staff from adopting these appropriate attitudes.
9. The implementation of Universal Infection Control Precautions in primary services.

Different staff groups will require further training

1. *For district nurses.* The necessary training to ensure competence – confidence for the administration of intravenous drugs.
2. *For health visitors.* To obtain a knowledge of:
   (a) the possible effects on the health of a pregnant woman infected with HIV and subsequently as a new mother;
   (b) the possible consequences to the unborn and new infant of a mother/father with HIV infection;
   (c) the district's community HIV policy for children under the age of five, and
      i the safe practices required when visiting any client and child at home and undertaking child health clinics
      ii immunization procedures for a baby who is HIV positive;
   (d) HIV and child sexual abuse;
   (e) monitoring health and development of a child who is HIV positive;
   (f) giving appropriate information about HIV transmission to groups and on a one-to-one basis.
3. *For school nurses.* To obtain knowledge for:
   (a) monitoring the health and development of a child who is HIV positive;
   (b) developing safe clinical practice for all children;
   (d) giving appropriate information about HIV to parents, teachers and school children.
4. *For family planning nurses.* To gain knowledge for:
   (a) health promotion in relation to HIV infection;
   (b) developing skills in discussing safer sexual practices with clients.
   (c) the implementation of Universal infection Control Precautions in Family Planning Settings.

Learning activities

1. Two day orientation programme designed specifically for community staff.
2. All staff to attend day one.
3. All district nurses to attend day two to receive theoretical education and training on the administration of IV drugs. (Practical experience will be arranged in the community).

4. Specific sessions wiil be arranged as appropriate to meet the particular needs of other groups of community staff.

Continuing education

Intended learning outcome

All qualified nurses will have an opportunity to extend their knowledge and skills in reference to caring for patients with HIV-related illnesses and will have space in which to explore their attitudes towards those infected with HIV.

Specific training will include:

1. The nature and cause of AIDS and AIDS-related conditions.
2. The clinical consequences of infection and basic skills needed to care for patients with AIDS and AIDS-related conditions.
3. The means of HIV transmission and the adoption of Universal Infection Control Precautions designed to protect patients and staff.
4. Basic health education skills designed to facilitate primary prevention.
5. Clarification of management/professional/ethical issues and exploration of attitudes which may hinder the deployment of confident, compassionate and competent nursing care.

Learning activities designed to achieve the intended learning outcomes:

1. A series of one-day seminars to be planned and implemented on an authority-wide basis which all qualified nursing personnel will be required to attend. This is to be completed within 12 months.
2. Existing orientation programmes to be extended by one day so that the above one-day programme can be included for all newly joined nursing personnel.
3. More in-depth, sophisticated programmes to be arranged for nursing personnel currently caring for patients, with HIV-related illnesses.
4. Staff support groups to be formed for nursing personnel working with patients with HIV-related illnesses and to meet on a regular basis
5. Managers to identify key employees who require more extensive training and to arrange for them to attend ENB course number 934 (The Care and Management of Persons with AIDS). This is to include nurse educationalists.
6. All departments within the Schools of Nursing to designate at least one teacher who will become an expert resource person for HIV education within their programme or department.
7. The subject of HIV-related illnesses to be comprehensively covered in all ENB post-registration clinical courses, ENB short development courses where clinical updating is appropriate and in all staff development programmes.

Midwifery services

Aims

The necessary education to ensure competence/confidence in counselling women regarding HIV.

To obtain a knowledge of:

1. The possible effects on the health of a pregnant woman with HIV infection and subsequently as a new mother.
2. The possible consequences to the unborn and new infant of a mother/father with HIV infection.
3. The district's community HIV policy for children under the age of five.
4. HIV and sexual abuse.
5. Monitoring health and development of a child who is HIV positive.
6. Giving appropriate information about HIV transmission to groups and on a one-to-one basis.
7. Health promotion in relation to HIV infection.
8. Developing skills in discussing safer sexual practices with women.
9. The legal and ethical considerations involved in serological screening of expectant mothers.
10. Pre- and post-test counselling skills.

For neonatal nurses/mid wives

1. The possible consequences to the unborn and new infant of a father/mother with HIV infection.
2. Monitoring the health and development of a child who is HIV positive.
3. Developing safe clinical practice for all infants.
4. Giving appropriate information about HIV to parents.
5. The district's community HIV policy for children who are under the age of five.
6. HIV and sexual abuse.
7. The legal and ethical considerations involved in screening neonates for markers of HIV infection.
8. Pre- and post-test counselling skills.

Appendix 7: Model Philosophy for Nursing

Reproduced from *Philosophy for Nursing*, 2nd edn (1990). Riverside Health Authority, London.

The purpose of nursing

To support people during the activities and events of life, from birth to death; using skills, strength and knowledge to enable people to maintain their own balance of health, and assist them in illness and disability towards greater understanding and return to autonomy or, at the end of life, to death.

Philosophy for Nursing

The nature of health and ill health

1. People are deeply rooted in the particular circumstances and events of their lives, and in their own social and economic circumstances, and have differing capacities to deal with life's events.
2. Health is multi-dimensional with interdependent physical, pyschological, social and spiritual aspects. Health and illness are normal states in life.
3. Health is a state of balance between self and the environment. In this instance the environment is taken to mean:
   (a) The physical requirements for living;
   (b) Relationships between family, friends, and neighbours;
   (c) Relationships within a wider societal role, which reflects a person's perceived value by society.
4. Disability, in the absence of illness or disease, is compatible with being healthy.

People's relationship to health and ill health

1. Adults are autonomous, independent and responsible for their own health. The responsibility for the child's health lies with the parents or parent substitute. However people can be overwhelmed by circumstances, lack sufficient resources or knowledge, skills and strength to take appropriate action. The individual may decide not to take the necessary steps. Social, economic, political and cultural factors may prevent appropriate action.
2. The service needs related to health and illness are not static but will vary over time with social, economic and cultural changes and differing expectations of people.
3. The prevention of ill health is achieved through people coming to know the causes and nature of health and illness and their own capacity to take charge of their own and dependants' health.
4. People have the capacity to heal themselves, but may not have the knowledge

to do so or be prepared to accept the responsibility. It is important for every individual to know how they perceive their own health and/or their child's health, illness and role in health care, in order to participate fully.

5. Healing does not necessarily mean the curing or eradication of disease or disability. Healing involves knowing and accepting one's strengths and weaknesses and, within these, leading a happy and fulfilled life.
6. People have rights when well or ill. They should be able to make informed choices and understand the consequences of their decisions. Adults have the right not to consent to treatment.
7. People have the right to privacy and confidentiality.
8. People have the right to receive an explanation of their own or child's condition in language they can understand.
9. Dying is a normal event in life. People should be able to participate in discussions about the management of their care, and to make decisions themselves. For children, the participation of the family is particularly important.

The nursing role in health and ill health

1. Nursing views health as a dynamic relationship between the individual, friends, family and the environment. The individual in health or illness is seen within this context. The professional relationship between nurses and people is one of equality, in which people take responsibility for their own health, and towards which nursing will contribute support which is jointly agreed.
2. The aim of nursing will be to assist people in the identification and fulfilment of their own health needs. This may be achieved by facilitating them to use their own resources, either independently from, or supported by, the specialist knowledge of nursing, or linking into the network of other health care professions.
3. To support people means working with them to agree the care appropriate to their needs. Care means assuming a sense of responsibility, being aware, showing interest, being alert to change, and not necessarily direct physical contact.
4. Nursing is concerned with caring for people who are ill, maintaining the health of those who are not ill, and with preventing ill health. It also seeks, through education, to promote knowledge and develop people's confidence in their own ability to effect their longer term health status.
5. The care given should be sensitive to the patient's own needs for autonomy and responsibility for independence.
6. Nursing care will be offered to anyone who is in need of It, regardless of age, sex, sexual orientation, race, religion, political persuasion or presenting illness. Any person who is accepted by the nursing service is owed a duty of care from which nurses may not withdraw.
7. Care will be assessed, planned, implemented and evaluated using an appropriate model of nursing and a systematic problem solving approach.
8. Planning should take into account the person's current medical condition and treatment as recorded in the patient's notes.
9. It is expected that nursing records will be comprehensive, accurate and written contemporaneously .
10. Nurses should ensure that treatment, its implications and the care required, is fully discussed with the individual, and where appropriate, his or her relatives or friends.

11 Any nurse whose conscience is offended by the way a person's nursing care or medical treatment is managed should make this known to the senior nurse manager.

12. In situations when a person is unable to defend or promote his own health needs the nurse may act as his or her advocate.

13. In meeting people's needs nurses have a responsibility to make the best use of finite resources. However there may be times when available resources will not meet assessed need and in these instances there is a responsibility to inform the senior manager.

14. Each registered nurse, midwife and health visitor is accountable for her or his practice, and in the exercise of professional accountability shall observe the code of conduct of the United Kingdom Central Council for Nursing, Midwifery and Health Visiting (U.K.C.C.).

People's needs

1. The need for support in health and illness can be defined by the person, the parent in the case of children, or nurse, and preferably will be jointly agreed. Where these needs are not agreed, the nurse should recheck the professional evaluation against the person's beliefs and capacity, their wishes and their need for dignity and independence.

2. How the support needed might be achieved should also be jointly agreed. There will be times when the need may be agreed but the support cannot be achieved.

3. The need for support may not necessarily be linked to an individual but could apply to a family, or a community of people.

4. In the situation of health and illness people have different levels of need which usually occur simultaneously, although one may dominate, and the nurse will have to use professional judgement to determine any priority.

5. **Physiological and survival needs.** These can be in response to physical, developmental, social, economic, psychological, emotional or spiritual distress.
    5.1. To live
    5.2. To be offered assistance
    5.3. To be given refuge or sanctuary
    5.4. To be comforted
    5.5. To be adequately fed

6. **Safety and security needs.** These are related to both physical and emotional safety and security.
    6.1. To be safe
    6.2. Not to be hurt
    6.3. To be guided through health and ill health
    6.4. To feel secure

7. **Belonging and affection needs.** These are met by the acknowledgement of the essential human being in every individual, even when the person is perceived as being unattractive, difficult or anti-social.
    7.1. To be accepted
    7.2. To belong
    7.3. For friendship
    7.4. To give and receive love

8. **Self-esteem or respect needs.** These needs will always be present, but may increase with the degree of vulnerability which is experienced.

8.1. To retain own identity as a unique human being
8.2. To have autonomy
8.3. To know and to understand
8.4. To be consulted
8.5. To be creative

Nurses' needs

1. Nurses have the same basic needs as others. Their need for survival, security, belonging, self-esteem and self-actualization must be met to enable them to meet the illness and health needs of people. Fulfilment of them is a joint responsibility of the individual and the Health Authority.
2. Nurses working within a caring environment which allows them to express their individual needs will be better able to provide optimum care.
3. In order to carry out their supporting role and responsibilities nurses must receive relevant education and training throughout their career. Learning in the clinical areas is aimed at integrating the theory and practice of nursing to enable all levels of registered and student nurses to achieve and maintain the competencies necessary for professional practice. Development of these competencies is the responsibility of the individual nurse. Creating the environment which fosters such professional growth is the joint responsibility of the clinical and educational staff.
4. Maximum use should be made of the wide range of experience within the District to develop and enhance the personal and professional development of nursing staff.
5. The ward sister is responsible for the provision of service to patients, towards which the student nurse usually makes an essential contribution. There is, within this situation, an inherent conflict between service and educational objectives particularly in the event of inadequate resources. It is expected that in the acknowledgement of these differing objectives resolution of problems can be achieved.
6. Where clinical experience is required for students, Nurse Management and the College of Nursing have a joint responsibility to identify the resources required for supervision, teaching and assessment and to monitor that these are adequate. Where resources are inadequate it is expected that nurse management and the College of Nursing will undertake joint action.

Inter-professional collaboration

1. People's needs are often multidisciplinary and health care plans will require input from other professionals. Nursing staff will expect to work, and participate fully, within a multidisciplinary setting.
2. Where the nursing assessment identifies the need for consultation with other health care professionals, the nurse has a responsibility to initiate this and monitor that the changing needs of the person are being met. Assessment of health care needs is best made jointly between the person, the parent/informal carer, the nurse and members of other professions prior to joint agreement on how it will be provided.
3. In a multidisciplinary situation, effective communication is essential to a successful outcome. Nursing, the role of which is continuous and central to the provision

of health care, has a particular opportunity to facilitate this.

4. In addition people quickly identify each role and select what is seen to be appropriate knowledge for each. Thus no one worker comes to see the whole picture. It is important that information is shared and this is probably best achieved through agreement on having a key worker or primary nurse.

5. All nurses have specialist knowledge, but the specialist nurse has the opportunity to keep abreast of changes in current practice and to develop a broad range of skills related to that practice. The role is both educational and advisory and offers support to colleagues, other health care professionals, people and families. They are also concerned with the development of resources and liaison between institution and community, health care and social services. Clinical care is given to facilitate learning.

6. The specialist nurse role requires that mutual understanding of, and respect for, others' roles and expertise is established. Where there is dual responsibility for care then entry into that care and withdrawal from it should be negotiated between professionals. This will clarify roles for client and worker and be in accord with a holistic approach to care.

7. Admissions for treatment should be arranged in the best interest of the people concerned, and should take into account their general and specialist nursing needs. People should be cared for within an environment which has the facilities and specialist skills to meet their particular identified nursing and medical needs.

8. The senior nurse on duty should ensure that nursing, medical and other staff are aware of agreed policies. The nurse can advise the appropriate professional manager if these are not followed.

9. Discharges must be planned in the best interest of people. Nurses have a duty, in liaison with medical, paramedical staff, and relatives/friends, to be satisfied that the conditions to which the person is returning are safe, and to state and document their views.

10. Nurses have a responsibility to ensure that discharge teaching has been carried out and is documented; and that the person and parent/informal carer/family have full understanding of what they have been taught.

Appendix 8: Model Policy Statements

Universal infection control precautions: HIV disease

The number of individuals in the community who are asymptomatically infected with HIV is increasing and it is likely that many patients/clients in hospital or the community, infected with HIV, are unaware of it. Consequently, we would also be unaware of their infection. The current trend is for the prevalence of asymptomatic HIV infection to continue to increase within our community.

It is not our policy to routinely screen all patients/clients. Serological testing for markers of HIV infection could not reliably detect all those who are infected as a negative test does not necessarily indicate that an individual is not infected with HIV.

Therefore, it is important that all nursing personnel take reasonable precautions against exposure to blood and body fluids from ALL patients, in ALL departments, ALL of the time, regardless of what is or is not known regarding their serological status in relation to HIV infection. This concept in infection control has become known as **Universal Infection Control Precautions.**

Universal Infection Control Precautions require that nursing personnel wear non-sterile, disposable latex or vinyl gloves whenever exposure to blood or body fluids is anticipated.

BLOOD IS THE SINGLE MOST IMPORTANT SOURCE OF HIV and other blood-borne pathogens (e.g., HBV, HBC, HTLV-1, etc.) in the occupational setting. The prevention of exposure to all blood and to body fluids is in line with current standards of nursing practice.

All nursing personnel should take precautions to prevent injuries caused by needles, scalpels and other sharp instruments.

Universal Infection Control Precautions are part of the routine infection control advice described in the 'Infection Control Manual.' For more detailed advice, nursing personnel should consult the senior nurses for infection control. **Inappropriate and over-zealous infection control precautions are to be discouraged.**

All nursing service personnel are obligated to comply with current infection control policies and procedures, including this advisory statement. All sisters/charge nurses and nurse managers must ensure that their nursing staff are familiar with this advice and that Universal Infection Control Precautions are incorporated into routine nursing practice.

Amendment 1
Universal Infection Control Precautions apply to blood and to other body fluids containing visible blood. Universal Infection Control Precautions also apply to tissues and to cerebrospinal (CSF), synovial, pleural, peritoneal, pericardial and amniotic fluids. These precautions also apply to semen, vaginal secretions and saliva in association with dentistry.

In addition, it is recommended that gloves should be worn for direct contact with other body fluids, excretions or secretions, e.g. faeces, urine, etc., and for contact with non-intact skin and mucous membranes. Please refer to the 'Infection Control Manual' for further information.

Amendment 2

Additional protective clothing, e.g. plastic aprons and eye protection should be worn whenever contamination of clothing with blood and/or body fluids is anticipated or during procedures that are likely to generate aerosol contamination.

Duty of care

The philosophy of nursing service embraces the concept that skilled nursing care is available to all individuals requiring it, regardless of their race, religion, age, sexual or political orientation or disease presentation.

Nursing personnel do not have the right to decide which patients they will care for and which patients they will not care for. Nursing personnel have a duty of care towards all patients and are professionally obliged to offer appropriate and meaningful care to those requiring it.

All nurses have an individual responsibility to remain clinically up-to-date and to be aware of the policies and procedures for caring for patients with HIV-related illnesses. Refusing to care for any patients will lead to disciplinary action by both the Health Authority and the United Kingdom Central Council for Nursing, Midwifery and Health Visiting.

Nurses are reminded that it is both the philosophy and intention of the nursing service to offer competent, compassionate and non-judgemental care to **all of our patients**.

Confidentiality

All nurses have both a legal and a professional responsibility to observe **The Code of Professional Conduct for the Nurse** published by the United Kingdom Central Council for Nursing, Midwifery and Health Visiting. One of the key statements (Clause 10) in this code concerns Confidentiality. It reads:

> Each registered nurse, midwife and health visitor is accountable for his or her practice and, in the exercise of professional accountability, shall:
>
> Respect confidential information obtained in the course of professional practice and refrain from disclosing such information without the consent of the patient/client, or a person entitled to act on his/her behalf, except where disclosure is required by law or by the order of a court or is necessary in the public interest.

It can be seen from the general description of the Code of Professional Conduct and the particular contents of Clause 10 that **breaches of confidentiality should be regarded as exceptional**, only occurring after careful consideration and discussion with senior nurse managers and other practitioners directly involved in the clinical care of the patient/client.

Clearly, it is impractical to obtain the consent of the patient/client every time that health care information needs to be shared with other health professionals, or other staff involved in the health care of that patient/client. Consent in these instances can be implied, provided that is known and understood by the patients/clients that such information needs to be made available to others involved in the delivery of his/her care. Patients/clients have a right to know the standards of confidentiality maintained by those providing professional care at their first point of contact.

When an individual practitioner considers that it is necessary to obtain the **explicit consent** of a patient/client before disclosing specific information, it is the responsibility of the practitioner to ensure that the patient/client can make as informed a response as possible as to whether that information can be disclosed or withheld.

It is essential that nurses, midwives and health visitors recognize the fundamental right of their patients or clients to information about them being kept private and secure. This point is sharply reinforced by only brief consideration of the personal, social or legal repercussions which might follow unauthorised disclosure of information concerning a person's health or illness.

The care of confidential information includes ensuring or helping to ensure that record keeping systems are not such as to make the release of information possible or likely. Neither technology nor management convenience should be allowed to determine principles. Each practitioner has a responsibility to recognise that risks exist, and to satisfy himself or herself in respect of the system for storage and movement of records operated in the health care setting in which he or she works, and to ensure that it is secure.

The practitioner should act so as to ensure that he/she does not become a channel through which confidential information obtained in the course of professional practice is inadvertently released. The dangerous consequences of careless talk in public places cannot be overstated.

Where access to the records of patients or clients is necessary so that students may be assisted to achieve the necessary knowledge and competence, it must be recognized that the same principles of confidentiality stated earlier extend to them and their teachers. The same applies to those engaged in research. It is incumbent on the practitioner(s) responsible for the security of the information contained in these records to ensure that access to it is closely supervised and occurs within the context of the teacher and student undertaking to respect its confidentiality and in knowledge of the fact that the teacher has accepted responsibility to ensure that students understand the requirement for confidentiality and the need to observe policies for the handling and storage of records. It is expected that the student or teacher who is active in giving care as a practitioner will apprise the patient of their role, thus enabling the patient who is so capable to control the information flow. Where deemed necessary, the recipient of confidential information from a patient/client will advise him/her that the information will be conveyed to the nurse, midwife or health visitor involved in his/her care on a continuing basis.

Confidentiality is a rule with certain exceptions

The needs of the community can, on occasions, take precedence over the individual's rights as, for example, when a Court order demands that a professional confidence be broken.

It is essential that before determining that a particular set of circumstances constitute such an exception, the practitioner is satisfied that the best interests of the patient/client are served thereby or the wider public interest necessitates disclosure.

In all cases where the practitioner deliberately discloses or withholds information in what he/she believes is the public interest, he/she must be able to justify the decision and may find it useful to consult with senior colleagues or seek advice from the relevant professional organization.

If confidential information is deliberately disclosed without the consent of the patient/client, he/she should be informed that this is being done and the recipient of the information should be informed that it is being given to them without the consent of the patient/client.

Summary of the principles on which to base professional judgement in matters of confidentiality

1. That a patient/client has a right to expect that information given in confidence will be used only for the purpose for which it was given and will not be released to others without their consent.
2. That practitioners recognize the fundamental right of their patients/clients to have information about them held in secure and private storage.
3. That, where it is deemed appropriate to share information obtained in the course of professional practice with other health or social work practitioners, the practitioner who obtained the information must ensure before its release that it is being imparted in strict professional confidence and for a specific purpose.
4. That the responsibility to either disclose or withhold confidential information in the public interest lies with the individual practitioner, that they cannot delegate the decision, and that they cannot be required by a superior to disclose or withhold information against their will.
5. That a practitioner who chooses to breach the basic principle of confidentiality in the belief that it is necessary in the public interest must have considered the matter sufficiently to justify that decision.
6. That deliberate breaches of confidentiality, other than with the consent of the patient/client, should be exceptional.

Consent for serological testing

Nurses must not take blood or collude with other professionals in obtaining blood for named serological testing for antibodies to HIV ('anti-HIV') or HIV antigens unless patients have given consent for this procedure.
Consent implies that the reason why the test is desired is carefully explained to the patient/client (in language they understand), the results are made known to the patient/client and that he/she agrees to this test and understands its significance.

Nurses and other health care professionals should ensure that they have the necessary expertise and training to engage meaningfully in pre- and post-test counselling, **both events being a requirement for testing clients.**

The United Kingdom Central Council for Nursing, Midwifery and Health Visiting have advised nurses that on the specific issue of taking blood for testing **without consent,** they expose themselves to the possibility of civil action for damages, of criminal charges of assault or a complaint to their regulatory body (the Council) alleging misconduct if they personally take the blood specimens, and of aiding and abetting such an assault if they cooperate in obtaining such specimens.

Additionally, those actions (like that of being party to any statements aimed at leading patients to believe that blood specimens taken for HIV testing were for some other purpose) expose nurses, midwives and health visitors to the possibility of complaints to their registration body, alleging misconduct, which would put their registration status and right to practise at risk.

If any nurse is **unsure** as to whether or not patient/clients are being asked for their consent to serological testing for anti-HIV or HIV antigens, they should discuss this initially with the medical staff who have ordered the investigation and, if necessary, seek professional advice.

There may be rare and exceptional circumstances when unconsented testing may legitimately occur. These circumstances must be justifiable as **in the interests of the particular patient at the operating time,** and for no other reason, and only where it is not possible to obtain consent. Additionally, **anonymous testing for the prevalence of HIV** is authorized on condition that the principles, elaborated by the UKCC and outlined in the following policy, are observed.

Unlinked anonymous testing for the prevalence of the human immunodeficiency virus (HIV)

Surveillance testing for the prevalence of the human immunodeficiency virus (HIV-1) has been conducted in several health facilities in the United Kingdom since 1989. These surveys, which were designed by the Medical Research Council at the request of the health departments and which are coordinated by the Public Health Laboratory Services, are intended to accurately determine the prevalence of HIV infection in the general population. Present data, collected from people who come forward voluntarily for HIV tests, do not give a complete picture and the actual number of infected individuals is thought to be higher than the number reported. More accurate data will assist the health departments in planning services for people with HIV disease and action to prevent the further spread of HIV.

Unlinked anonymous HIV surveys will use blood that has been taken from patients for specified diagnostic or treatment purposes (e.g. complete blood counts etc.). After the specified test has been carried out, the residual specimen will be stripped of any identifying factors (i.e. anonymized) and may then be tested for markers of HIV infection. It is 'unlinked' in the respect that the results of the tests will not be able to be associated with an identified individual. A further safeguard to anonymity is that the person who tests the batches of samples will not be the same as the person who anonymizes them.

This healthcare facility supports unlinked anonymous prevalence data testing for HIV infection **only if the following requirements are met:**

1. A specific research protocol for each test group (e.g. pregnant women, newborn infants, GUM clinic patients, etc.) must have been approved by the local research ethics committee of the health authority covering the territory within which the blood specimens are to be obtained prior to the commencement of any unlinked anonymous test programme.

2. The relevant providers of health care, as an associated part of the research approval, have considered and acted upon any resource implications for their professional staff and pronounced themselves satisfied.

3. No extra blood will be taken for HIV prevalence data testing; the amount of blood taken on any occasion should be only that which would normally be taken for the specific tests ordered by the patient's medical practitioner.

4. It is made known to those whose blood may be used (and in the case of children, their parents/guardians) that this surveillance programme is taking place, to explain it and to assure them of the absolute anonymity of the samples used. This is to be done by posters in clinics and units of service selected for prevalence data testing and by giving all patients a copy of the Department of Health leaflet (AHTI,

December 1989) entitled '**If You Are Having A Blood Test**' or, AHTI/E (1990) entitled: '**If You or Your Baby are Having a Blood or Urine Test**' in Pre-natal settings. Posters and leaflets must be available in the full range of relevant languages appropriate to the known patient/client population;

5. All nursing personnel assigned to clinics and units of service where prevalence data testing will take place will have received a copy of this **policy statement** and a copy of the Department of Health leaflet (AHT4, December 1989) '**Unlinked Anonymous HIV Surveys – Guidance For Health Service Staff**'. Nursing personnel must also be aware of guidelines from the Professional Conduct and Registration Division of the United Kingdom Central Council for Nursing, Midwifery and Health Visiting **Registrar's Letter, 4/1994 Annexe 2, (25 March 1994)** 'Anonymous Testing For The Prevalence of the Human Immunodeficiency Virus – (HIV)'. In addition, all nursing personnel will have had an opportunity of discussing the procedures for unlinked anonymous testing with their manager.

All registered nurses, midwives and health visitors assigned to units of service from which samples are being obtained for this prevalence testing programme must be made aware of that fact in order that

- they may answer honestly any questions put to them by patients and clients about the full range of purposes for which blood samples will or may be tested, and
- they may consider how best to act to protect the interests of any patients or clients whose transient or permanent condition results in an inability to consider and/or understand the available information literature.

All posters, leaflets and verbal advice given to patients/clients will clearly inform them of **their right to opt out of this screening programme**.

Any patient or client who objects to participation in the test programme must have his or her wishes respected fully and must not:

- be discriminated against in any way;
- be identified as being a higher risk than those who have not objected;
- have required treatment withheld or suffer any other detriment.

There must be no possible detriment to those whose blood is or is not screened as part of the unlinked anonymous testing programme. Other than noting on the routine request form that a particular specimen is not to be used for anonymous HIV testing, no other record will be kept.

If the patient or client wishes, a personal or named test for markers of HIV infection will be arranged, with the required pre- and post-test counselling.

The employment of nursing personnel infected with HIV

Guidelines have been issued by the Department of Health, the World Health Organization, the Department of Employment, the Health and Safety Executive and the United Kingdom Central Council for Nursing, Midwifery and Health Visiting.

1. The following guidelines are compatible with the above and seek to clarify the employment issues for nursing personnel infected with HIV.
2. Protection of the human rights and dignity of HIV-infected persons, including persons with AIDS, is essential for the prevention and control of HIV/AIDS.

3. The JKCC **Code of Professional Conduct** for the Nurse, Midwife and Health Visitor is a statement to the profession of the primacy of the patient's interest.
4. Nurses with HIV infection, who are healthy, should be treated the same as any other nurses. Nurses with HIV-related illness, including AIDS, should be treated the same as any other nurse with an illness.
5. It is the policy of this healthcare facility that members of staff who become HIV positive or develop AIDS shall retain their contractual rights of employment. The existence of HIV infection, and illness due to HIV infection, are not sufficient reasons in themselves for termination of employment.
6. Consequently, nursing personnel are encouraged to confide the nature of their HIV antibody status or illness to the Occupational Health Services. This will allow the nurse to be appropriately supported and cared for.
7. Nursing personnel who know they are HIV antibody positive or who have been diagnosed with an HIV-related condition must be under appropriate medical supervision. This can be undertaken by their own medical practitioner or the Occupational Health Department. There is available within this healthcare facility a comprehensive range of services and personnel with expertise in the care and support of individuals with HIV disease. Nursing personnel are encouraged to take advantage of these services and expertise, which can be accessed through the Occupational Health Department.
8. **Information disclosed to the Occupational Health Department is confidential.** Positive counselling by the Occupational Health Department will encourage and support nurses in being able to share information with their manager.
9. If a nurse confides confidential information to their manager, it may not be disclosed to other managerial colleagues without the express consent of the affected nurse.
10. The risk to a client of HIV transmission from a nurse infected with this virus is considered to be minimal. However, the small but possible risk which can exist is described fully in Department of Health guidelines ('**AIDS: HIV-Infected Health Care Workers: Guidance on the management of infected health care workers**', March 1994). In most cases the risk can be eliminated by judicious use of disposable gloves, waterproof dressings covering any open lesions and a high standard of personal hygiene (as discussed in the previous policy statement on '**Universal Infection Control Precautions: HIV Disease**' and current infection control policies). All nurses are required to comply with current control of infection policies and procedures.
11. A theoretical risk may exist in nursing practice, should an accidental injury to the nurse occur during a surgical invasive procedure, where blood to tissue contact could occur. If a nurse, midwife or health visitor, known to be infected with HIV, is practising in a post which involves contact with sharp instruments, sharp splinters or edges of bone, particularly when the hands are not completely visible, clinical re-assignment may be necessary. Consequently, any nurse, midwife or health visitor, who knows or suspects that they may be infected with HIV, must not continue to practise in this type of clinical area until they have received specialist medical advice as to the safety and appropriateness of their clinical responsibilities. This advice must be followed; failure to do so will be regarded as a contravention of the UKCC's guidance to Registered Nurses and may result in disciplinary action.
12. Nursing personnel with HIV disease may be susceptible to a wide range of illnesses which may affect their ability to work, including visual and mental impairment

and/or infectious disease. Should the Occupational Health Department advise that a member of staff is unfit to continue to work in a specific area, every effort will be made to provide alternative employment.

13. Nurses who are asymptomatically infected with HIV do not pose any special risk to clients of transmitting opportunistic or other non-HIV related infections. However, they should remain under regular medical supervision in order to ensure the early detection of infections such as tuberculosis, measles and varicella. These can be contained by the same provisions that apply generally to infectious diseases affecting any nurse.

14. Nurses infected with HIV may be more susceptible to infections such as tuberculosis, varicella or measles. The Occupational Health Department (in liaison with the infection control officer/consultant microbiologist and the nurse's own physician) will be able to advise whether exclusion from contact with clients with these infections is necessary.

15. Reasonable and appropriate alternative clinical assignments will be made available to those nurses who require it as per numbers 11, 12 and 14 of this policy statement.

16. Screening facilities exist in the GUM Services for any member of staff who wishes to be tested for HIV infection. The previous statements on '**Informed Consent**' and '**Confidentiality**' apply **equally** to the clients and employees of this healthcare facility.

17. Although there is no requirement for any employee to be screened for HIV infection, we strongly advise that those nursing personnel who consider, on the basis of the known means of transmission, that they may have been exposed to HIV, should seek immediate counselling and, if appropriate, diagnostic HIV antibody testing.

18. Nurses affected or perceived to be affected by HIV/AIDS will be protected from stigmatization and discrimination by colleagues and clients. This health care facility is committed to dealing effectively with all complaints of discrimination, victimization or harassment.

19. This organization is an equal opportunity employer and, as such, have a legal obligation to ensure that they, their employees and managers do not unlawfully discriminate.

20. Pre-employment HIV/AIDS screening is unnecessary and is not required. This refers to HIV antibody tests already taken. However, potential nursing personnel employees who know they are HIV antibody positive are encouraged to confide in the Occupational Health Service. This will enable them to access the support and care available and to obtain appropriate advice regarding clinical assignment and early intervention.

21. We are committed to offering the highest quality support and care to both our clients and employees and observance of these guidelines promotes that commitment.

Bibliography

Centers for Disease Control (1987). Recommendations for Prevention of HIV Transmission in Health Care Settings. *Morbidity and Mortality Weekly Report (MMWR)* **37**(24).

Centers for Disease Control (1988). Update: Universal Precautions for Prevention of

Human Immunodeficiency Virus, Hepatitis B Virus and Other Blood-borne Pathogens in Health-Care Settings. *Morbidity and Mortality Weekly Report (MMWR)* **37**(24).

Centers for Disease Control (1989). Guidelines for Prevention of Transmission of Human Immunodeficiency Virus and Hepatitis B Virus to Health-Care and Public-Safety Workers. *Morbidity and Mortality Weekly Report (MMWR)* **38** (S-6).

Department of Employment (1987). *AIDS and Employment.* HMSO, London.

Department of Health (1989). *If You Are Having A Blood Test.* AHTI, December, HMSO, London.

Department of Health (1989). *Unlinked Anonymous HIV Surveys – Guidance For Health Service Staff.* AHT4, December, HMSO, London.

Department of Health (1990). *Guidance for Clinical Health Care Workers: Protection against Infection with HIV and Hepatitis.* Expert Advisory Group on AIDS (EAGA), January, HMSO, London.

Department of Health (1994). *AIDS–HIV Infected Health Care Workers (Guidance on the Management of Infected Health Care Workers).* March, HMSO, London.

Department of Health (1990). *If You or Your Baby are Having a Blood or Urine Test.* AHT1/E, HMSO, London.

Heptonstall, J. and Gill, O.N. (1989). The legal and ethical basis for unlinked anonymous HIV testing. *Communicable Diseases Report,* 1 December, **89**(48) 3–6.

Sieghart, Paul (1989). *AIDS & Human Rights: A UK Perspective.* British Medical Association, Foundation for AIDS, London.

United Kingdom Central Council for Nursing, Midwifery and Health Visiting (1992). *Code of Professional Conduct,* 3rd edn. London.

United Kingdom Central Council for Nursing, Midwifery and Health Visiting (1994). (1) Acquired Immune Deficiency Syndrome and Human Immunodeficiency Virus Infection (AIDS) and HIV Infection), (2) Anonymous Testing for the Prevalence of the Human Immunodeficiency Virus (HIV). *Registrar's Letter,* 25 March, 4/1994, London.

UK Health Departments (1993). *AIDS–HIV Infected Health Care Workers: Practical Guidance on Notifying Patients.* Recommendations of the Expert Advisory Group on AIDS,, April, HMSO, London.

World Health Organization (1988). *Consensus Statement: WHO Consultation on AIDS in the Workplace.* WHO Press, Geneva.

World Health Organization (1988). *Guidelines for Nursing Management of People Infected with Human Immunodeficiency Virus (HIV).* WHO AIDS Series 3, WHO in Collaboration with the International Council of Nurses, Geneva.

Appendix 9: Technical Guidance on HIV Counseling

Reproduced from Centers for Disease Control (1993). *Morbidity and Mortality Weekly Report*, 15 January, 42(RR-2).

Summary

Human immunodeficiency virus counseling and testing services (HIV-CTS) have been recommended by CDC since 1985, when serologic tests became available to detect antibodies to HIV[1,2]. In August 1987, CDC published the Public Health Service Guidelines for Counseling and Antibody Testing to Prevent HIV Infection and AIDS[3]. These guidelines remain in effect today.

In December 1991, CDC convened a meeting of expert consultants to address the need for additional technical guidance on the subject of HIV counseling. As a result of that meeting, this document was developed to supplement the existing guidelines and distributed to state and local health departments in February 1992. This document updates the original guidelines to address: relevance of prevention messages; opportunities to provide and reinforce HIV prevention messages; messages tailored to behaviors, circumstances, and special needs of clients; development of individualized, negotiated HIV risk-reduction plans; barriers to return for post-test counseling; and appropriate, ongoing counselor training.

Introduction

In 1991, more than 2 million serologic tests to detect antibodies for human immunodeficiency virus (HIV) were performed at publicly funded HIV counseling and testing sites[4]. In addition to the provision of HIV counseling and testing services (HIV-CTS) at publicly funded sites, many private providers, including physicians, offer HIV-CTS[5].

CDC identifies the following as major functions of HIV-CTS: a) provide a convenient opportunity for persons to learn their current HIV serostatus; b) allow such persons to receive prevention counseling to help initiate behavior change to avoid infection, or, if already infected, to prevent transmission to others; c) help persons obtain referrals to receive additional prevention, medical-care, and other needed services; d) provide prevention services and referrals for sex and needle-sharing partners of HIV-infected persons[6].

To achieve the functions stated above and to address the specific HIV-prevention needs of each client, HIV counseling must do more than provide factual information in a didactic manner. This form of counseling – as the following recommendations define – should be 'client-centered' and based on consultation with expert HIV counselors, program managers, and other specialists.

Recommendations

HIV prevention messages

Counselors in programs that offer HIV-CTS should take advantage of all available opportunities to provide clients with HIV-prevention messages.

Clients manifest varying degrees of acceptance of HIV CTS. Some clients are highly motivated to learn their HIV serostatus, while others may be wary or suspicious of suggestions that they learn their HIV serostatus. Still others may not perceive themselves to be at risk for HIV infection and consider the test unnecessary. Changing high-risk behavior is not an 'all-or-nothing' process. Even after availing themselves of HIV-CTS, seronegative clients may continue to engage in behaviors that place them at risk for HIV infection.

Therefore, counselors should view all clinical encounters with clients as potential opportunities to provide and reinforce HIV-prevention messages. These messages should be clear and straight forward (e.g., 'If you are not infected with HIV, you should take steps to make sure you stay that way, and, if you are already infected, early treatment can preserve your health by delaying the onset of illness.')

Client-centered counseling

HIV counseling must be 'client-centered.'

To fulfill its public health functions, HIV counseling must be client-centered; i.e., tailored to the behaviors, circumstances, and special needs of the person being served. Risk-reduction messages must be personalized and realistic. Counseling should be:

- Culturally competent (i.e., program services provided in a style and format sensitive to cultural norms, values, and traditions that are endorsed by cultural leaders and accepted by the target population);
- Sensitive to issues of sexual identity;
- Developmentally appropriate (i.e., information and services provided at a level of comprehension that is consistent with the age and the learning skills of the person being served);
- Linguistically specific (i.e., information is presented in dialect and terminology consistent with the client's language and style of communication).

HIV counseling is not a lecture. An important aspect of HIV counseling is the counselor's ability to *listen* to the client in order to provide assistance and to determine specific prevention needs.

Although HIV counseling should adhere to minimal standards in terms of providing basic information, it should not become so routine that it is inflexible or unresponsive to particular client needs. Counselors should avoid providing information that is irrelevant to their clients and should avoid structuring counseling sessions on the basis of a data-collection instrument or form.

Client-risk assessment

HIV pretest counseling must include a personalized client-risk assessment.

A focused and tailored risk assessment is the foundation of HIV pretest counseling. Risk assessment is a process whereby the counselor helps the client to assess and take 'ownership' of his/her risk for HIV infection. Client acceptance of risk is a critical component of this assessment. Risk assessment is not a counselor's passive appraisal of the client's behavior, such as checking off risks from a written list, but an interactive process between counselor and client. Risk assessment should be conducted in an empathic manner with special attention given to the ongoing behaviors and circumstances (e.g., sexual history, sexually transmitted disease (STD) history, drug use) that may continue to place the client at risk for HIV infection/transmission. For example, clients who are being counseled in STD clinics, where they have come for the treatment of a symptomatic STD (other than HIV), should be advised that their current infection demonstrates that they are at increased risk for HIV.

Because the risk-assessment process serves as the basis for assisting the client in formulating a plan to reduce risk, it is an essential component of all pretest counseling.

HIV risk-reduction plan
HIV counseling should result in a personalized plan for the client to reduce the risk of HIV infection/transmission.

HIV counseling is more than providing routine information. Such counseling should also include the development of a personalized, negotiated HIV risk-reduction plan. This plan should be based on the client's skills, needs, and circumstances, and it must be consistent with the client's expressed or implied intentions to change behaviors; HIV counseling should not consist of the counselor 'telling' the client what he/she needs to do to prevent HIV infection/transmission, but instead should outline a variety of specific options available to the client for reducing his/her own risk of HIV infection/transmission. The counselor should confirm with the client that the risk-reduction plan is realistic and feasible – otherwise, it is likely to fail.

When negotiating a personalized risk-reduction plan, counselors should be especially attentive to information provided by the client – especially information about past attempts at preventive behaviors that were unsuccessful (e.g., intentions to use condoms but failure to do so) and those which were successful. Identifying and discussing previous prevention failures helps to ensure that the risk-reduction plan is realistic, attentive to the clients' prevention needs, and focused on actual barriers to safer behaviors. Identifying previous prevention successes (e.g., successful negotiation of condom use with a new sexual partner) offers the counselor the opportunity to reinforce and support positive prevention choices.

An interactive risk assessment and a personalized risk-reduction plan developed during pretest counseling ensure that clients receive adequate prevention information, even before they learn the results of their tests. Counselors can use the client's expectation of test results to facilitate the development of a personalized risk-reduction plan (e.g., 'What do you expect your test results to be? Why? What will you do if you are HIV seropositive? Is there anything different you will do if you are HIV seronegative?').

Post-test counseling
Programs should take active steps to address the problem of failure to return for post-test counseling.

Not all clients who receive pretest HIV counseling and testing return for post-test counseling and test results. In 1991, 31 state and local health departments recorded HIV counseling and testing data in such a way that analysis of individual post-test counseling return rates was possible. These project areas reported an average 63% return rate for post-test counseling. However, this rate ranged from 41% to 86% and varied by age, sex, race/ethnicity, self-reported risk behavior, service-delivery site, and HIV serostatus. Analyses indicate that adolescents, blacks*, and clients served in family-planning clinics and STD clinics, have lower return rates for HIV post-test counseling[7].

HIV-CTS programs should be active in addressing the problem of failure to return for HIV post-test counseling. Program managers should determine if specific operational barriers exist that prevent clients from returning for HIV post-test counseling (e.g., excessive waiting time). Counselors should stress the importance of receiving post-test counseling and should identify it as a specific component of the personalized risk-reduction plan. HIV-CTS programs should give priority to contacting seropositive and high-risk seronegative clients who have not returned to learn their test results and have failed to receive post-test counseling.

As part of a comprehensive quality-assurance program, publicly funded counseling and testing programs must monitor: a) blinded seroprevalence rates to assess the extent of client access and acceptance of recommended counseling, testing, referral, and partner-notification services (CTRPN); and b) the rates at which clients return to receive HIV-antibody test results and post-test counseling.

When < 50% of high-risk clients are receiving counseling and testing, or when low return rates (e.g., < 80% for seropositives and < 60% for high-risk seronegatives) are identified, documented 'action steps' must be initiated to determine the reasons for such low rates and to resolve barriers to clients in accessing services, learning their test results, and obtaining counseling and referral services[6].

Counselors should routinely assess whether clients require additional post-test counseling sessions.
Many HIV counselors have reported that some clients may require more than a single post-test counseling session. Seropositive clients are often disturbed by the realization that they have a life-threatening disease and often require additional counseling and support. Seronegative clients who are at increased risk for HIV infection or transmission may also require additional counseling to develop the skills needed to practice safer behaviors.

Although CDC does not require its funded programs to routinely provide repeated post-test counseling sessions, counselors and program managers should be aware that certain clients may require additional support and further counseling opportunities. If deemed appropriate, additional counseling should be provided on-site or through referral. In considering options for additional post-test counseling, program managers should work with local community-based organizations that might offer such services.

Programs should ensure that HIV CTS clients receive appropriate referrals.
Seronegative clients at continuing risk for HIV infection and HIV-infected clients often require additional primary and secondary HIV-prevention services that may not be available on-site. For example, clients whose drug use continues to place them at risk for HIV infection should be referred for appropriate drug treatment. HIV-infected clients should be provided (on-site or through referral) with immune system

---

*CDC's National Center for Prevention Services recognizes that a variety of terms are used and preferred by different groups to describe race and ethnicity. Racial and ethnic terms used in this document reflect the way data are collected and reported by official health agencies.

monitoring and a medical evaluation to determine the need for anti-retroviral therapy and prophylaxis for *Pneumocystis* pneumonia. Facilitating referrals for these services, as well as for tuberculosis (TB) and STD care as needed, are important aspects of HIV post-test counseling.

Identifying appropriate referral sites i.e., sites where appropriate services which meet acceptable standards of quality are offered in a timely manner) should not be the sole responsibility of the person performing HIV counseling. Program managers should take the lead in identifying referral sites and developing programmatic relations (e.g., contracts and memoranda of understanding) with those sites to facilitate needed client referrals.

Training and counselor feedback
Programs should provide training and counselor feedback to ensure the quality of HIV-CTS.

Counselors, as well as their supervisors, require adequate training in HIV-CTS. In addition to training on the scientific/public health aspects of HIV-CTS, training should address other relevant issues such as substance abuse, human sexuality, the process of behavior change, and the cultural perspectives of the clients being served.

Training for HIV counseling is not a one-time event – it should be an ongoing process. An important component of ongoing quality assurance and training for HIV counselors is routine, periodic observation during counseling sessions and subsequent feedback. When a trained supervisor is not available to perform this important function, routine observation should be done by trained peer counselors. Performance standards that define expectations for the content and delivery quality of counseling should be developed. (Note: observational supervision requires the consent of the client being counseled.)

Conclusion

Publicly funded HIV-CTS are a major component of the national HIV-prevention program[4]. Further, national health promotion and disease prevention objectives for the year 2000 target increases in the proportion of HIV-infected persons who have been tested for HIV infection and the number of health-care facilities (e.g., family-planning clinics, TB clinics, drug-treatment centers, primary-care clinics) where counseling and testing is provided[8].

These recommendations, which supplement existing guidelines[3], focus on the counseling portion of the HIV counseling and testing process – a cooperative endeavor that includes giving information and assisting the client in identifying his/her HIV-prevention needs, and in developing a strategy to address those needs[9]. These guidelines stress the importance of ensuring that HIV counseling is empathic, a quality known to be important in other clinical encounters[10].

By ensuring that counseling is empathic and 'client-centered,' counselors will be able to develop a realistic appraisal of the client's level of risk and assess at which stage the client has reached in the behavior change process[11,12]. Assessing the client's state of behavior change is important since intentions to reduce/modify risky behavior or initiate/ increase healthy behavior will vary among clients. The 'Stages of Behavior Change' model recognizes that persons usually pass through a series of steps before achieving consistently safe behavior – whether in terms of sexual or drug-use behavior[13,14]. These stages are: precontemplation (no intention to change one's behavior); contemplation (long-range intentions to change); ready for action (short-term intentions to change); action (attempts to change); maintenance (long-term consistent behavior change); and relapse (which can end the new behavior or restart the process)[11,12,14].

Assessing the client's stage of behavior change is necessary to ensure that prevention messages are individually relevant – a crucial consideration if HIV counseling is to effect behavior change. For instance, counseling messages that increase clients' intentions to reduce risky behaviors are different from those required to maintain safer behaviors and prevent relapse[15].

Cost-benefit analysis of HIV-CTRPN indicates that, even under conservative assumptions, CDC's expenditure on HIV-CTS results in a substantial net economic benefit to society[16]. Program managers and staff must have realistic expectations about HIV counseling and testing programs. Although it is unlikely that a single episode of HIV counseling will result in the immediate and permanent adoption of safer behaviors[17], client-centered HIV counseling and attendant prevention services (i.e., referral and partner notification) do contribute to the initiation and maintenance of safer behaviors.

References

1. CDC. Recommendation for assisting in the prevention of perinatal transmission of human T-lymphotropic virus type III/lymphadenopathy-associated virus and acquired immunodeficiency syndrome. MMWR 1985;34:721–32.
2. CDC. Additional recommendations to reduce sexual and drug abuse-related transmission of human T-lymphotropic virus type III/lymphadenopathy-associated virus. MMWR 1986;35:152–5.
3. CDC. Public Health Service guidelines for counseling and antibody testing to prevent HIV infection and AIDS. MMWR 1987;36:509–15.
4. CDC. Publicly funded HIV counseling and testing – United States, 1991. MMWR 1992;41:613–7.
5. CDC. Testing for HIV in the public end private sectors – Oregon, 1988–1991. MMWR 1992;41:581–4.
6. CDC. Cooperative agreements for human immunodeficiency virus (HIV) prevention projects, program announcement, and availability of funds for fiscal year 1993. Federal Register 1 992;57:40675–82.
7. Valdiserri RO, Moore M, Gerber AR, Campbell CH, Dillon BA, West GR. Retum rates for HIV posttest counseling: implications for program efficacy. Public Health Rep 1993;108:12–18.
8. Public Health Service. Healthy people 2000: national health promotion and disease prevention objectives – full report, with commentary. Washington, D.C.: US Department of Health and Human Services, Public Health Service, 1991;DHHS publication no.(PHS)91–50212.
9. Davis H. Fallowfield L, eds. Counseling and communication in health care. New York: John Wiley and Sons, 1991:23–5.
10. Bellet PS, Maloney MJ. The importance of empathy as an interviewing skill in medicine. JAMA 1991;266(13):1831–2.
11. Prochaska JO, DiClemente CC. Stages and processes of self-change of smoking: toward an integrative model of change. J Consulting Clin Psychol 1983;51:390–5.

12. Prochaska JO, DiClemente CC. Toward a comprehensive model of change. In: Miller W. Heather N. eds. Treating addictive behaviors. New York: Plenum Press, 1986:3–27.
13. Prochaska JO, DiClemente CC, Norcross JC. In search of how people change; applications to addictive behaviors. Am Psychol 1992;47(9):1102–14.
14. O'Reilly KR, Higgins DL. AIDS community demonstration projects for HIV prevention among hard-to-reach groups. Public Health Rep 1991;106:714–20.
15. CDC. Patterns of sexual behavior change among homosexual/bisexual men – selected U.S. sites, 1987–1990. MMWR 1991;40:792–4.
16. Holtgrave DR, Valdiserri R0, Gerber AR, Hinman AR. HIV counseling, testing, referral, and partner notification services: a cost-benefit analysis. Arch Intern Med (in press).
17. Higgins DL, Galavotti C, O'Reilly KR, et al. Evidence for the effects of HIV antibody counseling and testing on risk behaviors. JAMA 1991;266:2419–29.

Index

Abortion 88
Abscesses 135, 190, 347
  as AIDS indicator disease 96
  brain 91, 150
  injection site 80–1, 236
  intracerebral 146–7
  irrigation 395
  post-injection 122
  tubo-ovarian 100, 178–80, 357
Accidents 245, 299
Acetaminophen *see* Paracetamol
Acquired Immune Deficiency
  Syndrome *see* AIDS
Acyclovir 76–7, 90, 153, 180, 330, 334
Adenine arabinoside 154
Africa 92
  tuberculosis in 108, 111, 128, 223
AIDS
  in adolescents 72, 191
  'age of ' 341
  cause of **11–27**, 65, 227, 229, 348
  and community care 288, 296
  coordinating committee 316
  and cryptococcal infection 85
  definition of paediatric 189–91
  fear of 249
  Foundation, San Francisco 259
  and herpesviruses 88, 90
  a human disease 259
  indicator diseases 67, 77–90, 95–7,
    178, 223, 265
    surveillance case definition 344,
      360–1
    WHO staging system 368
  and individualized care 259–60
  MAC disease in 121
  with neoplasms 154–5
  and neuropsychiatric syndromes
    148–50
  a new disease 3

onset of 336
opportunistic infections 69–70, 77–94,
  103, 151–4
and PCP 78–9, 82–3
remission 94
standard IC precautions 213–16
stigma 254
stressors 255
surveillance case definition for 72, 95,
  97
a terminal illness 323
and TNF 114
with tuberculosis 208, 398
without HIV infection 102–3
AIDS Coordinating Group (Nursing)
  324–5
AIDS dementia complex (ADC) 96,
  150, 268, 347
AIDS-related complex (ARC) 3, 75, 95,
  148
Air contamination 400–1
Alcohol 150, 173, 206
  and antidepressants 256
  in nutrition 275
  sexual behaviour and 259
  and sleep 253
Alcoholism 128, 394
Allergies 54, 125–6, 128, 239
Ambulation 244, 247–8, 284, 414
American Society of Heating,
  Refrigerating, and Air Conditioning
  Engineers (ASHRAE) 400, 411–13
Amikacin 126
Amino acids 277, 279, 282, 284
Amoebiasis 85, 241
Amoxicillin 91
Amphotericin B 86–8, 152–4, 269
Ampicillin 91
Anaemia 245, 269, 330
Analgesia 146, 150, 172, 253

Anorexia 114
and anxiety 255–6
and malnutrition 268–9, 271
and nutrition 239, 275
Antacids 269
Anti-emetics 172, 240–1, 275
Antibiotics 1–2, 180, 237, 269
for bacterial infection 80
for candidiasis 90
for catheter infection 284
fungicidal and fungistatic 86
macrolide 84
Antibodies
in acquired immunity 49–54, 57–8
anti–HAV 167–8
anti–HCV 171
anti–HDV 170
in cell killing 45
classes of 53–4
for CMV 89
'core' 335
cytomegalovirus (CMV) 181
IgG 335–6, 340
IgM 334–6
and immune complexes 42–3
immunodeficiencies and 61
markers of acute infection 53
neutralizing 334
structure 51
Toxoplasma gondii 181
viral 337
Anticoagulants 124, 127
Anticonvulsants 84, 147
Antidepressants 253
monoamine oxidase inhibitors
(MAOI) 256
tetracyclic 256
tricyclic 256
Antidiarrhoeals 77, 85, 241, 274–5
Antifungals 76, 88, 123–4, 127, 179, 248
Antigens
in acquired immunity 54–8
Australia 169
bacteria 47, 52, 57
characteristics 47–8
core (p24) 334–5
cryptococcal 152–3, 181
detection 189, 356
epitopes 47, 52
extracellular 57
fragments 56
hepatitis B 169–70, 181, 226
HIV 74
human leucocyte 14
and immune complexes 42–3

intracellular 57–8
mycobacterial 118–19
purified protein derivative (PPD)
117–18
receptors, cell surface 47–9, 55–6
superantigens 68–9
viral 337
Antihistamines 82, 87, 153
Antipyretics 146–7, 172
Antiseptics 226
Anxiety 237, 252–6
acute 255
and death 261–2
nursing management and 317, 320
patient education 305, 311
testing and counselling 341
Appetite stimulants 275
Asia, tuberculosis in 108, 128, 223
Aspergillus 78, 83, 402
Aspirin 243
Autopsies 375, 391, 395
Azidothymidine (AZT) *see* Zidovudine

Bacilli, acid-fast (AFB) 119–20, 393,
397–8
respiratory precautions 135–40
smear positive 132–4
and tuberculosis control 411–12
Bacteraemia 53, 91
Bacteria
activators 43
antibacterial substances 40–1
antigens 47, 52, 57
cause of pneumonia 83
commensals 41
Gram-negative 44, 91
and killer cells 22
and mycobacteria 119
pyogenic 78, 96, 190, 347
resident 41
spores 204
Bags, plastic 298–300
Barbiturates 253
Bed pans/urinals 209, 242, 299
Bed-bath 248
Bell's palsy 148
Benzodiazepines 253
Beta-carotene 276
Biopsy 396
brain 84, 152–4
colposcopic 179
gastro-intestinal mucosa 85
open lung 81
transbronchial 79, 84
Bisexuals, HIV transmission 5, 30, 32–3,

359
Blood
  collection 298–9
  and community nursing 296
  contamination 296, 298–9, 321
  donation 31, 297, 389
  HIV transmission by 31–2
  and infection control 203, 205, 207–8,
    211–12, 215–18, 325, 370–9
  occupational HIV exposure 221–2,
    227–8
  pressure 237–9
  products 25, 31–3, 188
  tests 84, 87, 224, 227
  transfusions 32
  antiviral therapy 330
  and CMV 88
  and HIV in children 188
  HIV–contaminated 33
  nursing management and 319
  screening 337–8
  and women 177
  universal precautions 386–9
Body contact 310
Body fluids
  and community nursing 296
  contamination 321
  in HIV transmission 307
  and infection control 203–8, 211–12,
    215–18, 225, 325, 370–9
  occupational HIV exposure 221–2,
    228
  and tuberculosis 120
  universal precautions 386–9
Body hygiene 247–8
Body image 254–5, 258, 319
Body language 310–11
Body temperature 243–4, 271
Boredom 251
Breast feeding 297
Breast milk 29, 54, 170, 370
  banks 387
  and CMV 89
  and HIV in children 188
  universal precautions and 387
British Standards 209
Bronchoscopy 79–80
  fibre-optic 119
  in infection control 137, 208
  for tuberculosis 129–30, 395–6, 407–9
Brucellosis 22

Cachexia 60, 77, 114–15, 267, 275
  see also Wasting
Calories 277–8, 282–3

Cancer 46, 97–8
  invasive cervical 97, 100–2, 178–9, 361
  secondary 75, 95
  skin 403
Candida albicans 78, 150–1, 153–4, 238
Candida spp. 76, 333
Candidiasis 357–8
  buccal 268
  definitive diagnosis 351
  disseminated 248–9
  oesophageal 96, 178, 346, 348, 352,
    369
  oral 75–6, 90, 189–90, 369
  oropharyngeal 100
  systemic 154
  vulvovaginal 100, 178–9
Cannabis 275
Capreomycin 126
Carbohydrates 277, 282, 284
Catabolism 239–40, 244
Cataracts 403
Catecholamines 61
Catheter
  cardiac 373, 404
  central venous 279–82
  embolism 283
  external 242
  infection 283–4
  misplacement 283
  urinary 41
Cell(s)
  antigen-presenting (APC) 56, 58
  B lymphocyte 53–5, 58, 69
  CD4+ T lymphocyte (helper) 56–8,
    64–6, 70, 73
    in AIDS classification
      system 98–9, 101–3, 355–8
    and antiviral therapy 329–30
    categories 99–100
    killing mechanisms 67–8
    and nutrition 276
    paediatric HIV classification 192–3
    and pregnancy 180–1
    in testing and counselling 339
    in tuberculosis 112–15, 119
    WHO staging system 368
  CD8+ T lymphocyte (cytotoxic
    'killer') 21–2, 56–8, 60, 65, 67–8,
    70, 334
  death, programmed (apoptosis) 21,
    46, 68–9, 276
  follicular dendritic (FDC) 65
  invasion 20
  killing 45–6
  lysis 52

memory 49, 54–6
natural killer (NK) 46, 54, 59, 103
plasma 49, 55, 57, 65
T lymphocyte 54–6, 58
Center for Devices and Radiological
Health 390
Centers for Disease Control (CDC)
2–3, 72, 75
Adult and Adolescent Spectrum of
HIV Disease (ASD) project 360–1
AIDS surveillance case definition
100–2, 189–91, 371
expanded 178, 358–63
revision of 344–54
dentistry 297
guidance on HIV counselling 338
guidelines for prevention of
nosocomial tuberculosis
transmission 133
HIV classification system 94–8
paediatric 189, 191–2
revised 355–8, 362–3
infection control guidelines 135, 139
recommendations for the prevention
of HIV transmission 202
Central nervous system (CNS), and
HIV **145–66**, 257
Central Sterile Supplies Department
(CSSD) 204, 212, 215
Cerebrovascular disorders 145, 155
Chancroid 35
Chemoprophylaxis, post-exposure
227–8
Chemotaxis 52
Chemotherapy
anticancer 1, 79, 93, 101, 332
antituberculosis 134, 154, 408
following kidney transplants 1–2
interlesional 93
intravenous 319
and malnutrition 271
preventive 130
systemic 93
and tuberculosis control 398, 414–15
Children 336
acquired immunity in 47, 53–4
with AIDS 29, 195–7
and AIDS indicator disease 96
AIDS pandemic and 4, 6, 8
antituberculosis drugs and 125–6
at risk from infection 197
BCG vaccination 131–3
and CMV 88–9
death from AIDS 188
hepatitis A (HAV) in 167–8

and HIV 33, 175, **188–201**
immune dysfunction in 60–1
immunization 197–9
screening tests 336–7
and surveiilance case definition 344,
346–8, 350–1
tuberculosis in 113–15
Chlamydia trachomatis 179, 181
Chloramphenicol 91
Clarithromycin 126–7
Clindamycin 333
Clinics
dedicated 318–19
dental 376
medical 376
out–patient 319, 360
STD 361
Clofazimine 127
Clotrimazole 76, 179
Co–trimoxazole *see* Trimethoprim–
sulphamethoxazole
Cocaine 29, 189, 191
Coccidioides immitis 78, 91
Coccidioidomycosis 96, 190, 347, 351,
369
Cognitive dysfunction, subclinical 145,
149, 156
Colony stimulating factors (CSF) 60
Comfort 253, 258
Communicable Disease Surveillance
Centre (CDSC) 4, 220
Communication 304–5
barriers to 314
and expression 249–51
non–verbal 309–10
patient's bill of rights 322
press 320
skills 310
and testing 341
Community care 288, 292, 295–300,
299–300
Community nursing 298
night service 300
personnel 288, 293
services 290–2, 294–5, 297–8, 428–30
specialist care 300
Complement 41–5, 52–3, 55
Compliance/non–compliance 122–3,
128–30, 134, 398
Condyloma acuminata 76
Confidentiality 225–6, 228–9, 362–3,
438–40
and anxiety 253
in community nursing 297
nursing management and 320

patient's bill of rights 322
of tests 341, 381
Confusion 247, 250, 257, 261, 305
Consciousness 158, 161–3
Consent 249–50, 291, 293, 439
informed 226–8, 341
patient's bill of rights 322
for testing 381, 383
Contraception
barrier 181–2
injectable 183
intrauterine devices (IUDs) 177, 182
non-barrier 23
oral 124, 177, 183
spermicides 183
Control 253–4, 261
Convalescence 291, 294
Coping 253–4
Corticosteroids 61, 113
and amphotericin B 87
antituberculosis drugs and 128
and BCG vaccination 132
in neuropsychiatric syndromes 154
in toxoplasmosis 84
Coughing 134, 261
chronic 114
and infection control 137
suppressants 237
and tuberculosis 395–8, 404–8,
411–12, 414–15
Council of State and Territorial
Epidemiologists (CSTE) 344, 346, 358
Counselling 227–8
client–centred 447
dietary 272–4
discharge 293
feedback 450
guidelines for 338–41
HIV 256, 349, 446–52
lay 319
pre- and post–test 340–1, 448–50
pre-screening 319
services 319–20
for testing 380–3
and tuberculosis control 410–11
Crockery and cutlery 211, 216, 243, 296
Cryptococcosis
definitive diagnosis 351
extrapulmonary 96, 190, 346, 369
Cryptococcus neoformans 78–9
cause of pneumonia 83
community nursing and 296
and HIV disease 85–8
medical management 333
and neuropsychiatric syndromes

150–3
Cryptosporidiosis 85, 96
definitive diagnosis 350
and elimination 241
in paediatric AIDS 190
surveillance case definition 346
WHO staging system 369
Cryptosporidium spp. 78, 85, 269, 275
Cultures
biphasic 119–20
blood 122
bone marrow 122
CSF fluid 152–4
radiometric 119–20
sputum 130, 396–7
tissue 377
for tuberculosis diagnosis 116, 119–20
virus 189, 337
Cycloserine 126
Cytokines 42, 44
in acquired immunity 55–6, 58–60
in HIV 65
and malnutrition 268–9
in tuberculosis 112–16
Cytomegalovirus (CMV) 64, 235
and acute hepatitis 167
and AIDS 78–9, 88–9, 96
cause of pneumonia 83
definitive diagnosis 350
and diarrhoea 85
in early symptomatic HIV 75
and elimination 241
medical management 334
in neuropsychiatric syndromes 151,
153
in paediatric AIDS 190
presumptive diagnosis 352
surveillance case definition 346, 348
WHO staging system 369
Cytosine 154
Cytotoxicity, antibody-dependent cell-
mediated 54, 56

Dapsone 331–3
Day centre 293
Death
at home 300
causes of, in AIDS 78
children, from AIDS 188
counselling for 256
from tuberculosis 108, 110, 113
HIV and pneumonia 360
patient's needs 261–3
postnatal 88
Decontamination 137–8, 226

methods 204–6
and tuberculosis control 404–5, 409
Dehydration 238–9, 241, 243, 245, 247,
 261
Delirium 149, 156
Delusions 256
Dementia 150, 156, 257
Dentistry 228, 297
 employment of infected personnel
  320–2
 and infection control 370–5
 universal precautions for 388, 391
Department of Health and Human
 Services (DHHS) 407
Department of Health and Social
 Security (DHSS) 209
Depression 254–6, 271, 305
 clinical 253–4
Dermatitis, seborrhoeic 75–7
Desiclovir 76
Diabetes mellitus 113
Dialysis 375–6, 391
Diarrhoea 76–7, 82, 89, 149
 in AIDS 96, 121, 189
 body temperature and 244
 and elimination 241–3
 from dehydration 238
 in HIV disease 67, 85–6, 265
 idiopathic 85
 and infection control 207–8, 210, 216
 in malnutrition 268–9, 271
 and nutrition 239–41, 273–5, 277, 279
Didanosine 227, 330–1
Dideoxycitidine 327
Dideoxyinosine 327
Diet 239–40
 alternative 272
 and antidepressants 256
 balanced 272
 and body temperature 244
 counselling 272–4
 and elimination 242
 lactose-free 277
 macrobiotic 239–40
 nutritional assessment 271
 regular 276–7
 supplements 272, 276–7
Dietitian 239–40, 274, 276–7
Discharge **288–301**
 against medical advice 293
 co-ordinator 295
 date 294
 medication 304
 planning 288–95, 300, 318, 322
 policy 288–90

social history form 421–6
Disease
 Hodgkin's 61, 85, 132, 346
 liver 168, 171, 174
 neurological 190
 notifiable 164
 pelvic inflammatory (PID) 34, 100,
  177, 178–80, 357
 sexually transmitted (STD) 21, 34–5,
  183, 191, 361
 skin 190
Disinfection 204, 248, 274, 333
 chemical 205–6
 in community nursing 296–9
 and infection control 137–8, 209,
  212–13, 375–8
 in tuberculosis control 118, 395,
  404–5, 409, 414
 universal precautions 390
Disorientation 249, 257
Diuretics 154–5
DNA, and thymidine 327–9
DNA, virus 12–16, 20, 169, 174
Drug users, injecting 128, 360
 adolescent 191
 and AIDS pandemic 4–5
 hepatitis and 170, 172–3
 and HIV in children 188
 HIV transmission and 23, 28–9, 32–3,
  177–8
 support groups 319
 and tuberculosis 394
 women 176
Drugs 87, 368
 adrenergic neurone blocking 149
 antibacterial 248
 anticancer 61, 93, 154
 anticoagulant 124, 127
 antidiarrhoeals 77, 85, 241, 274–5
 antifungal 76, 88, 123–4, 127, 179, 248
 antihistamines 82, 87, 153
 antimycobacterial 122–8
 antipyretics 146–7, 172
 antiretroviral 77, 85, 222, 331–2
  and antituberculosis drugs 127
  for chemoprophylaxis 227–8
  in malnutrition 269
  in paediatric AIDS 195, 197
  toxicity 228
 antituberculosis 83, 108, 111, 122–8
 antiviral 76, 90, 153
  for CMV 89
  counterfeit 129
  for cryptococcal infection 85–8
  diabetic 124

dideoxynucleoside analogues 327
and discharge 292
in drug-resistant tuberculosis 125–6
fever 82, 125–6, 153, 237
hepatotoxic 172, 330
and immunodeficiencies 61
immunosuppressant 79
interactions 123, 125, 127
and malnutrition 268, 270
multiple 122
myelosuppressive 330
nephrotoxic 87, 330
for neuropsychiatric syndromes 158
and nutrient interactions 267, 269
nutrition and 265, 272, 274–5
over-the-counter (OTC) 330
for PCP 80–3
resistance 76, 122, 128
for septicaemia 91
and sexual behaviour 259
side-effects in CNS 150
in testing and counselling 339
for toxoplasmosis 84
Dying, psychological stages 262–3
Dysphagia 268
Dysphasia 238
Dysplasia, cervical 100–2, 178–9, 339, 357, 361

Eczema 126, 299
Education 317
continuing 430
health 178, 297, 300, 302–4, 320, 339
health care workers 131
in-service 134, 139–40, 163, 225–6, 229, 317–18
patient 36, 131, 236, 333
acute viral hepatitis 172
AIDS information 259–61
for discharge into community 297
evaluation 314
and infection control 136
nurse and **302–15**
nutrition 272–4, 284
tuberculosis 394
Electrolytes 150, 238–9, 275, 279, 282–3
Elimination, urinary and faecal 241–3
Embolism 283
Employment 251–2, 268
health care workers 318, 320–2, 442–4
and HIV disease 297
and tuberculosis control 410–11
Encephalitis 257
acute 72, 145–8
cytomegalovirus (CMV) 153

subacute 148
T. gondii 84, 332–3
Encephalopathy, hepatitis 171–2
Encephalopathy, HIV 96, 150–1, 190, 344, 347, 351, 369
Endorphins 61
Enkephalins 61
Entamoeba histolytica 78, 85
Environmental Protection Agency (EPA) (US) 376–8
Enzymes, complement 41–4
Enzymes, protein–digesting 51
Enzymes, viral 15, 17, 20
Epidemic
AIDS 22–3, 32, 35–6, 85, 224, 300, 321
hepatitis 168
HIV 363
Erythromycin 127
Escherichia coli 41
Ethambutol 125, 128
Ethionamide 125
Europe
AIDS classification system in 95, 102
and AIDS pandemic 4
HIV in adolescents 191
HIV transmission in 30–3
Kaposi's sarcoma (KS) 92
tuberculosis in 107, 114
women and HIV in 176
Exercise 244, 272
Expectorants 237
Extended care facilities 291

Factor VIII 21, 31
Family/friends/relatives 262, 299
admission and discharge 290–1, 295
anxiety and 257
and health education 302, 304
and HIV transmission 296
HIV-infected 136
and individualized care 249–51
as stressors 255
supportive care 195
Fats 277–9, 282–3, 285
Fatty acids, essential polyunsaturated (EFA) 276, 278
Fear 255, 261
Feeding, enteral 240–1, 272, 276–9
Feeding tubes 278–9
Fever 369
acute primary HIV 72
in AIDS 121, 189
and antiviral therapy 330
and body temperature 243–4
cryptosporidiosis 85

cytokines and 59
dehydration 238
and dying 261
haemorrhagic 22
Lassa 22
in malnutrition 269, 271
meningitis 146, 152
and neuropsychiatric syndromes 156
and nutrition 239, 273
pelvic inflammatory disease (PID)
    179
and self-care 248
and tuberculosis 115
Filters, high efficiency particulate air
    (HEPA) 135–6, 138–9, 400–3,
    406–8, 414
Fluconazole 76, 88, 123–4, 153–4, 248
for candidiasis 90, 179, 333
Flucytosine 88
Folinic acid 82, 84
Food
    contamination 273–4
    dairy 274
    frozen 273
    left-overs 274
    nutritionally complete 276–7
    poisoning 273
    preparation 273, 296, 333
    raw 273–4
    reduced intake 267–8
    safety 272–3
    shopping 273
    storage 273
Foscarnet 77, 89–90, 152–3, 180, 334
Free radicals 276
Fungi 83, 85–8, 90, 103, 204
    see also Infection

Ganciclovir 76–7, 89, 152–3, 180, 330,
    334
Gay Men's Health Crisis (GMHC)
    259–60
Gel electrophoresis 337
General practitioner (GP) 290, 295–6
Genes, human leucocyte antigen
    (HLA) 14, 58
Germicide, chemical 375–8
Giardia lamblia 78, 85
Giardiasis 85
Glasgow Coma Scale 158–60
Glycoproteins 49, 55, 335–6
Gonorrhoea 32, 35
Grief 254, 258, 263
Guilt 254, 256–9

Haemophilia 5, 31, 173
Haemophilus influenzae 78, 83, 96, 190,
    347
Haemoptysis 114, 117
Haemorrhage, postpartum 177
Handwashing 207, 212, 214, 217–18, 333
    and community nursing 296, 298
    and elimination 242
    food safety 273
    in infection control 137, 243, 373,
        375–6
    universal precautions 388–9
Health advisers 317, 319
Health care workers
    with AIDS 371
    HIV-infected 31, 220–9, 320–2, 382–3
    and individualized care 249–51
    and infection control 134–7, 173, 203,
        217
        HIV transmission 370, 372–5, 377,
            379
        universal precautions 208–9, 213–15
    invasive procedures and 373–4
    patient's bill of rights 322
    patients with mycobacterial diseases
        122–3
    pregnant 373
    resources for HIV patients 252
    and resuscitation 323
    risk of HIV 371–2
    support groups 319–20
    testing of 382
    and tuberculosis 129, 393–6
        control 400, 403, 405, 407, 409–12
Health Education Authority (HEA)
    259, 297
Health services, home 414–15
Health services, occupational 316
Health visitors 295, 429
Helicobacter pylori 85
Heparin 54
Hepatitis 88–9, 123–4
    A (HAV) 167–8
    acute **167–74**
    B (HBV) 75, 167, 169–74
        in children 194
        occupational exposure 223, 226, 228
        testing and counselling 339
        transmission 387–9
    C (HCV) 167, 171–3
        chronic 167, 170
    D (HDV) 167, 170, 173
    E (HEV) 167–8
    non-A, non-B 167–8, 171
    transmission

by insect bite 170
faecal-oral 167–8
parenteral 170–1
sexual 167, 170–1
vertical 170
Hepatomegaly 189
Herpes
genital 35
labialis 297–8
simplex 346, 369
and AIDS 78, 88, 96, 190
cause of pneumonia 83
definitive diagnosis 351
and HIV 75–7, 89–90, 178, 180
medical management 334
in neuropsychiatric syndromes 151, 153
occupational exposure 228
zoster 74, 76–7, 90, 369
and AIDS 78, 88, 100, 357
Heterosexuals and AIDS pandemic 4–5, 8, 170
Heterosexuals and HIV transmission 29–33, 176, 188–9, 371
Histamine 54
Histoplasma capsulatum 91
Histoplasmosis 91, 190, 347, 351, 369
HIV 15
and acute viral hepatitis **167–74**
in adolescents 191
AIDS without 102–3
asymptomatic 58, 65–6, 73–5, 114
antiviral therapy 329–30
infection control 202–3
screening tests 337–8
at risk of 5, 8
and BCG vaccination 132–3
biology of **11–27**
cell killing mechanisms 67–8
classification system 72, 75, 94–102, 191–5, 348
clinical consequences **72–106**
shape of HIV disease 72–94
community nursing and 300
and cytomegalovirus (CMV) 89
dedicated units 229
definition of pediatric 189–91
dementia 347, 351
effects of malnutrition 270
end-stage 116, 121, 188, 222, 267
health care problems for women 178–80
and herpes simplex 89–90
immunopathogenesis 64–5
indicator diseases 346–53

infected contacts 360
and malnutrition 276, 279
medical treatment 327–38
antiviral agents 227–32
counselling and testing 338–40
prophylaxis of opportunistic infections 332–4
screening for markers 334–8
microbicide 183–4
natural history 65–7, 355, 368
non-syncytium inducing (NSI) 68
occupational exposure 225–8
official designation 11
origins 22–3
pathogenesis 368
pathophysiology 18–22, 261
pathways of destruction **64–71**
patients 127, 206
antituberculosis chemotherapy 134
with hepatitis 171, 173–4
household contacts 388
with mycobacterial infection 120–8, 131
in psychiatric hospitals 164
standard IC precautions 213–16
with tuberculosis 116–20, 130, 133, 137–8
primary 65–6, 72–3, 99, 227
remission 94
resources for patients 251–2
risk factors for women 175–8, 182, 188–9
status 339
strains 222
survival in environment 377
symptomatic 329
early 75–7
late see AIDS
screening tests 337–8
syncytium inducing (SI) 67–9
syndrome, acute 66, 73
transmission **28–38**
accidental 222–3
bisexual 5, 30, 32–3, 359
by bites 388
by contaminated blood/body fluids 370
by drug use 28–9, 321
by infected health care workers 228–9
by tears 370
categories 32–3
and community nursing 296–7
domains of exposure 28–36
during invasive procedures 228–9

environmental considerations 376–9
heterosexual 29–33, 176, 188–9, 371
homosexual 29, 32–3, 35–6
iatrogenic 28, 31–2
in utero 197
modes of 8
nosocomial 164, 322, 371, 388–9
occupational 203, **220–32**, 321,
  386–7
perinatal 370, 373, 387
prevention 349, 447
in health care settings 370–85
  386–92
risk factors 34–5
sexual 28–35, 176–8, 191, 306–7,
  320, 370, 387
under natural conditions 22
vertical 24, 28–30, 188, 194
with tuberculosis 223, 360, 393–7, 405,
  414
virucide 183–4
in world population 5
HIV–1 15, 344
AIDS without 103
and antiviral therapy 329–30
cause of AIDS 11
ELISA/EIA tests for 336
epidemiology 175
occupational exposure 221
origins and spread 23–5
screening tests 336–7, 340
special characteristics 16–18
subtype O 25
variants 35
HIV–2 15–16, 344
AIDS without 103
cause of AIDS 11
ELISA/EIA tests for 336
epidemiology 175
origins and spread 23–4
screening tests 336–7, 340
variants 35
Hobbies and interests 251
Hodgkin's disease 61, 85, 132, 346
Home carers 295
Home helps 293, 296
Homelessness 109, 128, 223
Homophobia 259
Homosexuals 259
and AIDS 2, 4–5, 259, 359
anxiety 256
enteric infections in 85
and hepatitis B (HBV) 170
herpes simplex infection 89–90
HIV transmission 29, 32–3, 35–6

prejudice towards 259
visitors 249
Hospices 319, 413
Hospital
counselling services 319
dedicated units 324
general 317
infection control in 376
management 317
metropolitan 318
nursing personnel 288, 290–3, 295
psychiatric 163
testing and counselling in 340–1
and tuberculosis control 411–13
voluntary services 250
HTLV 15
HTLV–I 15–16
HTLV–II 15–16
HTLV–III 11, 15
Hydration 238–9, 242, 244
Hydrocortisone 76, 87
Hygiene 247–8, 295–7
Hyperglycaemia 236, 240, 284
Hypermetabolism 269
Hypertension 87
Hypnotics 253
Hypogammaglobulinaemia 132, 191,
  346
Hypoglycaemia 236, 240, 284
Hypotension 80–1, 87, 149, 236
Hypoxia, cerebral 150

Immune complexes 42–4, 49–51, 54–5
Immune system 60–1, 73, 103, 113
Immunity 114, 251
acquired 42, 47–60, 62, 70
cell–mediated 89, 97, 100, 118–19, 357
innate 41–7
natural 62
Immunization 386
active 168, 171, 173
hepatitis B (HBV) 172
HIV 197–9, 387
passive 168, 171
Immunization Practices Advisory
  Committee (ACIP) 382
Immunodeficiencies, secondary 61
Immunoglobulin, human normal
  (HNIG) 168, 197
Immunoglobulin *see also* Antibodies
Immunology **39–63**
acquired immunity 47–60
cell–mediated 55–60
humoral 48–55
immune dysfunction 60–1

innate immunity 39–47
  containment of invading pathogens
    41–6
  prevention of invasion 39–41
Immunosuppressants 61
Immunosuppression, iatrogenic 92
Immunosuppression and vaccination
  132, 173
Impotence 256, 275
Incontinence 156, 208, 241–3, 247, 261,
  299
Independence 244–5, 270
Indian subcontinent, tuberculosis in
  109, 132, 223
Infection
  AIDS-defining 95–7
  airborne 406
  bacterial 78, 83, 344, 369
    AIDS indicator diseases 96
    definitive diagnosis 351
    in paediatric AIDS 190
    recurrent 189
  carrier state 168, 170
  control *see* Infection control
  food-borne 273
  fungal 78, 85–8, 91, 333
  gastro-intestinal 269
  genito-urinary tract 41
  latent 89
  mycobacterial 79–80, 85, 97, 224
    tuberculosis 111, 114
  nosocomial 137, 224, 245, 247
  opportunistic 60, 62, 115, 276, 341
    in AIDS 69–70, 77–94, 98, 103,
      151–4
    paediatric 189, 195
    AIDS–defining 67, 223
    of CNS 145, 149, 151–4, 156, 164
    and community nursing 300
    control 206, 208–9, 212–14
    in early symptomatic HIV 75
    individualized care 233, 235, 241,
      243, 248–9, 257
    and malnutrition 267–71
    medical treatment 327, 329
    prophylaxis 332–4
    support groups 319
    terminal 94
    testing and counselling 339
    in women 178
  parasitic 54
  protozoal 78
  status 192–3, 225
  superinfection 170
  transmission 203–4, 297–8

unidentified 217
  viral 78, 88–90
Infection control 341
  acute viral hepatitis 173
  barrier precautions 372, 374, 386,
    388–9
  body substance isolation (BSI) 173,
    202–3, 225, 340
  a cause of isolation 202, 255, 373, 375
  and community nursing 298–300
  and death 263
  decontamination methods 204–6
  engineering 134, 138–9
  and individualized care 243, 248–50
  models 202–4, 224–5
  nosocomial 139, 173, 214
  nursing management and 317, 320
  in nursing practice **202–19**
  occupational exposure 226
  policies and procedures 134, 225,
    324–6, 414
  precautions 372–9
  primary prevention 36, 183–4
  and safety 247
  source-control methods 135–6
  standard precautions 213–16
  testing and counselling 340
  tuberculosis 224, 395–405, 410
  universal precautions 137, 173, 225,
    229, 297
    blood and body fluid 386–9
    and confidentiality 320
    HIV disease 372–3, 375–6, 379,
      437–8
    models 202–4
    in nursing practice 206–18, 340
Injections 209, 214, 298–9
Insemination, artificial 32
Instruments 212, 215, 375–6, 389, 404
Insulin 240, 284
Interferon 40–2, 46, 59, 268–9
  alpha 42, 44, 93, 172
  beta 42, 44
  gamma 42, 56
Interleukin 57, 59, 112
Interleukin-1 (IL–1) 42, 44, 56, 59,
  268–9
Interleukin-2 (IL–2) 56, 59
Invasive procedures 321–2, 370, 373–4,
  382, 391
Irradiation, germicidal ultraviolet 400,
  402–3, 412–14
Isolation 249, 251
  and community nursing 299
  and individualized care 316

and patient education 310
precautions, guidelines for 370
religion and 257
rooms 135–6, 138–9, 394
and tuberculosis control 396, 402–3,
  407–8, 411–12
through infection control 202, 255,
  373, 375
and tuberculosis control 398, 406,
  411–12
Isoniazid 108, 123–5, 128
Isospora belli 85, 91, 241, 269
Isospora spp. 78
Isosporiasis 85, 96, 190, 347, 350

Kanamycin 126
Kaposi's sarcoma (KS) 2, 369
  and AIDS 91–3, 96, 103, 190
  classic 92
  and CNS neoplasms 154
  definitive diagnosis 351
  and dehydration 238
  diarrhoea and 85
  and elimination 241
  endemic 92
  epidemic 92–3
  and infection control 206
  and malnutrition 268–9
  nutrition and 239
  and organic mental disorders (OMD)
    150
  and pneumonia 83–4
  presumptive diagnosis 352
  support group 319
  surveillance case definition 344,
    346–8
  transmission 34
Ketoconazole 76, 123–4, 127, 179, 331

Laboratories 207, 362, 413
  clinical 391
  infection control 375–6
  research 391
Lactose 277
Landmark 251
Landry-Guillain-Barré syndrome 145,
  149
LEAN 251
Legionella spp. 78
Leisure 251–2, 255
Lentiviruses 16
Leprosy 61, 111, 120, 127
Leucoencephalopathy, progressive
  multifocal (PML) 91, 96, 154, 190
Leukaemia 61, 132, 346

Leukoencephalopathy 347, 351
  progressive multifocal (PML) 369
Leukoplakia, hairy 75–6, 100, 357, 369
Linen 211, 215, 244, 296–7, 378
Listeria monocytogenes 78, 91
Listeriosis 91, 100, 357
Local authority 288, 296
  municipal services 293–5
Loneliness 251
Lymphadenopathy 72, 179, 346
  persistent generalized (PGL) 3, 74–5,
    95, 99, 368
  syndrome (LAS) 3, 74
Lymphocytopenia 74
  idiopathic CD4+ T (ICL syndrome)
    102–3
Lymphoma(s) 369
  B–cell 150, 154
  and BCG vaccination 132
  brain 96, 190
  definitive diagnosis 350
  non-Hodgkin's 94, 96, 191, 346–7
  systemic 154
  undifferentiated 94
Lysozyme 40–1

Macronutrients 265
Macrophages 22, 35
  in acquired immunity 52, 56–8, 60
  in innate immunity 42, 44–6
  and tuberculosis 112–14
  as virus targets 24
Malnutrition 239, 241, 265
  in early symptomatic HIV infection
    77
  interventions 272–85
  mechanisms 267–71
  and mobility 245
  protein-energy (PEM) 266–7
  risk factors 271–2
  types of 267
Meals service 293
Medical records 226, 362, 414
Medication 236–7
  anxiolytic 253, 255
  in individualized care 240–1, 243, 253
Meningitis 147, 154, 347
  AIDS indicator disease 96
  atypical aseptic 72, 145–9
  cryptococcal 85, 88, 147, 349
  fungal 91
  granulomatous 152
  listeriosis 91
  in paediatric AIDS 190
  pericardial 128

tuberculous 113, 128, 153
Meningoencephalitis 85
Menstruation 177
Mental disorders, organic (OMD) 145, 149–51, 156
Mental Health Act (1983) 163–4
Mental retardation 256
Methadone 330
Microbiologist 316
Micronutrients 265, 269, 276, 282–3
Microscopy, for tuberculosis diagnosis 116, 119–20
Microsporidia 85, 269
Midwifery 321–2, 430–1
Minerals 265, 276, 279, 282–4
Mobility 244–5, 261, 299
Models
  AIDS educational strategy for pre-registration nursing programmes 427–31
  behavioural 234
  consent, confidentiality and testing 341
  discharge policy 288–90
  of dying 262–3
  health education 302–4
  infection control 202–4, 224–5
  nursing care 263
  philosophy for nursing 433–6
  policy statements 438–45
  Riverside 323–6
  strategic nursing care 234
Mononeuritis multiplex 148
Mononucleosis 88–9
Mouth care 237–8, 247–8
Muscles 244–5, 267, 269
Mutation, virus 65
Mycobacteria 111, 347, 397
  antituberculosis drug-resistant 122
  atypical 120
  drug–resistant 128
  environmental 79, 83, 111, 118–20, 269
  and BCG vaccination 133
  in infection control 137–8
  and tuberculosis 120–2
  multiple drug–resistant 122
  in neuropsychiatric syndromes 153–4
  transmission 120
Mycobacteriosis 352, 369
Mycobacterium africaneum 111
Mycobacterium avium 96, 111, 119–21
Mycobacterium avium complex (MAC) 78, 83, 85, 121–2, 346
  CNS infection 151, 153–4

drug treatment 123, 126–7
infection control 135, 137–8
and malnutrition 269
in paediatric AIDS 190
and tuberculosis control 396–7
Mycobacterium bovis 111, 131
Mycobacterium chelonei 119–22
Mycobacterium fortuitum 121–2
Mycobacterium intracellulare 111, 121
Mycobacterium kansasii 78, 96, 119–21, 190, 346
Mycobacterium leprae 111, 120
Mycobacterium malmoense 121
Mycobacterium marinum 120, 122
Mycobacterium szulgai 121
Mycobacterium tuberculosis 42, 58, 347
  and AIDS 78
  cause of pneumonia 83
  destruction 204–5
  discovery and history 107–8
  epidemiology and aetiology 108–11
  and HIV 79, 115
  and infection control 135, 137–8, 214
  multi-drug resistant 393–4
  in neuropsychiatric syndromes 151, 153–4
  testing for 117–19
  transmission 111, 223–4, 394–5
  prevention 396–7
Mycobacterium ulcerans 120, 122
Mycobacterium vaccae 133
Mycobacterium xenopi 121
Mycoplasma penetrans 64
Myeloma, multiple 346
Myelopathy, vacuolar 145, 148, 156

National Health Service (NHS) 211
National Institute for Occupational Safety and Health (NIOSH) 407
Nausea and vomiting 85, 261
  and antiviral therapy 330
  from dehydration 238
  and malnutrition 268–9, 271
  medication side-effects 82, 237
  in meningitis 146, 152
  and nutrition 239–40, 274–5, 279
Neisseria gonorrhoeae 179, 181
Neoplasms 43, 91–3, 145, 150, 154–5, 235
Nephrotic syndrome 61
Nephrotoxicity 180, 237
Neurological disorders 237
Neuropathy
  autonomic 145, 149, 156
  peripheral 100, 123, 145, 148, 156,

244, 357
symmetrical sensorimotor 148
Neuropeptides 61
Neurotransmitters 61
Neutrophils 44–5, 52, 60
Night sweats 67, 115, 121, 243, 248
Nocardia asteroides 91
Nocardia spp. 78
Noise 253
Norton scale 242, 245–6
Nurse
  clinical specialist 316, 319
  community psychiatric 295
  as counsellor 338–41
  district 293, 295–300, 429
  educationalists 317
  as educator **302–15**
    assessing learning needs 304–5
    implementing patient education
      310–14
    planning educational response
      305–9
    teaching plan 309–10
  family planning 295, 429
  HIV infected 320
  infection control 316–18
  manager, senior 317
  neonatal 430–1
  practice 295
  school 295, 429
Nursing Advisory Committee (NAC)
  324–5
Nursing care
  AIDS counselling 338
  and AIDS medical management
    327–43
  assessment 234
  in the community 288, 295–300
  coordination 316–17
  duty of care 325–6, 438
  evaluation 237–8
  HIV
    individualized **233–64**
    patient needs 234–63
      associated with dying 235, 261–3
      body temperature control 234,
        243–4
      expression and communication
        234, 249–51
      expression of sexuality 235,
        258–61
      hydration 234, 238–9
      movement and mobilization
        234, 244–5
      nutrition 234, 239–41

personal cleansing and dressing
  234, 247–9
psychological equilibrium 235,
  253–7
respiration 234–8
rest and sleep 235, 252–3
safe environment 234, 245–7
urinary and faecal elimination
  234, 241–3
working and playing 235, 251–2
worship according to faith 235,
  257–8
individualized 428
management of **316–26**
  infection control in 206–18
  intensive 323
  long-term facilities 376
  neurological evaluation 157–8
  paediatric 195
  patient social history 288, 290
  patients with acute viral hepatitis
    171–2
  patient's bill of rights 322–3
  of patients with late, symptomatic
    HIV 94
  for patients with mycobacterial
    diseases 120–8, 131
  patients with neuropsychiatric
    syndromes 155–63
  philosophy 325
  policy statements 325–6
  prevention of malnutrition 270
  'state of the art' 318
  strategic 233–4
  terminal care 319
  TPN patients 279–84
  withdrawal 318
Nursing homes 413
Nutrients 265–8, 277
Nutrition 113
  deficiencies 276
  evaluation 270–1
  and HIV disease **265–87**
    defined 265
    interventions 272–85
    mechanisms of malnutrition 267–71
    risk factors 271–2
  oral 239–40
  overnutrition 265
  parenteral 279–85
    peripheral (PPN) 284–5
    total (TPN) 240, 272, 279–84
  side-effects 274–5
  supplements 277–9
  support 241

total 277–8
undernutrition 265–6

Occupational Safety and Health
  Administration (OSHA) 225, 407
Oedema, cerebral 150, 154–5
Oesophagitis, candidal 90, 248
Oliguria 241
Opiates 256
Opsonins 45, 52
Orientation, reality 250
Osmolality 277–8
Ototoxicity 126
Out patients 290, 319, 373, 380, 414
Oxidants 276
Oxygen 235–6, 247

Pain 305
  acute primary HIV 72
  chest 114
  and dying 261
  and malnutrition 268, 271
  in neuropsychiatric syndromes 156
  and nutrition 273
  in peripheral neuropathy 148
  relief 292
  and sleep 252–3
  women and HIV 179
Pandemic, AIDS **1–10**, 22–3, 33, 140,
  188
Pandemic, dual 109
Panic 255
Papovaviruses 78, 91, 151, 154
Paracetamol 87, 172, 243, 330
PAS (para–aminosalicylic acid) 108, 125
Pathogens
  acquired immunity against 47
  antibiotic–resistant 41
  bloodborne 202–3
    in infection control 206, 225, 370,
      372–4, 376, 379
    occupational exposure 223
    universal precautions 386–9
  containment of 41–6
  extracellular 22
  and immune dysfunction 60
  and individualized care 235, 257
  in infection control 204, 212–14, 216
  innate immunity to 39
  new 22
  non-bloodborne 387
  nosocomial 387
  and nutrition 274
  opportunistic 77–8, 103
  parasitic 296

pelvic inflammatory disease (PID)
  179
  protection against 39–41
Pentamidine 1–2, 80–2, 236, 238, 269
  aerosolized 136, 180–1, 237, 332,
    407–8
Peptides 277
Pethidine 256
Phagocytes 44–5, 52
  in acquired immunity 54, 56, 58, 60
  polymorphonuclear (PMN) (killer)
    45–6
Phagocytosis 44–5, 53
Phenothiazines 256
Photophobia 152
Physiotherapy 236, 244
Pneumococcus 78, 96, 190
Pneumocystis carinii see pneumonia
Pneumocystosis *see* pneumonia,
  Pneumocystis carinii
Pneumonia
  bacterial 135, 360
  in HIV 83–4
  lymphoid interstitial 96, 344, 346, 348,
    352
  pneumococcal 339
  Pneumocystis carinii 1–2, 78–83, 135
    and AIDS 96, 103
    classification system 355
    definitive diagnosis 350
    diagnosis 79
    and individualized care 235
    in paediatric AIDS 190
    presumptive diagnosis 352
    prophylaxis 332
    surveillance case definition 344–5,
      347–8
    symptoms 79
    terminal opportunistic infection
      94
    treatment 80–3
    WHO staging system 369
  in women 178
  recurrent 97, 100–2, 360–1
  and toxoplasmosis 84
Pneumonitis, lymphoid interstitial (LIP)
  189–90
Pneumothorax 283
Polypeptides 40–1
Posture 311
Prednisolone 123, 128
Pregnancy 123
  antiretroviral drugs in 197, 227
  and antituberculosis drugs 125–6, 128
  and BCG vaccination 132

hepatitis infection in 168
and HIV 177, 180–1, 188, 373
nutrition in 275
Prejudice 259, 318
Pressure area care 242, 245–6, 248, 253
Pressure sores 156, 242–5, 261
Prisons 413
Protective clothing 210, 216–18
    in community nursing 296–300
    in individualized care 236, 243
    and infection control 136–7, 203,
        207–9, 213–16, 372–5
    for last offices 263
    and medical management 333
    PCP patients 79, 81
    and tuberculosis control 400, 403–4,
        412
    universal precautions 386
Protein
    acute phase 40–1, 43
    antigens 47
    depletion 61
    in nutrition 277–9, 282
    viral 337
Protozoa 83–5, 91
Proviruses 20
Pseudomonas aeruginosa 83
Psychiatrist 293
Psychologist, clinical 255–6, 260, 319
Psychosis 123, 126, 128, 164
Public Health (Control of Diseases)
    Act (1984) 163–5
Public relations 320
Pyrazinamide 124, 128
Pyrexia 150, 244, 283
Pyrimethamine 333

Quality assurance 134, 139–40, 295, 318
Quality of care 300, 323
Quality of life 270, 279, 329
Quinolones, fluorinated 125

Radiation 61, 93, 132, 139, 154
Rape 176, 178
Rashes, medication side–effects 236–7
Rehydration 238–9, 242, 319
    therapy, oral (ORT) 275
Rejection 251, 255
Relaxation 255, 257
Religion 257–8, 305
Remission 94
Research, medical 227
Residential homes 293
Respiration 235–8
Rest 252–3

Resuscitation 323
Retrovirus(es) 14–16
    AIDS–associated (ARV) 11, 15
    genomes 17–18, 20
    LAV–2 23
    non–pathogenic 22
Rifabutin 127
Rifampicin 124, 127–8
RNA, and thymidine 327–8
RNA, virus 12–16, 20–1, 167–8, 327–8
Rubbish 211, 215–16, 296

Safety, environment 245–7
Salicylic acid 76
Salmonella 85, 91, 269, 347
    septicaemia 91, 369
Salmonella typhimurium 78
Salmonellosis, definitive diagnosis 351
San Francisco AIDS Foundation 259
Sarcoidosis 61
Scanning, computerized tomography
    (CT) 84, 146–7, 152–4, 351–2
Scanning, magnetic resonance imaging
    (MRI) 152, 351–2
SCID (severe combined immune defi-
    ciency) 1, 60, 191
Screening 319
    blood 177, 183
    cervical cancer 102
    disadvantages 339–40
    of donor blood 31
    of donors for AI 32
    gynaecological 179
    for HIV 31–2, 321
        markers 334–8
    prenatal 180
    serological 203, 217, 333
    tests 334–8, 340, 349–50, 356, 380
    tuberculosis 102, 117–18, 339, 394,
        396
        prevention 405, 407–11, 414–15
Sedation 150, 253
Seizures 150, 152, 154–6, 245
Self–care 163, 234, 247–9, 270
Self–esteem 254
Self–reproach 256
Septicaemia 91, 96–7, 150, 190, 347, 369
Seroconversion 73, 95
    and infection control 380–1
    in neuropsychiatric syndromes 145,
        147
    and occupational HIV exposure 222
    testing and counselling 224, 256, 340
Serotonin 54
Sex industry 33, 176, 178, 183

Sex tourism 178
Sexual abuse 176, 188
Sexual behaviour 172, 176, 341
  high risk 32, 189, 191, 259, 304, 306
  modifying 258, 261
  risk factors 34
  safer 305–7
Sexual expression 258–61, 306–7
Sexual orientation 249, 305
Sexual partners 227, 259
Sexual practices 177–8
  high risk 259–60
  safer 183, 258–60, 297, 305–7, 339
Sexual relationships 176
Sharps 173, 211, 214–15, 217, 404
  in community nursing 298–9
  and infection control 207, 209–10,
    373–4, 376
  occupational HIV exposure and
    221–2
  universal precautions 387–9
Shigella 85, 91
Shigella flexneri 78
Sinusitis, chronic 190
Skin, care 242–3
Skin, turgor 238–9
Sleep 252–3, 255–6
Social relationships 299
Social services 290, 293, 359
Social workers 251, 262, 317, 319
  and discharge 291, 293
  hospital 294
Socialization 255
Specimens 207, 216
Splenomegaly 75, 189
Sputum
  conversion 122
  and individualized care 235, 237
  induction 79–80, 129–30, 395, 407–9
  and infection control 135–7
  in tuberculosis control 397–8, 411–12,
    415
  for tuberculosis diagnosis 119
Staphylococcus aureus 40, 43
Starvation 61, 266–7
Sterilization 395, 404–5
  ethylene oxide gas (EOG) 205
  heat 204
  hot air 205
  in infection control 137–8, 374, 376–7,
    409
  instrument 212
  surgical 181
Steroids 61, 76, 128
Stevens–Johnson syndrome 125, 332

Stillbirth 88
Streptococcus 78, 96, 190, 347
Streptococcus pneumoniae 83, 334
Streptomycin 108, 124–6, 128
Stress 61, 113, 227, 272
  and anxiety 253, 255
  and malnutrition 267–9
Strongyloides stercoralis 85
Suicide 256
Sulphaziadine 333
Sulphonamides 333
Support
  bereavement 319
  discharge 291
  groups 250, 256, 319–20
  non-nursing 299
  psychosocial 338
  social 254
  testing and counselling 341
Suppositories 275
Surfaces 212, 375–8, 405
Surgery 221, 320–2, 381
  transplant 339
Surveys, serologic 23
Surveys, seroprevalence 23
Sympathetic nervous system (SNS) 61
Syncytia 67–8
Syphilis, primary 35

Tars 76
Terence Higgins Trust 250–1, 259–60,
  297, 319
Tests
  anonymous prevalence data 341
  antigen 334, 336, 338, 350
  ß$_2$-microglobulin 338
  blood 84, 87, 224, 227
  CD4+ T lymphocyte counts 338
  confirmatory 336–7
  drug susceptibility 119–20
  EIA (enzyme immunoassay) 336–7,
    340, 379–81
  ELISA (enzyme linked immunosor-
    bent assay) 189, 336–7, 340, 350
  guidelines 338–41
  Heaf 117–18
  HIV antibody 116, 224, 229, 348–50,
    410
  home 337
  IFA (immunofluorescence assay) 152,
    154, 189, 336, 350, 356
  magnetic resonance imaging (MRI)
    152, 351–2
  Mantoux 117–18, 181, 359, 397
    and tuberculosis control 405,

409–10
monitoring 338–9
Papanicolaou (PAP) smears 179
PCR (polymerase chain reaction)
189, 337, 340
procedures 359
rapid method 337–8
Sabin-Feldmann dye inclusion 152
screening 334–8, 340, 349–50, 356, 380
HIV antibody 349–50
serological 152, 189, 335–6
consent for 440–1
for HIV 32, 224, 226, 228, 341
and infection control 379–83
supplemental 349, 356, 379–80
tine 118
tuberculin skin 113, 116–19, 181,
359–60
and BCG vaccination 132
for tuberculosis control 396–7, 405,
407–10, 414
unconsented 341
unlinked anonymous prevalence
441–2
Western blot 189, 337, 350, 356,
379–81
Ziehl–Neelsen (ZN) technique 119
Tetracycline 91
Thiacetozone 124
Thrombocytopenia 74
Thrombosis 244–5, 275, 279, 283
Thymidine 327–30
Thyroxine 61
Tinea cruris 75–6
Tinea pedis 75–6
Tinea spp. 78
Toxoplasma gondii 78, 296
abscesses 146–7
cause of pneumonia 83–4
medical management 332–3
and neuropsychiatric syndromes
150–2, 154
Toxoplasmosis 84, 257, 347–8, 369
and AIDS 96, 190
definitive diagnosis 351
presumptive diagnosis 352
Trace elements 276, 282–4
Transcriptase, reverse 327–31
Transplantation, kidney 92
Transplantation, organ 32, 58
Transplantation surgery 79
Transplantation, tissue 58
Trimethoprim–sulphamethoxazole 74,
81–2, 237
against *T. gondii* 333

for diarrhoea 85
in pneumonia prophylaxis 332
for *Shigella* infection 91
Tropism 14–15
Tuberculomas 153
Tuberculosis 229
active 112–14, 118–19
BCG vaccination 132
control 134–7, 139, 202, 396–7,
408–10, 415
identification and treatment
396–7, 405–6
occupational exposure 223–4
risk of 412–13
and tests 119
transmission 393–4
classification system 359
definition 112
drug-resistant 412, 415
epidemiology and aetiology 108–11,
394–5
extrapulmonary 97, 112, 115–16, 360,
369
control 135, 398
high risk for 396
historical background 107–8
and HIV disease 9, **107–44**
immunopathology 114
infectiousness 397–8
laryngeal 134
miliary 61
multi–drug resistant 128–31, 133,
223–4
occupational exposure 223–4
pathogenesis 112–14, 394–5
primary infection 112–13
pulmonary 97, 114–15, 369
AIDS classification system 100–1
AIDS surveillance case
definition 360–1
contagious 112
control 397–8, 405–6, 411–13
and HIV disease 107
infection control 134–5, 208,
211, 214, 216
screening 339
spinal 107
symptoms 396–7
transmission 111, 115, 394–6
airborne 415
environmental factors 395
nosocomial 116, 129, 131,
133–40, 223, 393, 395
prevention 393–420
in health care settings 393–420

source control methods
398–400
risk of 402, 405, 407
surveillance 409–11
Tumour necrosis factor (TNF) 60, 114,
116, 268–9

United Kingdom
AIDS pandemic 4–5
BCG vaccination 131–3
classification system for HIV
infection 95
dentistry 297
hepatitis 167, 170
HIV in adolescents 191
immunization 199
infection control 202, 211
occupational HIV exposure 220–2,
229
Project 2000 302
resources for HIV patients 251–2
safer sex information 259–60
screening tests 337
transmission categories 32
tuberculosis in 109, 118
United States 102
AIDS pandemic 1–3, 5
dentistry 297
HIV in adolescents 191
immunization 198–9
infection control in 202, 225
Kaposi's sarcoma (KS) 92
occupational HIV exposure 220, 229
P. carinii 79
paediatric AIDS 197
safer sex information 259
transmission categories 32–3
tuberculosis in 107, 109, 114, 118, 128,
223, 394
women and HIV 176

Vaccination 382, 409
polyvalent pneumococcal 334
Vaccines 368
active 198, 382
against HIV 341
BCG 108, 119, 131–3, 199
biological 227, 334
cholera 199
diphtheria, tetanus, pertussis (DTP)
198
H. influenza type–b conjugate (HbC)
199
hepatitis B (HBV) 199, 226, 386
inactivated virus 168, 198

influenza 198–9
measles, mumps, rubella (MMR) 198
meningococcal 199
new 133
pneumococcal 199
polio (OPV/IPV) 198
preventive 334
testing and counselling 339
therapeutic 334
typhoid 199
yellow fever 198–9
Ventilation 138–9
engineering 406
general 400–1
local exhaust 399–400
mechanical 395
and tuberculosis control 411–14
Vertigo 245, 255
Vidarabine 90
Vinblastine 93, 154
Vincristine 154
Viomycin 126
Viraemia 65–6, 73, 89
Virus(es)
activators 43
active and inactive 64–5
antigenic characters 14
antigens 47, 57–8
budding 12, 21, 65, 67
cause of pneumonia 83
characteristics 11–13
chickenpox 52–3
DNA 12–16, 20, 169, 174
encephalitis due to 150
endemic 168
Epstein-Barr (EBV) 75, 78, 88, 90,
167
fragility of 204–6
hepatitis *see* Hepatitis
hepatotropic 167
herpes *see* Herpes
human immunodeficiency *see* HIV
human immunodeficiency type 1 *see*
HIV-1
human immunodeficiency type 2 *see*
HIV–2
human papilloma (HPV) 75, 179
human T-cell leukaemia *see* HTLV
isolation 356
lentiviruses 16
lymphadenopathy–associated (LAV)
11, 15
papovaviruses 78, 91, 151, 154
progenitor 22
proviruses 20

replication 20–1, 42, 64–5, 67, 227, 332
retroviruses *see* Retrovirus(es)
RNA 12–16, 20–1, 167–8, 327–8
simian immunodeficiency 16, 22–3
variants 35
see also Infection
Visitors 249–50, 252–3, 323
and infection control 209, 211, 216
nutrition and 239–40
Vitamins 241, 265, 276, 279, 282–4
Voluntary organizations 252

Wards 206–8, 216, 292–4
dedicated 318–19
Warts, anogenital 179
Waste, infective 378–9
Waste management 390
Wasting
cachexia 60, 77, 114–15, 267, 275
distal atrophy 148, 156
and malnutrion 77, 266–7, 269
muscle 244–5
syndrome 97, 344, 347, 351, 369
Weight loss 121, 239, 369
in HIV disease 67, 265–7, 269, 271–2
involuntary *see* Wasting
and nutrition 241, 275
Wills 262
Wiskott–Aldrich syndrome 191
Women 339
and AIDS pandemic 4, 8
and HIV **175–87**
postmenopausal 177
World Health Organization (WHO)
AIDS epidemiology 175–6
and BCG vaccination 133
classification system 359

clinical staging system for HIV 102,
368–9
Global Programme on AIDS 5, 8
immunization policy 198–9
sponsored biomedical research 184
transmission categories 33
and tuberculosis 108–11, 223

X–rays 84
abdominal 278
chest 79–80, 113, 130, 134, 352
for tuberculosis 116–17, 396–8,
410
treatment, deep (DXT) 154–5

Yeasts 78, 86

Zalcitabine 227, 330–1
Zidovudine
and antituberculosis drugs 124, 127
in antiviral therapy 327–32
for CMV 89
and cryptosporidiosis 85
for Kaposi's sarcoma (KS) 93
in malnutrition 269
in meningitis 146
in occupational HIV exposure 222,
227
in organic mental disorders (OMD)
151
in paediatric AIDS 197
in peripheral neuropathy 148
and remission 94
side-effects 330
in testing and counselling 339
women and HIV 181
Zoonosis 22